Treating Opioid Use Disorder in General Medical Settings

Sarah E. Wakeman · Josiah D. Rich
Editors

Treating Opioid Use Disorder in General Medical Settings

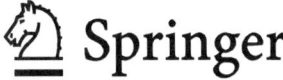 Springer

Editors
Sarah E. Wakeman
Department of Medicine
Massachusetts General Hospital
Charlestown, MA
USA

Josiah D. Rich
Brown University
The Miriam and Rhode Island Hospitals
Providence, RI
USA

ISBN 978-3-030-80817-4 ISBN 978-3-030-80818-1 (eBook)
https://doi.org/10.1007/978-3-030-80818-1

This Springer imprint is published by the registered company Springer Nature Switzerland AG
The registered company address is: Gewerbestrasse 11, 6330 Cham, Switzerland

Preface

This book is an attempt to demystify and encourage the treatment of opioid use disorder (OUD) in general medical settings, like any other health condition. This change is long overdue. For over a century, OUD has been perhaps the most stigmatized medical condition. During a raging overdose crisis which claimed a predicted 95,230 lives in the past 12-months alone, a majority due to opioids, integration of OUD treatment in medical settings remains uncommon [1, 2]. In the midst of the COVID-19 pandemic, deaths from opioid overdose are accelerating with disproportionately high overdose mortality among Black and Latinx/Hispanic people serving as a brutal reminder of the health harms of structural racism. Despite being exceedingly treatable, the diagnosis and treatment of OUD still is largely not taught in medical school and residency training.

Even when effective treatment for this deadly disease with methadone was discovered in the pivotal studies by Dole and Nyswander in the 1960s and 1970s, it was relegated to tightly federally regulated programs, mostly disconnected from the rest of medicine [3]. These regulations have left methadone treatment siloed and tethered by strict program-centered requirements, which limits access for patients. Patients who are treated in opioid treatment programs also live with the implied or real threat of having their medication dose decreased or stopped to enforce compliance with whatever the program needs, as opposed to what the patient thinks they need. This presents a tremendous challenge to developing and nurturing a therapeutic alliance. With the Drug Addiction Treatment Act (DATA) of 2000, passed nearly 2 decades ago, an opportunity to incorporate treatment for OUD in general medical settings was created through obtaining an X-waiver to prescribe buprenorphine. However, despite free trainings and efforts to incentivize participation, this opt-in model of providing OUD treatment has resulted in less than 7 percent of prescribers waivered, leaving huge swaths of the country without access to effective office-based OUD care [4, 5]. In addition, racism has deeply impacted access to buprenorphine, which has been more available to white, commercially insured individuals and in segregated, white neighborhoods [6–9].

With the National Academy of Medicine report on OUD, it is now abundantly clear that a dramatic expansion of capacity of high-quality care using medication treatment for OUD is needed to address the overdose crisis [10]. The lack of understanding of OUD by most medical practitioners left us, and ultimately, our patients, vulnerable to the current overdose crisis. The onset of the first wave of three waves of the current overdose crisis (prescription opioids to heroin to illicit synthetic fentanyl) was driven by the greed and deception of certain members of the pharmaceutical industry coinciding with a rising tide of social despair. The healthcare system not only enabled this disaster, but also turned its back on patients who developed OUD and on those with chronic pain. Our lack of collective understanding of OUD also fueled often inadequate approaches to address the crisis, relying heavily on racist models of interdiction and criminalization, abruptly denying care to patients with pain, and continuing to funnel patients into an ineffective and costly model of OUD care centered on harmful short-term "detox" and omnipresent calls for more residential treatment beds, with little to no evidence to justify this approach.

This book is an attempt to shine a light on these fallacies and provide the tools to expand OUD treatment into general medical settings where it belongs. People living with OUD are patients with a complex health condition akin to many others managed effectively in medical settings, and we never should have sent them away to another disconnected part of the healthcare system in the first place. The best way to both deal with this current deadly overdose epidemic and to minimize the risk of future crises is to embrace and disseminate care for people with OUD in general medical settings. Addressing the overdose crisis effectively is also not possible without acknowledging and repairing the harms caused by the racist "War on Drugs" which resulted in mass incarceration of Black and Latinx/Hispanic Americans long before the softer, gentler narrative of treatment began to emerge as more white, middle class communities were impacted.

This book begins with three chapters on care models, followed by seven chapters on different care settings and strategies, a chapter on training, and the final four chapters addressing additional unique aspects of caring for people with OUD. The first chapter is an eloquent description of patient centered care and why and how it should be used in the treatment of patients with OUD. Chapter 2 offers an analysis of the historic context of the currently available medication treatments for OUD and the different regulatory structures which sheds light on the various players and divergent interests that have shaped the current treatment environment. Chapter 3 describes the latest evidence for integrated treatment models in primary care. The fourth chapter highlights how to capitalize on the all too often missed "reachable moment" of hospitalization to diagnose, engage, and link to medication treatment for OUD care after discharge. Emergency Departments can serve as a primary linkage site for initiation of treatment for OUD, described in the fifth chapter, which includes strategies to identify, assess, initiate medication, refer, and provide harm reduction and pain management for people with OUD. Because of our drug policies, many individuals with OUD experience criminal legal system involvement and incarceration. Chapter 6 describes the current state of OUD treatment in corrections, the need for advocacy for expanded treatment and linkage post incarceration, and ideally reducing criminal legal involvement through decriminalization of substance use and expanding access to quality treatment with medications for OUD. Chapter 7 describes the use of Project ECHO in detail as a novel model of care expansion for OUD care. Chapter 8 expands the discussion of care of people with OUD to include interprofessional teams. It describes a successful inpatient consult team model that uses a range of disciplines to offer patients a holistic treatment approach that addresses the biological, psychological, and social components of addiction. Recovery coaches, described in Chapter 9, are an exciting addition to the range of options for recovery support, and are a promising innovative intervention that can be integrated into the medical team. Chapter 10 provides a detailed description of harm reduction strategies that should be incorporated as a critical component of care for people with OUD. Training the next generation of care providers is critical to the long-term success of treatment for people with OUD. Chapter 11 articulates how this can be done at each level of medical education. Chapter 12 makes the strong case for "reverse integration," that is, incorporating comprehensive medical care into opioid treatment programs to improve outcomes and patient satisfaction while reducing healthcare costs. Racial equity is a pervasive challenge in the field of addiction treatment. Chapter 13 articulates a race equity framework tailored to treatment for OUD. Chapter 14 explores the unique challenges of caring for pregnant and post-partum people with OUD, and the critical need to align public health and policies with the evidence and turn back a disturbing trend towards punitive approaches. Lastly, chapter 15 offers the patient perspective from two experienced journalists, themselves people with a history of addiction, weaving lived experience with a nuanced review of the evidence supporting medication treatment for OUD and not short-term "detoxification" or psychosocial treatment alone.

Among the many tragic tolls of the COVID-19 pandemic has been the marked increase in opioid overdoses in much of the country. This underscores the tremendous need to treat OUD in general medical settings as quickly and effectively as possible. This work is feasible, and importantly it is also deeply rewarding. As internists who are also addiction specialists, we both treat a range of illnesses across the spectrum of medicine. Hands down the most rewarding and among the most treatable conditions we care for is OUD. We hope that this book will provide a roadmap as readers experience the privilege and reward of providing this lifesaving medical care.

Boston, MA, USA   Sarah E. Wakeman
Providence, RI, USA   Josiah D. Rich

References

1. Centers for Disease Control. Provisional drug overdose death counts. Available online at https://www.cdc.gov/nchs/nvss/vsrr/drug-overdose-data.htm Accessed on 26 August 2021.
2. Agency for Healthcare Research and Quality. Blacks Experiencing fast-rising rates of overdose deaths involving synthetic opioids other than methadone. 2020. Publication No. 20-0032-1.
3. Dole VP, Nyswander ME. Methadone maintenance treatment. A ten-year perspective. JAMA. 1976;235(19):2117–9. PMID: 946538.
4. Ghertner R. U.S. trends in the supply of providers with a waiver to prescribe buprenorphine for opioid use disorder in 2016 and 2018. Drug Alcohol Depend. 2019 Nov 1;204:107527. https://doi.org/10.1016/j.drugalcdep.2019.06.029. Epub 2019 Aug 30. PMID: 31525570.
5. Langabeer JR, Stotts AL, Cortez A, Tortolero G, Champagne-Langabeer T. Geographic proximity to buprenorphine treatment providers in the U.S. Drug Alcohol Depend. 2020;213:108131. https://doi.org/10.1016/j.drugalcdep.2020.108131. Epub ahead of print. PMID: 32599495.
6. Lagisetty PA, Ross R, Bohnert A, Clay M, Maust DT. Buprenorphine treatment divide by race/ethnicity and payment. JAMA Psychiat. 2019;76:979–81.
7. Goedel WC, Shapiro A, Cerdá M, Tsai JW, Hadland SE, Marshall BDL. Association of racial/ethnic segregation with treatment capacity for opioid use disorder in counties in the United States. JAMA Netw Open. 2020;3(4):e203711.
8. Hansen H, Siegel C, Wanderling J, DiRocco D. Buprenorphine and methadone treatment for opioid dependence by income, ethnicity and race of neighborhoods in New York City. Drug Alcohol Depend. 2016;164:14–21. https://doi.org/10.1016/j.drugalcdep.2016.03.028. Epub 2016 May 4. PMID: 27179822; PMCID: PMC5539992.
9. Hatcher AE, Mendoza S, Hansen H. At the expense of a life: race, class, and the meaning of Buprenorphine in Pharmaceuticalized "Care". Subst Use Misuse. 2018;53(2):301–310. https://doi.org/10.1080/10826084.2017.1385633. Epub 2017 Nov 21. PMID: 29161171; PMCID: PMC5901978.
10. National Academies of Sciences, Engineering, and Medicine. 2019. Medications for opioid use disorder save lives. Washington, DC: The National Academies Press. https://doi.org/10.17226/25310.

Contents

Contributors

Jacqueline Bango Addiction Consult Team (ACT), Massachusetts General Hospital, Boston, MA, USA

Judy Bartlett Bartlett Evaluation, Albuquerque, NM, USA

Prabhat Chand Centre for Addiction Medicine, Department of Psychiatry, National Institute of Mental Health and Neurosciences (NIMHANS), Bangalore, India

Edouard Coupet Jr Department of Emergency Medicine, Yale School of Medicine, New Haven, CT, USA

Chinazo Cunningham, MD, MS Department of Medicine, Albert Einstein College of Medicine, Bronx, NY, USA

Gail D'Onofrio Department of Emergency Medicine, Yale School of Medicine, New Haven, CT, USA

Honora Englander Division of Hospital Medicine, Department of Medicine, Oregon Health & Science University, Portland, OR, USA

Caroline G. Falker Department of Psychiatry, VA Connecticut Healthcare System, West Haven, CT, USA

Jessica Isom Codman Square Health Center/Boston Medical Center, Dorchester, MA, USA

Ayana Jordan Department of Psychiatry, Yale University School of Medicine, New Haven, CT, USA

Martha T. Kane Department of Psychiatry, Massachusetts General Hospital, Boston, MA, USA

Stephen Hayward Keizer Bridge Clinic & Addiction Consult Team (ACT), Boston, Massachusetts General Hospital, MA, USA

Miriam Komaromy Grayken Center for Addiction, General Internal Medicine, Boston Medical Center, Boston University, Boston, MA, USA

Elizabeth E. Krans Obstetrics and Gynecology, University of Pittsburgh, Pittsburgh, PA, USA

Walter Ling Department of Family Medicine, David Geffen School of Medicine, University of California, Los Angeles, CA, USA

Tiffany Lu, MD, MS Department of Medicine, Albert Einstein College of Medicine, Bronx, NY, USA

Caitlin E. Martin Obstetrics and Gynecology, Virginia Commonwealth University, Richmond, VA, USA

Caridad Ponce Martinez Department of Psychiatry, University of Massachusetts Medical School, Worcester, MA, USA

Angela Mason REACH Health Services, Institutes for Behavior Resources, Inc., Baltimore, MD, USA

Kenneth L. Morford Program in Addiction Medicine and Section of General Internal Medicine, Department of Internal Medicine, Yale School of Medicine, New Haven, CT, USA

Yngvild Olsen REACH Health Services, Institutes for Behavior Resources, Inc., Baltimore, MD, USA

Ashish Premkumar Obstetrics and Gynecology, Northwestern University, Chicago, IL, USA

Darius A. Rastegar Division of Addiction Medicine, Johns Hopkins Bayview Medical Center, Baltimore, MD, USA

Josiah D. Rich Brown University, The Miriam and Rhode Island Hospitals, Providence, RI, USA

Windia Rodriguez Department of Psychiatry, Massachusetts General Hospital, Boston, MA, USA

Elizabeth A. Samuels Department of Emergency Medicine, Alpert Medical School of Brown University, Providence, RI, USA

Madeleine Sedlack Institute of Health Professions & Addiction Consult Team (ACT), Massachusetts General Hospital, Boston, MA, USA

Christopher J. Shaw Addiction Consult Team (ACT), Substance Use Disorder Initiative, Massachusetts General Hospital, Boston, MA, USA

Steve Shoptaw Department of Family Medicine, Department of Psychiatry and Biobehavioral Sciences, David Geffen School of Medicine, University of California, Los Angeles, CA, USA

Zachary Siegel Health in Justice Action Lab, Northeastern University School of Law, Boston, MA, USA

Rachel Simon Department of Medicine, Massachusetts General Hospital, Boston, MA, USA

Kimberly L. Sue, MD, PhD Harm Reduction Coalition, New York, NY, USA

Maia Szalavitz New York, NY, USA

Mishka Terplan Friends Research Institute, Baltimore, MD, USA

Jeanette M. Tetrault Program in Addiction Medicine and Section of General Internal Medicine, Department of Internal Medicine, Yale School of Medicine, New Haven, CT, USA

Sarah E. Wakeman Department of Medicine, Massachusetts General Hospital, Boston, MA, USA

Zoe M. Weinstein General Internal Medicine, Boston University, Boston, MA, USA

Patient-Centered Care in Opioid Use Disorder Treatment

Darius A. Rastegar

What Is Patient-Centered Care?

Patient-centered care has been defined as "care that is respectful of and responsive to individual patient preferences, needs and values" [1]. Patient-centered (or "person-centered") care contrasts with the traditional biomedical model of "doctor-centered" or "illness-centered" care that has defined the practice of medicine. The main objectives of patient-centered care are effective communication, partnership, and health promotion [2]. Although a universally accepted definition is lacking, characteristics of patient-centered care include [3, 4] the following:

1. Respect for patient's values, preferences, beliefs, and expressed needs – that is, recognizing the patient as a person.
2. Shared power and responsibility between patient and clinician.
3. Care that is accessible, continuous, coordinated, and integrated.
4. High-quality information and education for patient and family.
5. Focus on physical comfort and emotional support.
6. Involvement of friends and family when appropriate.

Why Provide Patient-Centered Care?

Providing patient-centered care upholds the fundamental bioethical principles of autonomy, beneficence, and justice. Simply put, patient-centered care is the right thing to do. Therefore, patient-centered care should be the default care model even if it has not been shown to improve outcomes; the burden of proof should be on

D. A. Rastegar (✉)
Division of Addiction Medicine, Johns Hopkins Bayview Medical Center, Baltimore, MD, USA
e-mail: drasteg1@jhmi.edu

© Springer Nature Switzerland AG 2021
S. E. Wakeman, J. D. Rich (eds.), *Treating Opioid Use Disorder in General Medical Settings*, https://doi.org/10.1007/978-3-030-80818-1_1

approaches that are not patient centered. Nonetheless, studies suggest that patient-centered care has many benefits. Behaviors consistent with patient-centered care are associated with increased trust in physicians [5] and with improved health outcomes and reduced health care utilization [6]. Moreover, patient-centered attitudes are associated with a reduction in ethnic and racial disparities in care [7] and hold the promise of doing the same for individuals with substance use disorders (SUD).

How Can Patient-Centered Care Be Applied to Treatment of Individuals with Opioid Use Disorder?

Traditionally, treatment for SUD has been provided by "programs" that are dedicated to addiction treatment and separate from the rest of the health care system. Table 1.1 provides examples of the ways in which "program-centered care" differs from "patient-centered care."

Historically, addiction treatment has been "program-centered" in that individuals with SUD were expected to seek help in locations dedicated to addiction treatment, demonstrate that they were "ready" for treatment, and agree to the rules and expectations of the program. The treatment itself was generally provided in a group setting with a predetermined treatment protocol and duration of treatment. Failure to follow rules or meet expectations was met with sanctions and could lead to discharge from the program. The goal of treatment was abstinence from illicit substances and, in many programs, abstinence from all drugs – including opioid agonist

Table 1.1 Comparing program-centered with patient-centered care for substance use disorders

Program-centered	Patient-centered
Treatment initiation	
Patients must approach the program and prove that they are ready.	Patients are offered help in a variety of health care and community settings.
Patients may be forced into treatment.	Treatment is voluntary.
Patients must agree to rules and expectations prior to starting treatment.	There are no pre-conditions for starting treatment.
Treatment duration	
Patients complete treatment after a pre-determined time period or course of treatment.	There is no pre-determined duration of treatment or endpoint.
Patients are discharged from the program if they do not follow rules or meet expectations.	Patients are provided help for as long as they need it.
Treatment approach	
Treatment is provided in a group setting with a fixed approach.	Treatment plan is tailored to patients' needs.
Treatment entails confrontation and breaking down resistance.	Treatment is supportive and encourages positive changes.
Treatment outcomes	
Treatment goals are set by the program.	Treatment goals are flexible and decided upon in collaboration with patients.
Focus is on drug abstinence.	Focus is on risk reduction, health promotion, improved functioning and quality of life.

therapy. In these settings, patients would "graduate" once they completed the predetermined duration or stages of treatment.

There are a number of ways in which the principles of patient-centered care can be applied to the treatment of individuals with opioid use disorder (OUD). The first is to make treatment easier to access – this can be done by offering treatment in a variety of settings, including community settings and in a range of health care settings from emergency departments to inpatient units and primary care – that is, "meeting patients where they are" rather than waiting for them to find and engage with specialized treatment programs. The treatment of OUD in hospitals, emergency departments, correctional settings, and general medical care are discussed further in Chaps. 4, 5, 6, and 15.

Another important principle of patient-centered care is that it is voluntary. There is a long tradition of forcing or coercing individuals into drug treatment, with pressure being applied by the criminal legal system, social service agencies, employers, and family members [8]. "Drug courts" are the coercive instrument that has been most studied; while mandated drug treatment is arguably more humane than incarceration and evidence suggests court-mandated treatment is marginally better than incarceration (or probation) with no treatment [9], evidence for long-term impact is lacking [10, 11]. Notably, individuals involved in drug courts are often there because of drug use or possession and this approach has never been scientifically compared with voluntary, supportive, patient-centered treatment. Moreover, coercive treatment is fundamentally at odds with a patient-centered approach and there is some evidence that it may be harmful, particularly when individuals are forced into "drug-free" treatment [12].

OUD treatment can also become more patient-centered by providing help and support for affected individuals without preconditions – that is, "low-threshold treatment" [13]. This would include offering harm reduction services, including syringe distribution/exchange, safe consumption sites, naloxone distribution, and pre-exposure prophylaxis for HIV [14]. Harm reduction is covered in more detail in Chap. 10. Another example of low-threshold treatment is opioid agonist treatment on demand (sometimes referred to as "medication first approach"), where opioid agonist medication is provided without preconditions and is only discontinued if there is evidence of harm [15]. Studies have shown that providing methadone [16] or buprenorphine [17] without any additional services dramatically reduces illicit drug use. Moreover, forcing individuals receiving methadone or buprenorphine into counseling and other forms of treatment (i.e., using the medication to "assist with treatment") has not been evident to provide significant benefits [18] and may be harmful if it creates a barrier to receiving life-saving medication [19].

Patient-centered care focuses on outcomes that are important to the patient. Traditionally, drug treatment programs have focused on abstinence from illicit substances and sometimes even certain prescribed medications (i.e., buprenorphine and methadone) as their primary treatment goal. In these settings, any use was labeled as a set back and "relapse." For patients with OUD, patient-centered care would mean developing flexible goals that are decided upon in collaboration with patients and focus on risk reduction, health promotion, improved functioning, and quality of life rather than drug use. As noted earlier, harm-reduction measures take this approach.

A final patient-centered measure is to use "person-first language" when speaking to and about individuals with SUD. For example, referring to a "person with opioid use disorder' instead of "opioid addict" or "opioid abuser." Studies have shown that patients with opioid use disorder prefer person-first language when referring to them [20] and that using person-first language helps to mitigate explicit and implicit biases against this stigmatized population [21].

Why Provide Patient-Centered Care for Opioid Use Disorder?

As noted earlier, the primary reason to provide patient-centered care is because it is the right thing to do. Patient-centered care upholds the ethical principles of autonomy (allowing patients to choose), beneficence (offering any and all treatments that would help), and justice (treating patients with substance use disorder like other patients).

Patient-centered care should be provided because this is what patients want. In a study of patients with OUD receiving buprenorphine in a primary care setting, patients reported valuing a number of patient-centered aspects of care, including physicians adopting an accepting rather than confrontational attitude, flexibility in decision-making, and personalized treatment plans and goals developed in collaboration with the patient [22]. In another study of patients receiving buprenorphine in a primary care setting, fewer required visits and briefer counseling was associated with increased satisfaction with care [23].

There is also some evidence that patient-centered care can improve outcomes for individuals with OUD. It is difficult to summarize the evidence for (or against) patient-centered care because of the heterogeneous interventions that can be considered patient-centered but are not generally labeled as "patient-centered care." As noted earlier, harm reduction strategies are a form of patient-centered care and there is abundant evidence that shows that these strategies help reduce the risks associated with substance use. In addition, developing a therapeutic alliance is a measure that is consistent with patient-centered care; a 2005 review concluded that therapeutic alliance early in treatment is associated with improved engagement and retention in SUD treatment [24]. Flexibility in treatment is also consistent with the patient-centered approach; studies in methadone maintenance programs found that more flexibility in dosing was associated with decreased illicit drug use [25] and improved retention [26]. A 2019 systematic review of patient satisfaction and experience indicators of patient-centered care for people receiving specialist treatment for SUD concluded that "there appeared to be a significant positive relationship between indicators of patient-centered care and improved outcomes" [27].

In one of the few studies that explicitly set out to investigate patient-centered care for OUD, subjects in two methadone programs were randomly assigned to "patient-centered care" or "treatment as usual" [28]. Individuals assigned to patient-centered care were not required to attend counseling sessions and their counselors served solely as therapists and did not enforce rules. The primary outcome was opioid-positive urine drug tests at 12-month follow-up. There was no significant difference in the primary outcome measure; however, two secondary measures were significantly different: Quality of Life Global score was higher among those assigned to patient-centered care (mean of 3.7 vs. 3.5) and they received significantly lower methadone doses (mean of 71 vs. 77 mg). A limitation of this study was that the "treatment as usual" was more patient-centered than traditional programs and did not discharge individuals from treatment if they did not adhere to rules and expectations. Although this was a "negative" study, the primary outcome was not patient-centered and one could argue that quality of life would have been a more appropriate outcome to focus on. Moreover, this study shows that requiring attendance at counseling sessions and having counselors enforce rules does not improve outcomes.

Are There Any Risks or Limitations to Patient-Centered Care for Opioid Use Disorder Treatment?

Addiction treatment has traditionally relied on the carrot and stick approach of providing rewards for desirable behavior and sanctions for undesirable behavior. An example of the "stick" approach are drug courts, which was discussed earlier. There is some evidence that behavioral approaches such as providing the "carrot" of positive incentives (i.e., contingency management) are modestly effective at reaching certain goals (usually abstinence from a specific drug) in the short term (while incentives are offered), but evidence for long-term effectiveness is lacking [29]. The behavioral approach runs contrary to patient-centered care principles. Despite this, it is possible that some individuals respond to behavioral approaches and a patient-centered approach focusing on shared decision-making may not be as effective at reaching certain goals. Research comparing these approaches is needed to answer this question. There may be a middle ground of "nudges" toward positive changes through measures such as scheduling more frequent visits when an individual is not doing well. However, more drastic or coercive measures such as discharge from treatment or discontinuation of pharmacotherapy are more likely to be harmful than beneficial.

Patient-centered care and the pursuit of shared decision-making may lead to an attitude where "the patient is always right" and where practitioners acquiesce to patient demands, even those that are potentially harmful. There are situations where a clinician should do what is best for the patient even if this is contrary to the patient's requests or demands. For example, an individual who is being prescribed opioids for chronic pain may wish to continue receiving these medications after an overdose, but giving in to this demand could put them at risk for further harm and it may be more appropriate to offer a safer alternative such as buprenorphine, even if they are resistant to making this change.

Another potential barrier to patient-centered care when applied to SUD treatment is that decision-making and judgment may be impaired when an individual is intoxicated, withdrawing, or having a strong craving for a substance. This does not absolve clinicians from providing compassionate and effective care, but makes the process of shared decision-making more difficult.

Patient-centered care fits best in the primary care setting where a practitioner is dealing one-on-one with a patient and the care plan can be open-ended and tailored to the patient's values and needs. It is more difficult to apply this approach in the group setting and sometimes the needs of the group may take priority over the needs of an individual. For example, if an individual in a recovery house is using illicit substances, making that person leave would not necessarily be the best for that individual, but may help others in the house maintain a therapeutic community. Despite these competing demands, there are ways in which group treatment can be made more flexible and patient centered.

Conclusion

In summary, health care is moving toward a patient-centered approach. Patient-centered care carries the promise that treatment of individuals with OUD can become more compassionate, ethical, and effective. Treatment of SUD in general has lagged behind this trend and there is a need for efforts to provide treatment that is more patient centered and for evidence to support this transformation.

Acknowledgments The author would like to thank Jarratt Pytell for his helpful comments and feedback during the drafting of this chapter.

References

1. National Research Council. Crossing the quality chasm: a new health system for the 21st century. Washington, DC: National Academies Press; 2001.
2. Constad MK, MacDeermid JC, Bello-Haas VD, Law M. Scoping review of patient-centered care approaches in healthcare. BMC Health Serv Res. 2014;14:271.
3. Mead N, Bower P. Patient-centeredness: a conceptual framework and review of the empirical literature. Soc Sci Med. 2000;51:1087–110.
4. Barry MJ, Edgman-Levitan S. Shared decision making – the pinnacle of patient-centered care. N Engl J Med. 2012;366:780–1.
5. Fiscella K, Meldrum S, Franks P, et al. Patient trust: is it related to patient-centered behavior of primary care physicians? Med Care. 2004;42:1049–55.
6. Stewart M, Brown JB, Donner A, et al. The impact of patient-centered care on outcomes. J Fam Pract. 2000;49:796–804.
7. Beach MC, Rosner M, Cooper LA, Duggan PS, Shatzer J. Can patient-centered attitudes reduce racial and ethnic disparities in care? Acad Med. 2007;82:193–8.
8. Wild TC. Social control and coercion in addiction treatment: towards evidence-based policy and practice. Addiction. 2006;101:40–9.
9. Gottfredson DC, Kearley BW, Najaka SS, Rocha CM. The Baltimore City Drug Treatment Court: 3-year self-report outcome study. Eval Rev. 2005;29:42–64.

10. Wittouck C, Dekkers A, DeRuyver B, et al. The impact of drug treatment courts on recovery: a systematic review. ScientificWorldJournal. 2013;2013:493679.
11. Kearley BW, Cosgrove JA, Wimberly AS, Gottfredson DC. The impact of drug court participation on mortality: 15-year outcomes from a randomized controlled trial. J Subst Abus Treat. 2019;105:12–8.
12. Rafful C, Orozco R, Rangel G, et al. Increased non-fatal overdose risk associated with involuntary drug treatment in a longitudinal study with people who inject drugs. Addiction. 2018;113:1056–63.
13. Snow RL, Simon RE, Jack HE, et al. Patient experiences with a transitional, low-threshold clinic for the treatment of substance use disorder: a qualitative study of a bridge clinic. J Subst Abus Treat. 2019;107:1–7.
14. Walley AY, Stancliff S, Perez-Urbano I. Harm reduction, overdose prevention, and addiction medicine. In: Miller SC, Fiellin DA, Rosenthal RN, Saitz R, editors. The ASAM principles of addiction medicine. 6th ed. Philadelphia: Wolters Kluwer; 2019. p. 473–81.
15. Winograd RP, Presnail N, Stringfellow E, et al. The case for a medication first approach to the treatment of opioid use disorder. Am J Drug Alcohol Abuse. 2019;45:333–40.
16. Schwartz RP, Highfield DA, Jaffe JH, et al. A randomized controlled trial of interim methadone maintenance. Arch Gen Psychiatry. 2006;63:102–9.
17. Sigmon SC, Ochalek TA, Meyer AC, et al. Interim buprenorphine vs. waiting list for opioid dependence. N Engl J Med. 2016;375:2504–5.
18. Amato L, Minozzi S, Davoli M, et al. Psychosocial combined with agonist maintenance treatments versus agonist maintenance treatments alone for opioid dependence. Cochrane Database Syst Rev. 2008;8(4):CD004147.
19. Bentzley BS, Barth KS, Back SE, Book SW. Discontinuation of buprenorphine maintenance therapy: perspectives and outcomes. J Subst Abuse Treat. 2015;52:48–57.
20. Pivovarova E, Stein MD. In their own words: language preferences of individuals who use heroin. Addiction. 2019;114:1785–90.
21. Ashford RD, Brown AM, Curtis B. Substance use, recovery, and linguistics: the impact of word choice on explicit and implicit bias. Drug Alcohol Depend. 2018;189:131–8.
22. Fox AD, Masyukova M, Cunningham CO. Optimizing psychosocial support during office-based buprenorphine treatment in primary care: patients' experiences and preferences. Subst Abus. 2016;37:70–5.
23. Barry DT, Moore BA, Pantolon MV, et al. Patient satisfaction with primary care office-based buprenorphine/naloxone treatment. J Gen Intern Med. 2007;22:242–5.
24. Meier PS, Barrowclough C, Donmall MC. The role of the therapeutic alliance in the treatment of substance misuse: a critical review of the literature. Addiction. 2005;100:304–16.
25. Havassy B, Hargreaves WA, De Barros L. Self-regulation of dose in methadone maintenance with contingent privileges. Addict Behav. 1979;4:31–8.
26. White JM, Ryan CF, Ali RL. Improvements in retention rates and changes in client group with methadone maintenance streaming. Drug Alcohol Rev. 1996;15:83–8.
27. Davis EL, Kelly PJ, Deane FP, et al. The relationship between patient-centered care and outcomes in specialist drug and alcohol treatment: a systematic review. Subst Abuse. 2020;41:216–31.
28. Schwartz RP, Kelly SM, Mitchell SG, et al. Patient-centered methadone treatment: a randomized clinical trial. Addiction. 2016;112:454–64.
29. Ainscough TS, McNeill A, Strang J, Calder R, Brose LS. Contingency management interventions for non-prescribed drug use during treatment for opiate addiction: a systematic review and meta-analysis. Drug Alcohol Depend. 2017;178:318–39.

Opioid Use Disorder Pharmacotherapy: A Historical Perspective on How We Practice, and Why

2

Walter Ling and Steve Shoptaw

Even if history doesn't repeat itself, those who ignore its lessons will still suffer.

—Mama Ling

Introduction

The introduction of methadone maintenance treatment in the 1960s ushered in the modern era of pharmacotherapy for opioid use disorders (OUD) [1]. Four opioid-based medications have since been approved and marketed: methadone, L-alpha-acetylmethadol (LAAM), naltrexone, and buprenorphine [2]. LAAM is not currently available because the manufacturer has discontinued its supply; naltrexone is available in an oral and an injectable form; and buprenorphine is available in several buccal formulations, a subdermal implant, and several subcutaneous injections. In the United States, methadone's availability is limited to highly regulated specialized opioid treatment clinics. Therefore, the available medications for treatment of OUD in general medical settings in the US consist of two formulations of naltrexone and several formulations of buprenorphine. Still, since methadone had played a pivotal role in heralding in the era of modern opioid pharmacotherapy, and, more importantly, its historical evolution continues to determine how we practice OUD pharmacotherapy today, it is where our story begins. In addition, since we are concerned here primarily with the historical events that shaped our current practice, we will

W. Ling (✉)
Department of Family Medicine, David Geffen School of Medicine, University of California, Los Angeles, CA, USA
e-mail: lwalter@ucla.edu

S. Shoptaw
Department of Family Medicine, Department of Psychiatry and Biobehavioral Sciences, David Geffen School of Medicine, University of California, Los Angeles, CA, USA
e-mail: SShoptaw@mednet.ucla.edu

© Springer Nature Switzerland AG 2021
S. E. Wakeman, J. D. Rich (eds.), *Treating Opioid Use Disorder in General Medical Settings*, https://doi.org/10.1007/978-3-030-80818-1_2

limit ourselves to providing only brief discussions of the clinical pharmacology of these medications, emphasizing those historical events that are relevant to our discussion.

Methadone

Invented by German scientists during World War II (WWII), methadone is a synthetic opioid analgesic with properties similar to morphine. It is quickly absorbed and slowly eliminated after oral administration, with an onset of action within 30 minutes of ingestion and an elimination half-life of about 18–24 hours. After WWII, the pharmaceutical company Eli-Lilly marketed methadone under the trade name Dolophine, used widely as an analgesic in clinical practice in this country.

In the late 1940s, studies at the Addiction Research Center in Lexington, Kentucky, found that methadone prevented symptoms of opioid withdrawal and reduced craving in people with opioid use disorder (OUD). Its long half-life allowed for once daily dosing. Tapering dosages of methadone were commonly given for the management of opioid withdrawal for "detoxification" [3], and by the 1950s, a small number of physicians in several cities were using methadone maintenance as an experimental treatment for heroin addiction, typically conducted under an Investigative New Drug (IND) application except for research work done in New York City by Dr. Vincent Dole and Dr. Marie Nyswander [1]. They were not the first to use methadone as a maintenance treatment, but they were the first to assert that treating heroin addiction with methadone was a legitimate medical practice and did not require an IND. Dole and Nyswander have been rightfully credited with the introduction of methadone maintenance treatment for OUD in this country, subsequently adopted by the rest of the world.

By the early 1970s, several thousand patients were receiving methadone maintenance treatment, notably in cities like New York and Chicago. Contrary to popular belief, many patients with OUD wanted treatment, and methadone stabilized their lives, allowing them to not use illicit opioids and other drugs, maintain employment, and stay out of jail—by not having to commit acquisitive, drug-related crimes. One such program was the State of Illinois's Drug Treatment Program in Chicago led by Dr. Jerome Jaffe.

Meanwhile, a pilot program in the District of Columbia showed that methadone maintenance significantly reduced street crime [3–5]. That caught the attention of the Nixon administration.

In 1967, the "Summer of Love" when the media began to focus on the youth bohemian counterculture known as the hippy movement, was a period accompanied by significant drug use. In addition, this era was marked by the Vietnam War and the protests against it. In Vietnam, many American soldiers were using heroin and some developed addiction, creating problems when they returned to the US for the military and for the Veterans Affairs Service. The confluence of these events, corresponding with President Richard Nixon running for a second term promising to be a law and order president and to reduce crime, gave rise to the idea to treat heroin addiction as a means of crime reduction. These political forces led to the establishment of the presidential-appointed cabinet-level Special Action Office for Drug Abuse Prevention (SAODAP), with Dr. Jerome Jaffe as its Director.

Under Dr. Jaffe's leadership, SAODAP initiated the US national methadone treatment system, which continues to be a major treatment modality for patients with OUD. SAODAP's effort has undoubtedly benefited more patients with OUD in the US and worldwide than any other single event in addiction medicine. Many countries adopted the US methadone treatment system and adapted it according to their own understanding and approach toward caring for people with OUD. In 2005, methadone was added to the World Health Organization's list of essential medications. Unlike the adaptations made to this model in other countries, the US system has unfortunately remained an entrenched industry. The history of SAODAP's effort to implement methadone treatment offers many lessons still relevant to our addiction medicine practice today.

From the beginning, methadone had its detractors: some in the recovery community, particularly those running therapeutic communities; law enforcement; and the medical establishment itself. When Jaffe proposed using methadone to treat heroin addiction, the National Institute of Mental Health did not support it. Instead, they wanted to expand psychotherapy, despite the fact that everybody interested in the subject already knew that psychotherapy did not work as treatment for OUD [3, 4].

With opposition coming from multiple quarters, SAODAP had to make compromises to protect methadone maintenance treatment so that it could thrive and be available to patients who wanted treatment. Up until that time, except for the Dole and Nyswander program, the administration of methadone to treat opioid addiction was mostly conducted under IND applications issued by the Food and Drug Administration (FDA), exempting the practice from policies of the Bureau of Narcotics, which considered it illegal to provide any opioid to people addicted to opioids.

Before 1970, the criteria for granting these INDs were rather loose, and in time concerns arose as to whether those applying were all legitimate addiction treatment researchers. Were some of them just money-making outfits exploiting patients? The major concerns were related to fears about the risk of methadone street diversion, accidental poisoning, and iatrogenic methadone addiction. Under mounting pressure from the community and Congress, the FDA proposed new rulings for issuance of INDs in 1970, imposing stringent requirements for treatment admission, limits on dosage, and duration of treatment. These presented serious barriers for patients with OUD seeking treatment.

Given the broader context at the time when SAODAP was proposing to expand methadone treatment throughout the country, it is not surprising that compromises were made just to garner support to move the project forward. Methadone clinics had to agree to urine testing and mandatory counseling that remain as required components of methadone treatment today. Dose limits on medications and limiting the length of treatment are still with us as well.

Urine Drug Testing

The first large-scale urine drug testing was put in place to detect heroin use in soldiers returning from Vietnam; those who tested positive had to stay behind and undergo medically supervised withdrawal. When Jaffe first proposed the idea of using urine drug testing to reduce heroin use among servicemen in Vietnam, there was strong opposition. At a meeting at the Pentagon, the generals were adamant that forcing soldiers to provide a urine sample was out of the question. Dr. Jaffe was reported to have said in response, "I cannot believe that the mightiest army on earth can't get its troops to piss in a bottle." That seemed to have won the argument [5, p. 110]. Testing demonstrated that the rate of heroin addiction among the soldiers was much lower (3–4%) than then believed (10–15%), and that many who dabbled in it could stop when they had reasons to do so.

Clinical urine drug testing began as an assurance to prevent methadone street diversion that could lead to accidental overdoses deaths in people not tolerant to opioids or be sold on the street and theoretically create new OUD. As time would show, accidental overdose rarely occurs, and virtually all the diverted street methadone was bought by people with OUD who wouldn't, and shouldn't, have had to do so if treatment had been made, as Jaffe had hoped, available to all those who wanted it. Iatrogenic methadone addiction simply did not exist. The two major arguments for drug testing did not stand the test of time.

Unfortunately, these findings over time did not make the treatment system rethink and limit drug testing to what would be clinically useful. Instead, urine drug testing has grown into a thriving industry of its own. More and more drugs are added to the list tested with little clinical considerations. Test results are often used to blame and punish patients instead of helping them. Billions are spent with little added therapeutic value except to enrich the industry. This is not to say that drug testing is useless, but rather that its practice today is largely unjustified and unhelpful.

Required Counseling

Counseling by counselors who themselves had a history of addiction was based on the premise that counselors' shared life experiences could uniquely help patients enter into recovery. This hypothesis was never tested or proven true, despite becoming a routine component of treatment. Instead of serving to extend patient care, counseling grew into a parallel service often in conflict with the physician's treatment goals. It also, unfortunately, provided the treatment industry excuses to reduce physician's time with patients by delegating the major therapeutic responsibility to the counsellor. Clinic operators constantly tried to negotiate less required physician time by promoting counselor time. Thus, the counselor became the patient's gatekeeper of physician access and often exercised control over patients, to their detriment. In a clinical study of buprenorphine plus counselling, most patients rated medications as very helpful, yet only 1% of patients rated counselling as helpful [6]. Yet counseling remains a required part of treatment today. No other medical practice has such a requirement. Although psychosocial treatments can be helpful, they are most so when they are in service to patients—not just filling a requirement to access medication [6, 7]. Many people in methadone who are recovering from OUD need help with health care, with getting (or keeping) a job, with housing instability, and with managing other life stressors like the burden of correctional supervision. For the most part, these are not what most counselling provides. So, most patients who have jobs and are engaging in prosocial lives experience the requirement for counseling in methadone treatment as a burden—not unlike that experienced by individuals without OUD when dropping their kids off for daycare who are mandated to have a session with the daycare administrator.

LAAM; Levo-alpha-acetylmethadol

L-alpha-acetylmethadol (LAAM), a congener of methadone with similar opioid activities, is often mistakenly called "long-acting methadone" (LAAM) by methadone patients because the terms sound alike. Its similarity to methadone, however, is far more complex than being clinically "long-acting." LAAM is a prodrug that is metabolized in the liver into two active metabolites, Nor-LAAM and Di-nor-LAAM, each more potent than the parent compound. Together, a single dose of LAAM can provide an opioid effect similar to methadone that lasts up to 48 hours, about twice that of methadone. It can thus be administered three times a week, with a higher dose on Friday, to achieve similar clinical effects of daily doses of methadone.

LAAM also was synthesized by German scientists during WW II, and became available to US investigators after the War. Early work by Fraser and colleagues had shown that LAAM possesses opioid analgesic properties and can alleviate the opioid abstinence syndrome and block the effects of subsequently administered opioids. Research in its analgesic use was abandoned, however, when it was discovered that the required repeated dosing for analgesia led to accumulation of metabolites that caused respiratory depression, nausea, vomiting, mental confusion, and, in some cases, coma [8, 9].

In the 1960s, a number of studies showed that LAAM could be a treatment for heroin addiction. Dr. Jaffe was familiar with this work when he was appointed to head SAODAP. He decided to roll out methadone immediately to meet the clinical demands and to undertake careful research to show LAAM's safety and efficacy, and then to bring on LAAM to replace or augment methadone. Since LAAM can be given three times a week, it would alleviate the patient's need to attend clinic daily for a prolonged period of time, at least for months, during a period critical to their rehabilitation [10–12].

SAODAP supported a number of large-scale clinical studies of LAAM's safety and efficacy compared to methadone, notably the multicenter VA Cooperative Study [13], the SAODAP Cooperative Studies [14, 15], the Goldstein Cohort Study [16], and others. By 1980, sufficient data had been accumulated to consider application of a New Drug Application. Unfortunately, the first application was deemed insufficient because of technical issues.

Meanwhile, the political climate shifted. The nation became preoccupied with cannabis, and we were into Mrs. Reagan's "Just say no" years. There was great fear that cannabis would be a gateway drug that leads to serious addiction with other hard drugs. It was not, and it did not. What did happen was a brewing serious cocaine problem, which exploded into a deadly epidemic with the introduction of crack cocaine in the 1980s.

Efforts to address opioid addiction thus took a back seat until another change in administration and the establishment of NIDA's Division of Medication Development. With renewed effort and several additional studies, a LAAM NDA application was successful in 1993, 20 years after SAODAP's concerted effort to bring it to clinical use.

Even so, LAAM's clinical implementation was fraught with difficulties. Chief among these was that Drug Enforcement Administration (DEA) mandated that dispensing of LAAM must occur within opioid treatment programs. The hard lessons from this chapter of the development of an opioid pharmacotherapy is worth remembering. Why was LAAM not a clinical success despite its research proven safety and efficacy? The answer lies not in the medication itself, but in its timing, the social political climate, and the regulatory process.

To bring LAAM to the marketplace required regulatory approval by multiple governmental bodies at the state and local levels. Since the use of opioids was regulated by the states, this means the manufacturer had to repeat this process at every state. Clinical uptake was so slow that 3 years after its approval, just over 800 patients were receiving LAAM treatment in only 62 of the 750 licensed opioid treatment programs [3].

Meanwhile, there were the usual oppositions from skeptics, law enforcement, and the abstinence-oriented recovery communication. By this time, methadone treatment had grown into an industry and those who were benefitting from it wanted to maintain the status quo.

Roxane, which owned LAAM at that point, made an application to the European Union's Drug commission for approval. When asked to provide additional data on a small number of cases of possible drug-related deaths, it did not respond, which led to LAAM's removal from European countries. This removal is often mistakenly said to be for toxicity, but it was in fact for failure to respond to the inquiries.

In the US, concerns about prolonged QTc, largely overblown, led to the FDA's issuance of a "black box" warning.

Facing so many obstacles to implementation, and realizing its period of exclusivity was running out, the manufacturer saw little incentive to maintain its interest in the marketplace and decided to discontinue LAAM's manufacturing and distribution. It was not withdrawn by the FDA for reason of safety; rather it was killed by bureaucracies and self-interests.

Thus, an effective medication that was methodically and systematically studied, and proven clinically safe and efficacious, was never given the opportunity to benefit patients not because it doesn't work, but for reasons unrelated to its pharmacology, and it could be said, precisely because it had been shown to work.

Buprenorphine

Buprenorphine's discovery was part of the systematic search for a non-addicting morphine-like analgesic that could selectively retain its desired analgesic properties while shedding the undesirable ones.

The discovery of nalorphine, a morphine antagonist with analgesic properties, heralded in the era of agonist/antagonist analgesics that included compounds like butorphanol, nalbuphine, and pentazocine, thought to be antagonist at the mu receptor and agonist at the kappa receptor. They were subsequently found to be partial agonists at both receptors. The exception was buprenorphine, uniquely different in being a partial agonist only at the mu receptor and an antagonist at the kappa receptor [17].

First synthesized in the 1960s, buprenorphine, a highly effective analgesic with potency 25–40 times that of morphine, was introduced into clinical use as a parenteral analgesic in 1978, and shortly thereafter as sublingual tablets and in the 1990s as a transdermal patch. In the United States, buprenorphine had been available as an injectable analgesic long before its use in treating OUD [3, 17].

Buprenorphine entered as candidate for treating OUD in the 1970s with studies by Jasinski and his colleagues [12]. Early work in inpatient settings had shown that buprenorphine diminished self- administration of heroin [18, 19], blocked the effects of subsequently administered doses of morphine [20], and on abrupt discontinuation, due to its tight binding to the opioid receptor, resulted in a slow onset, long-lasting, milder abstinence syndrome compared to that seen in morphine [21].

Dr. Jasinski postulated that buprenorphine might just be the right medication to treat patients with OUD since it possessed properties like those of both methadone and naltrexone. He hypothesized that patients would not mind taking it because it alleviated symptoms of withdrawal, but it also blocked subsequently administered opioids and therefore could prevent relapse. He was right.

A series of controlled clinical trials comparing buprenorphine to methadone, buprenorphine to placebo, and buprenorphine in ascending doses, confirmed its safety and efficacy for treatment of OUD, leading to its final approval by the FDA. And, with the passage of the Drug Addiction Treatment Act (DATA) in 2000, it became the first opioid-based medication available to treat OUD in physicians' normal practice setting for a century [22]. That effort had to overcome many oppositions, including those from people whose mission was to provide care for OUD patients, such as the methadone industry, the therapeutic community or "rehab" industry, and law enforcement. It literally took an act of Congress to make buprenorphine available to physicians in the general medical setting. Even so, it came with strings [4].

Under the provisions of DATA 2000, qualified physicians in the medical office and other appropriate settings outside the opioid treatment program system may prescribe and/or dispense Schedule III, IV, and V opioid medications for the treatment of opioid addiction, if such medications have been specifically approved by the Food and Drug Administration (FDA) for that indication. In practice, that means buprenorphine alone.

Physicians must obtain special designation on DEA registration, which requires certain qualifications relevant to addiction medicine—training, certification, or experience conducting research—and undergo an 8-hour training or submit a notice of intent under new practice guidelines. They can only treat a certain number of patients, must provide or make provision for counseling, perform required urine drug testing, and keep a list of patients for DEA inspection. Dose and time limits continue to loom in the background, often required by insurance plans. A most frequently asked question is when patients can get off buprenorphine. And of course, the right answer of when to stop a medication used to treat a chronic disease is when there is significant stability in medical health, in psychological and social functioning, in regular work, and in spiritual peace. Discontinuing buprenorphine absent this stability reliably increases risks for return to drug use.

The introduction of buprenorphine is the most notable watershed event in addiction medicine since the introduction of methadone. For the first time in nearly a century, physicians are able to use an opioid medication to treat OUD in their regular places of practice. Its significance lies not in the availability of a new, safe, and effective medication, but in the fact that the care of patients with OUD is returned to the hands of the physician. This calls for a new treatment philosophy, which requires changes in attitude and practice on the part of the physicians, which is to say physicians must themselves change before they can change the lives of their patients [22, 23].

Naltrexone

Research in opioid antagonists began as part of the effort to find non-addicting opioid analgesics dating from the 1930s. Nalorphine, a narcotic antagonist, was found to have analgesic properties and can prevent and abolish the actions of morphine [24, 25]. There were also Cyclazocine and Naloxone before Naltrexone [24–28].

Nalorphine was tried therapeutically but its use was limited by its short duration of action. Cyclazocine has longer duration of action but still requires daily dosing. Its side effects—dysphoria, vivid imagery, and anxiety, and its limited supply—hampered its search efforts [26]. Naloxone is similar but five to eight times more powerful than nalorphine; an oral dose of 100 mg blocks the effects of 20 mg heroin for up to 10 hours. However, its poor oral absorption, short duration of action, and high cost made naloxone a difficult choice for further development.

Naltrexone, a potent opioid antagonist, was first synthesized by scientists in the Endo laboratories in 1967. Naltrexone seems to possess all the desirable characteristics of an ideal antagonist and none of its drawbacks [27]. It completely blocks the euphoric effects of opioids like heroin and morphine—an oral dose of 50 mg blocks the effects of 25 mg heroin for up to 24 hours. It has low agonist effects of its own, does not cause physical dependence, does not show tolerance to its antagonist effects with chronic use, has no serious side effects even in chronic administration, and is easily administered orally.

Using an opioid antagonist for OUD had its rationale based on Dr. Abraham Wikler's postulate of extinction. Animals trained to self-administer opioids who were given an opioid antagonist that blocks the reward of the opioids would stop opioid self-administration. The lack of reward thus serves to extinct the drug use behavior. It was believed that humans would do the same [28, 29].

More specifically, naltrexone could be useful for the prevention of relapse based on the theory of addiction being a conditioned response, which posits that persons with addiction respond to stressful stimuli in life by seeking out drugs [29]. In time, tolerance develops to the rewarding aspects and increasing doses are needed to satisfy the desire. When drugs are not available, withdrawal is experienced and even after cessation of use and abatement of withdrawal symptoms, the individual experiences triggered withdrawal from environmental cues, leading to drug use—relapse—as a learned conditioned response. In this postulation, repeated use of heroin without the anticipated subjective effects would lead to extinction of the learned drug-seeking behavior.

There was great enthusiasm in using opioid antagonists as therapy for opioid addiction in the early 1970s. In 1970, barely 4 years after its synthesis, Congress designated it a high priority and gave specific funding for President Nixon's SAODAP to develop its use in treating OUD. As the Director of SAODAP put it, "SAODAP really had no choice in the matter."

Early clinical trials showed that it was very difficult to get patients who were maintained on methadone tapered off methadone and to stay off opioids long enough to be inducted onto naltrexone [30, 31]. People who were under threat, like physicians fearing loss of medical license to practice, people under correctional supervision taking naltrexone as a condition for a day pass to work, and people who were given money for coming to the clinic, found naltrexone acceptable, and those who took it stopped using heroin. Without the motivational lever, though, most people reject naltrexone. For example, parolees who received naltrexone while on parole stopped taking naltrexone as soon as they got off parole [30].

The responsibility to develop naltrexone, when SAODAP was phased out, fell to the newly established National Institute on Drug Abuse (NIDA), which coordinated several groups of studies for its safety and efficacy. It was approved for treatment of OUD in 1984, based on the laboratory evidence that it can block the effects of heroin. However, there was little data on its efficacy in clinical use.

Subsequent roll out of naltrexone was met with poor patient acceptance except for "highly motivated" people under threat of one kind or another, or those incentivized to take it. Most patients, given a choice, opted for another treatment. One of naltrexone's virtues, it was said, was that when you take it, it makes you feel like you have taken nothing. Apparently, no one had thought to ask patients with OUD whether they wanted to take medications that makes them feel like they have taken nothing; the answer, as it turned out, appears to be no.

Despite its low patient acceptance, NIDA continued to search for a longer-acting formulation of naltrexone which might improve patient adherence [32–34]. An injectable formulation with a 1-month duration of action became available but recruiting patients to participate in clinical trials proved to be difficult in the US where patients had choices of other medications. Eventually, a study conducted in Russia where agonist treatments were not available, generated sufficient data for the FDA's approval of depo-naltrexone for the treatment of OUD. Thus, ironically, a US product depended on data generated in Russia to obtain approval for its clinical use in the US [35].

The use of depo-naltrexone remains limited and controversial today. Induction on to the medication continues to prove difficult for those actively using opioids—who most need treatment. The manufacturer's promotion of the product has invited scrutiny by authorities, and the interpretation and propagation of certain research data have raised questions of propriety. In a clinical trial comparing buprenorphine to depo-naltrexone, the investigators found a large number of patients assigned to naltrexone failed naltrexone induction. Nevertheless, they selected to consider only patients who succeeded in getting on to the medication to conclude that since the subsequent performance of the two surviving groups were not different, the two medications are equally effective [36].

Success in induction onto a medication, and benefiting subsequently from it, is both critically important to the patient's success in recovery from OUD. In research, that means intent to treat analysis. There are no other acceptable measures of clinical effectiveness.

Comments and Conclusions

The lessons from history are many and some of them bring suffering; every reader comes away with her own insight. We here highlight our own biases.

The methadone story shows our society's ambivalence toward addiction and people with addiction. We simultaneously say that these patients are sick and need help, yet our policies and practices treat them as if they are sinners and need to suffer. We study addiction as a disease but treat patients with addiction as if they are just behaving badly. We are entrenched in our belief that patients with addiction cannot be trusted. We insist on their proving to us that they will take their medications faithfully, not sell them on the street to cause accidental overdose deaths, and create new opioid addiction. When follow-up data showed that our concerns were unfounded, we ignored the data and kept the practice.

The LAAM story reminds us that a medication with proven safety and efficacy does not necessarily succeed in the marketplace, even if it is superior to existing treatments. There has to be a champion that can garner support from the regulators and treatment providers, and a message that can reach the patients and patient advocates who are skeptical about the motives of the treatment system. The political climate has to be conducive. There needs to be sufficient financial incentives for the manufacturer, and not a threat to those already in control of the treatment system. In the end, LAAM's lessons largely call our attention to the competing interests of different parties. Treatment goals are not the same for patients, physicians, society, regulators, and the treatment industry. Everybody talks about serving patients, but everybody looks for ways to serve their own interests first.

The history of buprenorphine in this country shows the tremendous barriers which can be imposed by governmental regulation of clinical practice. We are left saddled with a cumbersome, inefficient, and irrationally conservative approach to using buprenorphine, often to the detriment of patient care: outdated training, overly elaborate and drawn-out induction schedules, and concerns about nonexistent hypersensitivity. This was all largely the result of the governmental agencies caving into the demands of the treatment industry. In his book *The Axemaker's Gift*, James Burke, with Ornstein, tells us that every gift, like the axe, is double edged. The regulatory agencies have become partners with what they regulate, and their own survival depends on it. While some of the people in charge of the treatment apparatus may have patients' best interest in mind, too often they give priority to their own interests.

Both the methadone and buprenorphine experience also remind us that perhaps God's greatest creation isn't Adam and Eve, but how easily humans get used to things. Remember the joke about Eve, after they had been in the Garden of Eden for a while, said to Adam "Adam, is this it?"

What about us? Is it not time to have a citizens' work group to address the rational use of buprenorphine?

Finally, the naltrexone story shows how we Americans act based on what we *believe* instead of what is demonstrated to be true. Our love for naltrexone, in all its formulations, can be traced to our long-held irrational belief that OUD recovery means taking no opioids. We do not want to give an opioid to any person with OUD despite the favorable treatment outcome. We believe irrationally that taking an agonist medication is swapping one drug for another, not true recovery, and we want everyone to be "drug free."

Let us tell the naltrexone story like it is. Its clinical effectiveness is limited by difficulties in induction onto the medication and by poor patient acceptance. And it is not equally effective as buprenorphine in clinical practice.

References

1. Dole VP, Nyswander M. A medical treatment for diacetylmorphine (heroin) addiction. A clinical trial with methadone hydrochloride. JAMA. 1965;193:646–50.
2. Ling W, Rawson RA, Compton MA. Substitution pharmacotherapies for opioid addiction: from methadone to LAAM and buprenorphine. J Psychoactive Drugs. 1994;26(2):119–28.
3. Campbell ND, Lovell AM. The history of the development of buprenorphine as an addiction therapeutic: Campbell & Lovell. Ann N Y Acad Sci. 2012;1248(1):124–39.
4. Jaffe JH, O'Keeffe C. From morphine clinics to buprenorphine: regulating opioid agonist treatment of addiction in the United States. Drug Alcohol Depend. 2003;70(2 Suppl):S3–11.
5. Massing M. The Fix [Internet]. 1998 [cited 2020 Jan 12]. Available from: https://www.goodreads.com/work/best_book/1095104-the-fix.
6. Ling W, Hillhouse M, Ang A, Jenkins J, Fahey J. Comparison of behavioral treatment conditions in buprenorphine maintenance. Addiction. 2013;108(10):1788–98.
7. Schwartz RP, Kelly SM, Mitchell SG, Gryczynski J, O'Grady KE, Gandhi D, et al. Patient-centered methadone treatment: a randomized clinical trial. Addict Abingdon Engl. 2017;112(3):454–64.

8. Fraser HF, Isbell H. Actions and addiction liabilities of alpha-acetylmethadols in man. J Pharmacol Exp Ther. 1952;105(4):458–65.

9. Fraser HF, Nash TL, Vanhorn GD, Isbell H. Use of miotic effect in evaluating analgesic drugs in man. Arch Int Pharmacodyn Ther. 1954;98(4):443–51.

10. Jaffe JH. The maintenance option and the Special Action Office for Drug Abuse Prevention. Psychiatr Ann. 1975;5:12–42.

11. Jaffe JH. The history and current status of opiate agonist treatment; 1997. p. 19–25.

12. Jasinski DR, Pevnick JS, Griffith JD. Human pharmacology and abuse potential of the analgesic buprenorphine: a potential agent for treating narcotic addiction. Arch Gen Psychiatry. 1978;35(4):501–16.

13. Ling W, Charuvastra C, Kaim SC, Klett CJ. Methadyl acetate and methadone as maintenance treatments for heroin addicts. A veterans administration cooperative study. Arch Gen Psychiatry. 1976;33(6):709–20.

14. Ling W, Klett CJ, Gillis RD. A cooperative clinical study of methadyl acetate. I. Three-times-a-week regimen. Arch Gen Psychiatry. 1978;35(3):345–53.

15. Ling W, Klett JC, Gillis RD. A cooperative clinical study of methadyl acetate. II. Friday-only regimen. Arch Gen Psychiatry. 1980;37(8):908–11.

16. Judson BA, Goldstein A. Levo-alpha-acetylmethadol (LAAM) in the treatment of heroin addicts I. Dosage schedule for induction and stabilization. Drug Alcohol Depend. 1979;4(6):461–6.

17. Cowan A, Lewis JW, Macfarlane IR. Agonist and antagonist properties of buprenorphine, a new antinociceptive agent. Br J Pharmacol. 1977;60(4):537–45.

18. Mello NK, Mendelson JH. Buprenorphine suppresses heroin use by heroin addicts. Sci New Ser. 1980;207(4431):657–9.

19. Mello NK, Mendelson JH, Kuehnle JC. Buprenorphine effects on human heroin self-administration: an operant analysis. J Pharmacol Exp Ther. 1982;223(1):30–9.

20. Bickel K, Stitzer L, Johnson E, Bigelow E, Liebson A, Jasinski R. Buprenorphine: dose-related blockade of opioid challenge effects in opioid dependent humans. J Pharmacol Exp Ther. 1988;247:47–53.

21. Kosten TR, Morgan C, Kleber HD. Treatment of heroin addicts using buprenorphine. Am J Drug Alcohol Abuse. 1991;17(2):119–28.

22. Ling W. Buprenorphine for opioid dependence. Expert Rev Neurother. 2009;9(5):609–16.

23. Ling W. A perspective on opioid pharmacotherapy: where we are and how we got here. J Neuroimmune Pharmacol. 2016;11(3):394–400.

24. Unna K. Antagonistic effect of N-allyl-normorphine upon morphine | J Pharmacol Exp Ther [Internet]. 1943 [cited 2019 Dec 10]. Available from: http://jpet.aspetjournals.org/content/79/1/27.

25. Houde R. Analgesic effectiveness of the narcotic agonist-antagonists. Br J Clin Pharmacol. 1979;7(S3):297S–308S.

26. Fink M, Freedman AM, Zaks A, Resnick RB. Narcotic antagonists another approach to addiction therapy. Am J Nurs. 1971;71(7):6.

27. Martin WR, Jasinski DR, Mansky PA. Naltrexone, an antagonist for the treatment of heroin dependence: effects in man. Arch Gen Psychiatry. 1973;28(6):784–91.

28. Martin WR. Naltrexone, an antagonist for the treatment of heroin dependence: effects in man | JAMA Psychiatry | JAMA Network [Internet]. 1973 [cited 2019 Dec 1]. Available from: https://jamanetwork.com/journals/jamapsychiatry/article-abstract/490912.

29. Wikler A. Conditioning factors in opiate addiction and relapse. In: Psychology in the Schools [Internet]. 1966 [cited 2019 Dec 1]. p. 21–9. Available from: https://onlinelibrary.wiley.com/doi/abs/10.1002/1520-6807%28196610%293%3A4%3C375%3A%3AAID-PITS2310030419%3E3.0.CO%3B2-L.

30. Hollister LE, Schwin RL, Kasper P. Naltrexone treatment of opiate-dependent persons. Drug Alcohol Depend. 1977;2(3):203–9.

31. Ling W, Wesson DR. Naltrexone treatment for addicted health-care professionals: a collaborative private practice experience. J Clin Psychiatry. 1984;45(9 Pt 2):46–8.

32. Comer SD, Sullivan MA, Yu E, Rothenberg JL, Kleber HD, Kampman K, et al. Injectable, sustained-release naltrexone for the treatment of opioid dependence: a randomized, placebo-controlled trial. Arch Gen Psychiatry. 2006;63(2):210–8.
33. Colquhoun R, Tan DYK, Hull S. A comparison of oral and implant naltrexone outcomes at 12 months. J Opioid Manag. 2005;1(5):249–56.
34. Comer SD, Collins ED, Kleber HD, Nuwayser ES, Kerrigan JH, Fischman MW. Depot naltrexone: long-lasting antagonism of the effects of heroin in humans. Psychopharmacology. 2002;159(4):351–60.
35. Krupitsky E, Nunes EV, Ling W, Gastfriend DR, Memisoglu A, Silverman BL. Injectable extended-release naltrexone (XR-NTX) for opioid dependence: long-term safety and effectiveness. Addiction. 2013;108(9):1628–37.
36. Lee JD, Nunes EV, Novo P, Bachrach K, Bailey GL, Bhatt S, et al. Comparative effectiveness of extended-release naltrexone versus buprenorphine-naloxone for opioid relapse prevention (X:BOT): a multicentre, open-label, randomised controlled trial. Lancet. 2018;391(10118):309–18.

Principles of Integrating Opioid Use Disorder Treatment in Primary Care

3

Tiffany Lu and Chinazo Cunningham

Introduction

Over the last two decades of rising opioid-related overdoses in the United States, the integration of treatment for opioid use disorder (OUD) in primary care has been an important approach to expanding access to care. National survey data highlights a substantial treatment gap for OUD, with less than 20% of an estimated 2 million people with OUD receiving treatment in the past year [1]. Primary care as a site for integration of OUD treatment is crucial for several reasons. First, the demand for integrated treatment in primary care is high for people with OUD who are not in treatment [2]. Second, primary care is a common touchpoint within the healthcare system for people with substance use disorders [3, 4]. Third, primary care settings are well suited to integrate treatment of OUD as a chronic condition, where proactive, team-oriented management of chronic medical illnesses is already being implemented [5].

The integration of OUD treatment in primary care is extensively described and evaluated in the literature. Successful integration centers around the availability of medications for OUD, namely buprenorphine and injectable naltrexone. Unlike methadone, buprenorphine is a partial opioid agonist that can be prescribed outside of federally regulated opioid treatment programs by clinicians who complete the required training and receive a special waiver. The literature is robust in demonstrating the feasibility, acceptability, and effectiveness of buprenorphine treatment in primary care [6–9]. Injectable naltrexone is an opioid antagonist that can be prescribed for OUD in general medical settings without requiring a special waiver. However, studies demonstrating the effectiveness of injectable naltrexone have not focused on primary care settings [10–12]. In addition, based on studies comparing OUD treatment outcomes and mortality between injectable naltrexone and

T. Lu (✉) · C. Cunningham
Department of Medicine, Albert Einstein College of Medicine, Bronx, NY, USA
e-mail: tlu@montefiore.org

© Springer Nature Switzerland AG 2021
S. E. Wakeman, J. D. Rich (eds.), *Treating Opioid Use Disorder in General Medical Settings*, https://doi.org/10.1007/978-3-030-80818-1_3

buprenorphine, practical challenges with providing injectable naltrexone treatment, and treatment guidelines for primary care settings, buprenorphine is generally a preferred treatment option over naltrexone [11–15]. Therefore, in this chapter, we focus on integrating OUD treatment in primary care with buprenorphine.

In this chapter, we describe principles of integrating OUD treatment in primary care, with focus on evidence-based approaches to addressing integration barriers. Principles of integration include the organization of care, assessing and preparing patients for treatment, buprenorphine formulations, initiating treatment, maintaining treatment, and addressing concerns for diversion. Although OUD treatment can be offered through individual primary care providers (PCPs), we center our discussion at the level of a primary care practice. Integration approaches vary from practice to practice, depending on the internal and external clinic system. We draw on experiences and findings from diverse primary care practices, including hospital-based clinics, academic primary care clinics, federally qualified health centers, community health centers, as well as urban and rural locations.

Organization of Care

Treatment Team

The integration of OUD treatment in primary care starts with structuring the treatment team. The optimal composition of the treatment team depends on the existing capacity and environment of the primary care setting. The most common type of OUD treatment team in primary care is *multidisciplinary*, which consists of two or more different types of health professionals working together to deliver OUD treatment [8]. The multidisciplinary team can be organized to promote *care coordination* between patients and their PCPs. The multidisciplinary team can also be organized to promote *shared care*, where the PCP may work with other clinical disciplines to comanage patients with OUD.

In the multidisciplinary team, the PCP is responsible for medical evaluation and medication management for OUD. PCPs currently need to be waivered under the Drug Addiction Treatment Act 2000 in order to prescribe buprenorphine treatment for OUD. PCPs are typically trained in general internal medicine or family medicine, and do not require specialty training in addiction medicine in order to treat OUD in primary care [16–20]. At academically affiliated primary care practices, resident physicians can provide buprenorphine treatment under the supervision of waivered PCPs [21–23]. Physician assistants and nurse practitioners in primary care practices can also be waivered to prescribe buprenorphine treatment under the Comprehensive Addiction and Recovery Act 2016 [24, 25].

Care coordinators are an essential part of the multidisciplinary team for integrated OUD treatment in primary care. Care coordinators are nonphysician health professionals who are responsible for supporting patients in OUD treatment and facilitating medical and behavioral health needs. Care coordinators may include nurses, pharmacists, or social workers who are trained in OUD treatment.

One well-studied type of care coordinator is nurse care managers, who are registered nurses that perform patient assessments and provide patient education in collaboration with PCPs [26, 27]. Hiring and training nurse care managers for collaborative care of OUD in primary care has been particularly successful in Massachusetts, where nurse care manager services in community health centers are billable to Medicaid, in addition to usual reimbursement for PCP visits and medications [7]. Pharmacists can also function as care coordinators, which is important in primary care practices where PCPs have varying levels of experience in medication initiation and maintenance for OUD [19, 28]. In primary care practices with integrated behavioral health care, social workers can take on the role of care coordinator [29]. The added benefit for social workers as care coordinators for OUD treatment is the ability to offer on-site psychosocial counseling, in addition to brief psychosocial counseling provided by the PCP.

Specialists can be part of the multidisciplinary team such that OUD treatment is delivered through *shared care* between PCPs and specialists. Addiction medicine specialists who are often also trained as generalists can be co-located in the primary care clinic to deliver and supervise integrated OUD treatment [22]. Psychiatrists are another type of specialist who can comanage medications for OUD and also evaluate and treat comorbid mental illness. Co-located psychiatrists have been important part of OUD treatment teams in primary care clinics that provide integrated HIV treatment [30, 31]. Psychiatrists do not have to be co-located in primary care to deliver *shared care*; for primary care clinics in rural settings, remotely located psychiatrists can be integrated to deliver OUD treatment through telemedicine [32]. Clinical psychologists can also facilitate *shared care* in the multidisciplinary team, albeit with a focus on providing psychosocial counseling and not medication management [33–35].

In addition, peer recovery coaches can be essential nonclinical members of the multidisciplinary team for OUD treatment. Peer recovery coaches are individuals with lived experience of substance use disorder who can provide outreach, navigation, and support for patients with OUD. Peer recovery coaches in nonprimary care settings have been found to improve treatment engagement and substance use outcomes [36]. The inclusion of peer recovery coaches as a part of the multidisciplinary team is feasible and promising for integrated OUD treatment in primary care [9].

Treatment Visits

OUD treatment in the primary care setting can be delivered through in-person visits or telemedicine visits. Under DATA 2000, office-based buprenorphine treatment requires the clinician to be waivered and to have the capacity to refer for appropriate counseling services; however, the organization of treatment visits are not regulated. The Ryan Haight Act of 2008, however, stipulates that clinicians prescribing controlled substances need to conduct at least one in-person medical evaluation of each patient, with the exception of clinicians who otherwise meet federal and state requirements to practice telemedicine. In this context, OUD treatment in primary care generally relies on in-person visits, at least initially.

National guidelines on office-based opioid treatment (OBOT) provide a roadmap for planning treatment visits [37, 38]. At the level of the primary care practice, OBOT consists of individual visits with the waivered PCP at the minimum. For primary care practices that utilize a multidisciplinary team, OBOT entails individual visits with the PCP, care coordinator, and/or co-located specialist. For example, the care coordinator may conduct the initial visit to gather information about a patient's substance use, comorbid illnesses, and treatment goals, while the PCP conducts a subsequent visit to confirm the diagnosis of OUD and tailor the treatment plan. In general, OBOT engages and retains patients through in-person visits.

While individual visits are typical, group visits are an emerging approach to expand access to OUD treatment in primary care. In group-based opioid treatment (GBOT), patients engage with the treatment team through group visits, where medical management along with group counseling are provided for multiple patients at the same time [39–41]. GBOT is feasible and acceptable for patient populations who need intensified psychosocial supports, including people experiencing homelessness as well as people with ongoing illicit opioid use [42, 43]. For primary care settings where there are a limited number of PCPs and/or co-located specialists waivered to prescribe buprenorphine, GBOT can address barriers of provider shortage for OUD treatment.

Telemedicine visits are also possible in primary care-based OUD treatment, but have historically been more common in rural health settings, where patients and PCPs access remotely located addiction specialists [32, 44]. More recently, federal regulations limiting telemedicine for buprenorphine treatment initiation were waived under the declaration of public health emergency for Coronavirus Disease 2019 (COVID-19). Telemedicine visits for OUD treatment have since been adopted widely in nonrural health settings, but at the time of this chapter's writing, have not been rigorously evaluated [45, 46]. Still, telemedicine visits can facilitate greater access and convenience for patients with OUD, as well as more flexibility in care delivery in the primary care setting [47–49]. Future use of telemedicine visits for OUD treatment depends on regulatory and reimbursement changes beyond the duration of COVID-19 pandemic.

Treatment Referrals

Patients with OUD may be referred to OUD treatment in primary care in various ways.

Patients may self-refer for treatment based on word of mouth or by searching for waivered providers listed on publicly available buprenorphine treatment locators [50]. More often, treatment referrals originate from clinicians within the primary care practice or affiliated medical center, as well as from local substance use treatment programs [18, 20, 30, 50]. The treatment referral process between specialty substance use treatment and primary care can be formalized through hub-and-spoke models, where patients initiate treatment in opioid treatment programs then transfer to primary care clinics for continue treatment [51, 52]. Treatment referrals can also be formalized between acute care settings and primary care settings. Buprenorphine treatment can be initiated in the emergency department with linkage to ongoing treatment in primary care [53, 54]. Patients who initiate OUD treatment during an inpatient admission may also be referred to primary care for both medical follow-up and OUD treatment [55–57]. Finally, treatment referrals from within the primary care practice can be expanded by implementing screening protocols for OUD [29, 58, 59]. Although patients with suspected OUD may be identified and counseled about treatment options with this approach, the effectiveness of screening, brief intervention, and referral to treatment for OUD is not clear in the primary care setting.

Assessing and Preparing Patients for Treatment

Following treatment referral, the next step is to ensure patients are comprehensively assessed to determine whether they are appropriate for OUD treatment in the primary care setting. The initial assessment also forms the basis of the treatment plan and establishes a baseline for measuring a patient's response to treatment. Components of the initial assessment include discussing current opioid use and patterns, other substance use, prior treatment, and experiences; identification of comorbid medical conditions and mental illness; assessing social supports and social needs; and determining readiness and goals to engage in treatment [37, 60]. Patients who are appropriate for OUD treatment in primary care should have a diagnosis of OUD, be interested in treatment, and able to demonstrate informed consent about risks and benefits of treatment.

During the initial assessment, the treatment team should consider patient-level factors that can increase the risk of adverse events while receiving medications for OUD, such as comorbid use of alcohol, sedatives, hypnotics, and anxiolytics. Historically, national guidelines listed concurrent alcohol or benzodiazepine use disorder as contraindications to office-based treatment of OUD [37, 61]. With continued worsening of the opioid overdose epidemic in the US, updated guidance now encourages individualized risk–benefit analysis and acknowledges the risk of withholding treatment for patients with comorbid alcohol or benzodiazepines use [62]. In general, for primary care practices that are in the early stages of integrating OUD treatment, focus on patients without significant comorbid use disorders who are likely to have optimal treatment outcomes with few complications may be more manageable for a novice care team. However, once the treatment team gains more experience, providing OUD treatment to patients who are more complex is warranted.

Beyond comorbid alcohol and/or benzodiazepine use, polysubstance use should not be a contraindication to OUD treatment in primary care. "High threshold and low tolerance" models for OUD treatment that require patients to be abstinent from nonopioid substances are associated with poor outcomes during treatment linkage, when patients are referred and assessed but have not yet initiated treatment [20, 63, 64]. In contrast, lowering the threshold for OUD treatment in primary care by not excluding patients with co-occurring substance use is not associated with worse outcomes [65, 66]. For example, patients with OUD who use cocaine experience similar buprenorphine treatment retention and illicit opioid use reduction compared to those who do not use cocaine [67]. Thus, patients with polysubstance use are appropriate for OUD treatment in primary care, taking into account that medications for OUD are not expected to treat other substance use disorders, and that treatment plans can be tailored on an individual basis to reduce harms from polysubstance use.

Other comorbid medical and mental health conditions should guide the initial assessment and treatment planning. Chronic pain often co-occurs with OUD and influences options of medications for OUD (e.g., injectable naltrexone may interfere with adequate analgesia). Patients with chronic pain, however, do not fare worse in primary care–based OUD treatment [68]. Depression and anxiety are also common in patients with OUD; patients with OUD requiring psychoactive medications for depression and anxiety can be successfully managed in primary care [69]. Serious mental illness with active suicidal ideation or psychosis, however, should prompt the treatment team to connect patients with specialized mental health care. In addition, national guidelines outline considerations for special populations that engage with OUD treatment in primary care, including pregnant persons, adolescents, and criminal-legal system–involved persons [61]. Coordinated care with specialty medical and mental health care as well as community-based supports is a critical part of primary care–based OUD treatment for these special populations.

Clinical tools to help assess and prepare patients for treatment should be adapted and implemented by the treatment team. Standardized intake forms help organize the many different components of the initial assessment. For patients who are ready to initiate treatment, treatment agreements may be used to delineate patient goals, risks and benefits of treatment, and expectations for both the patients and the treatment team [8].

Buprenorphine Formulations

Formulations of buprenorphine that are approved by the US Food and Drug Administration for the treatment for OUD are growing. As of July 2020, buprenorphine-containing medications approved for OUD treatment include buprenorphine and buprenorphine/naloxone sublingual tablets, buprenorphine/naloxone sublingual films, buprenorphine subcutaneous injections, and buprenorphine subdermal implants. In this chapter, we focus on the most widely used formulations of buprenorphine for OUD treatment—buprenorphine/naloxone tablets or films. Few studies have examined integration of buprenorphine injections or implants into primary care settings. While the use of these medications may expand in the future, in this chapter we do not discuss the unique challenges or issues that are associated with integrating these formulations of buprenorphine treatment into primary care.

When considering buprenorphine versus buprenorphine/naloxone tablets or films, the risk of misuse is greater with buprenorphine monoproducts than buprenorphine/naloxone products. In addition, there are few indications for buprenorphine monoproduct tablets or films; these include pregnancy and an allergy to naloxone. While we are not aware of data reporting the prevalence or incidence of allergies to naloxone, in our experience of providing buprenorphine treatment in primary care for over 15 years, allergies to naloxone are extremely rare. Therefore, we focus on the treatment of OUD with buprenorphine/naloxone tablets or films when discussing treatment initiation and maintenance below.

Initiating Treatment

When initiating buprenorphine treatment, goals include reducing or stopping illicit or misused opioids, reducing opioid withdrawal, and reducing opioid craving. Initiating buprenorphine treatment can be challenging due to its pharmacologic properties. Buprenorphine has a high affinity for the mu opioid receptor and is a partial opioid agonist; therefore, the first dose of buprenorphine can lead to acute precipitated opioid withdrawal. In this scenario, individuals with OUD who recently used a full opioid agonist (e.g., heroin, oxycodone, or fentanyl) then take buprenorphine, which displaces the full opioid agonist from the mu opioid receptor. Buprenorphine activates the mu opioid receptor, but as a partial agonist rather than a full agonist. This relative difference between full and partial opioid agonism manifests as acute precipitated opioid withdrawal. For that reason, individuals with OUD typically must experience symptoms of opioid withdrawal prior to buprenorphine initiation. When in opioid withdrawal from full opioid agonists, the risk of worsening opioid withdrawal is minimized, such that taking buprenorphine improves symptoms of withdrawal. Although precipitated opioid withdrawal is an exceptionally uncomfortable experience for patients, it is generally not dangerous or life-threatening.

Because of this challenge in initiating buprenorphine, national guidelines had initially called for initiation of treatment to occur under observation in clinical settings [37, 61]. However, several studies have demonstrated that unobserved treatment initiation (e.g., initiating treatment at home) has similar outcomes to observed initiation, and is common, feasible, acceptable, safe, and effective [70–73]. Therefore, initiating buprenorphine treatment in observed clinical settings or in unobserved settings, like home, are appropriate, which is reflected in recent treatment guidelines [13, 62]. Choosing the optimal treatment initiation strategy depends on patient experience, comfort, and preference, and account for provider experience and practice capacity. Clinical guides to conduct observed and unobserved treatment initiation are publicly available and also referenced at the end of this chapter [60, 70, 74]. Figure 3.1 shows an example patient guide for unobserved treatment initiation that has been effectively implemented in the primary care setting [71, 75].

For some individuals with OUD who may not be able to tolerate opioid withdrawal, low-dose buprenorphine initiation, sometimes call "microdosing", is an

STARTING BUPRENORPHINE ("Bupe" or "Suboxone")
Congratulations on starting treatment!

WHAT TO START WITH?

✓ 4 Buprenorphine ("Bupe") pills or films (8 mg)
(**There are many different brand names and generic forms of Bupe. Some are shown below.)

☐ 6 Ibuprofen pills (200 mg) – for body pain, take 1-2 pills every 8 hours as needed
☐ 6 Clonidine pills (0.1 mg) – for anxiety, take 1 pill every 8 hours as needed
☐ 6 Imodium pills (2.0 mg) – for diarrhea, take 1 pill after each episode of diarrhea. Max 6 pills per day

---

WHEN AM I READY TO START BUPE?

✓ Use the list of symptoms below to see when you are ready to start Bupe.
✓ Wait until you have **at least 5 symptoms** to start Bupe. If you don't have 5 symptoms, wait a bit longer and review the symptoms again. It is very important that you wait until you feel at least 5 symptoms before starting Bupe! To be sure that you are ready to start, it's best to have at least 1 of the 5 symptoms in the grey shaded area.

Symptoms	Do I have this?
I feel like yawning	☐ Yes
My nose is running	☐ Yes
I have goose bumps	☐ Yes
My muscles twitch	☐ Yes
My bones & muscles ache	☐ Yes
I have hot flashes	☐ Yes
I'm sweating	☐ Yes
I feel unable to sit still	☐ Yes
I am shaking	☐ Yes
I feel nauseous	☐ Yes
I feel like vomiting	☐ Yes
I have cramps in my stomach	☐ Yes
I feel like using	☐ Yes

THINGS _NOT TO DO_ WITH BUPE

✗ DON'T use Bupe when you are high—it will make you dope sick!
✗ DON'T use Bupe with alcohol –this combination is **not safe**.
✗ DON'T use Bupe with benzos (like Xanax ("sticks"), Klonopin, Valium, Ativan) unless prescribed by a doctor who knows you are taking Bupe.
✗ DON'T use Bupe if you are taking pain killers until you talk to your doctor.
✗ DON'T use Bupe if you are taking more than 60 mg of methadone.
✗ DON'T swallow Bupe – it gets into your body by melting under your tongue.
✗ DON'T lose your Bupe – it can't be refilled early.

Fig. 3.1 Patient instruction sheet for buprenorphine "home induction" or unobserved treatment initiation. Adopting clinical tools for primary care–based OUD treatment is important to supporting evidence-based practices such as unobserved buprenorphine treatment initiation. This patient instruction sheet was developed and implemented as part of an overall home-induction tool kit at a large community health center [71, 75]. It contains six sections that explain the typical contents of an initiation medication regimen, when to start taking buprenorphine, things not to do, how to take buprenorphine, plans to guide treatment initiation and facilitate follow-up, and a log to track medications taken

HOW TO TAKE BUPE

    ✓   **Before** taking Bupe, drink some water.
    ✓   Put Bupe **under** your tongue.
    ✓   Don't eat or drink anything until the Bupe has **dissolved completely**.

PLAN
- Use your last heroin / methadone / pain pill: _____
- When you have at least 5 symptoms from the list, then you are ready to start.
- Start with _____ pill or film under your tongue.
- Wait _____ minutes.
- If you feel the same or just a little better, then take another_____ pill or film
- Wait 2 hours – if you still feel sick or uncomfortable, take another _____ pill or film.

PROBLEMS? QUESTIONS?
- Call _____ at _____.
- Call _____ if you still feel sick after taking a total of _____ pills or film (____ mg).

NEXT STEPS
- Appointment with _____ at _____
- Appointment with Dr. _____ at _____

WHAT I TOOK

	Time	Amount of pills or films
Day 1	_____am / pm	_____
	_____am / pm	_____
	_____am / pm	_____
	_____am / pm	_____
Day 2	_____am / pm	_____
	_____am / pm	_____
	_____am / pm	_____
	_____am / pm	_____
Day 3	_____am / pm	_____
	_____am / pm	_____
	_____am / pm	_____

Fig. 3.1 (continued)

emerging method for buprenorphine initiation, particularly in the context of comorbid chronic pain or transitioning from high-dose methadone [76–78]. Details on low-dose buprenorphine initiation is outside the scope of this chapter.

Maintaining Treatment

When maintaining buprenorphine treatment, goals typically include reduction or cessation of illicit or misused opioids, OUD recurrence prevention, retention in primary care, improvements in other health conditions (e.g., HIV or hepatitis C viral infection), and improvements in psychosocial circumstances. There is no ideal duration for the treatment of OUD. Studies have not determined the optimal duration of treatment; however, the longer the duration of OUD treatment, the better are the outcomes. Patients who discontinue buprenorphine treatment are at very high risk of recurrence of OUD and overdose, particularly in the 2-week period following discontinuation [79].

Visits during buprenorphine maintenance are typically more frequent (e.g., weekly to monthly) at the beginning of treatment, and less frequent (e.g., monthly or every 2–3 months). after patients have been stable for some time. There are no data to support any specific interval of visit frequency. Manualized "medical management" of buprenorphine maintenance visits, which has been included in studies, can be delivered by physicians or nurses, typically takes 20 minutes to deliver, and focuses on recent drug use, efforts to achieve abstinence, mutual-help group activities, review of urine toxicology results, and support and advice for reducing or abstaining from drugs [34]. While delivering a manualized treatment plan during maintenance visits may be cumbersome and not feasible for many providers, addressing these elements while also supporting patients to develop and use healthy coping strategies is warranted and similar to care management for other chronic conditions in primary care.

OUD is a chronic condition, and recurrence of opioid use is common and an expected part of OUD. In primary care settings, at 6–12 months, approximately half to two-thirds of patients are retained in buprenorphine treatment, and ongoing opioid use occurs in up to one quarter of patients [27, 65, 71, 80, 81]. While many sociodemographic and clinical characteristics are associated with improved treatment retention, importantly, higher dose of buprenorphine/naloxone (12/3 mg and higher) is associated with longer treatment retention [82, 83]. With most chronic medical conditions, when patients experience poorly controlled disease, providers modify or intensify treatment. Treatment of OUD is no different. Therefore, when patients have recurrence of active use, modifying or intensifying OUD treatment is an appropriate response (rather than terminating treatment). Intensification can take many forms, including more frequent visits, adding or increasing psychosocial counseling, adding or increasing outpatient drug treatment programs or mutual-help activities, addressing mental health conditions, and potentially increasing the dose of buprenorphine/naloxone.

Although patients who discontinue buprenorphine treatment are at very high risk of recurrence and overdose [14], if patients have a strong desire to taper buprenorphine/naloxone and stop buprenorphine treatment, providers should discuss and evaluate the patient's reasons for wanting to do so. Many patients experience stigma of taking an opioid agonist for OUD treatment [84]. If stigma plays a role in patients' desire to stop buprenorphine treatment, providers should ensure that patients understand that OUD is a chronic illness that requires long-term management. If a decision is made to taper buprenorphine treatment, providers should provide education and counseling to address the risks of recurrence of use and overdose due to decreased opioid tolerance and offer a slow taper over several months. While studies have not adequately examined the optimal speed and duration of tapering buprenorphine/naloxone, compared to a fast taper, a slow taper is likely to lead to less severe opioid withdrawal symptoms and may be more tolerable. In addition, ensuring patients know that they can resume buprenorphine or increase their dose for reemergence of craving, withdrawal symptoms, or use is critical.

Psychosocial Counseling

Patients receiving buprenorphine treatment should be assessed for the need for psychosocial counseling and offered psychosocial counseling. However, data do not support *requiring* patients to receive counseling beyond what is delivered by primary care providers during routine visits; consequently, patients should not be excluded from receiving buprenorphine treatment because of lack of participation in psychosocial counseling [85]. In studies examining extensive versus brief psychosocial counseling among patients receiving buprenorphine treatment, outcomes were no better in those receiving extensive counseling [34, 86, 87]. Still, because many patients who have OUD also have mental health comorbidities, it is important that these patients receive appropriate treatment for co-occurring psychiatric illness. Mutual-help groups, such as 12-step support programs, have not been shown to be effective in rigorous randomized trials; however, many patients find these programs to be useful, and therefore can play an important adjunctive role to buprenorphine treatment [18]. When patients receive psychosocial counseling, depending on available resources, a patient-centered treatment plan may include treatment by an on-site behavioral health provider in the primary care setting or referral for treatment at an off-site location [81].

Toxicology Tests

Similar to other chronic illnesses, obtaining objective clinical information about patients' progress toward their goals can be helpful. When treating OUD, urine or oral fluid toxicology tests may provide important information. However, thoughtful use of toxicology in a way that is patient-centered rather than punitive is crucial. Toxicology tests can be an important tool to detect use of prescribed medications, along with detection of other substances that may be used by patients. Despite its potential importance, many providers have limited knowledge on interpretation of toxicology results, and toxicology testing can be challenging [88, 89]. In addition, because there are racial disparities in providers' approach to ordering toxicology testing [90], to minimize biases, it is important to have standardized approaches to ordering and interpreting toxicology tests.

Although an in-depth discussion on urine or oral fluid toxicology testing interpretation is beyond the scope of this chapter, it is important to note key approaches to toxicology tests. One key issue is to understand the different types of urine and oral fluid toxicology tests, including their indication, test characteristics, and cost. An appropriate first step is ordering a "screening" toxicology test in which results are reported as negative/positive often for a class of substances (e.g., using an enzyme-linked immunosorbent assay [ELISA] to detect opiates). Then, depending on results, a follow-up confirmatory test may be appropriate in which results are reported as levels of specific metabolites (e.g., using gas chromatography/mass spectrometry [GC/MS] to determine the level of oxycodone or morphine). It is critical to recognize that for opioids, many synthetic opioids require ELISA tests that are specific to the opioid – for example, methadone, buprenorphine, and fentanyl are not detected as "opiates," but require specific ELISA tests for each of them. Guidance on urine and oral fluid toxicology interpretation is available in the published literature and publicly accessible websites, and should be part of the clinical toolkit for OUD treatment in primary care [91, 92].

A second key issue is to have a clear understanding and transparent discussion with patients about how toxicology tests might be beneficial as a component of their treatment plan and also any ways testing could cause unintentional harm, for example, in the case of pregnant, birthing, or parenting people or people under correctional supervision. For all patients, it is important to establish what the clinical response is likely to be for a toxicology result suggesting recurrence of opioid use or other substance use. Using harm reduction principles, in those situations, patients are likely best suited by intensifying treatment, rather than terminating treatment. This should be clarified for the patient, who may have had prior treatment experiences which were more punitive. Additionally, it is helpful to address how urine tampering, which is not uncommon, will be handled [93, 94]. Having clear discussions and expectations about handling surprising results is important for providers and patients. For both providers and patients, it is important to frame the goal of treatment as being clinical and functional improvement in the treated person's life, which toxicology is an imperfect measure of.

Diversion

Because buprenorphine treatment involves prescribing a controlled substance to people with OUD, many providers are concerned about the potential for diversion (sharing or selling medication) [95, 96]. Among people with OUD, diversion with buprenorphine does occur; however, it occurs to a similar degree as within the general populations with other medications such as antibiotics [97–99]. Relative to other opioids which are nearly all full opioid agonists, studies suggest that diversion with buprenorphine, a partial opioid agonist, is less common [100, 101]. In addition, diversion often occurs because of the lack of availability of buprenorphine treatment. For example, many individuals who do not receive OUD treatment report taking diverted buprenorphine to self-treat symptoms of opioid withdrawal [102].

Therefore, it is important to understand motivations as to why diversion may occur [102–104].

Several strategies can be implemented in attempts to minimize diversion. Treatment agreements are a standardized way to explicitly discuss expectations of buprenorphine treatment, as well as consequences to specific behaviors. Treatment agreements can include important key tools such as the role of toxicology tests and pill counts, along with concerns about diversion [8]. As discussed above, toxicology tests can detect whether metabolites of buprenorphine are present in the urine or oral fluid, indicating that buprenorphine medication is taken. In addition, mobile health to monitor adherence, short duration between visits, and prescriptions for a small amount of medication may be all be additional tools if concerns for diversion arise [49, 105, 106]. While there is no foolproof way to ensure that patients do not divert their medication, addressing diversion through harm reduction principles and a standardized approach is likely to lead to overall patients' benefits outweighing harms. Lastly, given that most diversion is related to limited access to OBOT or high threshold or unwelcoming OUD treatment models, a crucial strategy to address diversion is to expand access to buprenorphine treatment, including in primary care.

Conclusion

The integration of OUD treatment in primary care is critical to addressing rising overdose deaths and glaring gaps in treatment access that underlie the opioid overdose epidemic. Successful integration ensures that primary care providers are trained to initiate and maintain medication treatment for OUD, and that patients with OUD can modify or intensify treatment through the course of their chronic illness.

The organization of care for OUD treatment can be tailored to the primary care practice, including but not limited to inclusion of care coordinators, specialists, and/or peer recovery coaches in a multidisciplinary treatment team, utilizing telemedicine visits and group visits where appropriate, and formalizing treatment referrals from the local health system. Patients with OUD who are informed about treatment options and ready to reduce or stop opioid use can safely initiate medication treatment – namely sublingual buprenorphine – in the primary care setting through unobserved treatment initiation strategies.

As OUD is a chronic condition, maintaining OUD treatment requires that a patient-centered approach is consistently used to inform the components and intensity of the treatment plan, as well as the dosing and duration of medication treatment. Toxicology tests can be important to monitoring treatment adherence and substance use, but their utility in informing the treatment plan must be approached in a standardized manner using harm reduction principles. Similarly, diversion of buprenorphine is not uncommon in OUD treatment and requires a standardized approach that balances harms with the benefits of ongoing access to medication.

Future directions for strengthening the integration of OUD treatment in primary care are numerous. These include rigorous evaluations of the quality and safety of telemedicine use for OUD treatment, as well as the effectiveness of incorporating peer-delivered recovery support services specific to the primary care setting. Further research is needed to evaluate the effectiveness of mobile health applications and other innovative strategies that improve engagement and retention in primary care–based OUD treatment.

References

1. Substance Abuse and Mental Health Services Administration. Key substance use and mental health indicators in the United States: results from the 2018 National Survey on Drug Use and Health; 2019.
2. Barry CL, Epstein AJ, Fiellin DA, Fraenkel L, Busch SH. Estimating demand for primary care-based treatment for substance and alcohol use disorders. Addiction [Internet]. 2016;111(8):1376–84. Available from: http://doi.wiley.com/10.1111/add.13364.
3. Wu L-T, McNeely J, Subramaniam GA, Brady KT, Sharma G, Van Veldhuisen P, et al. DSM-5 substance use disorders among adult primary care patients: results from a multisite study. Drug Alcohol Depend [Internet]. 2017;179(3):42–6. Available from: https://linking-hub.elsevier.com/retrieve/pii/S0376871617303277.
4. Lapham G, Boudreau DM, Johnson EA, Bobb JF, Matthews AG, McCormack J, et al. Prevalence and treatment of opioid use disorders among primary care patients in six health systems. Drug Alcohol Depend [Internet]. 2020;207(May 2019):107732. Available from: https://doi.org/10.1016/j.drugalcdep.2019.107732.
5. McLellan AT, Starrels JL, Tai B, Gordon AJ, Brown R, Ghitza U, et al. Can substance use disorders be managed using the chronic care model? Review and recommendations from a NIDA Consensus Group. Public Health Rev [Internet]. 2014;35(2). Available from: http://www.ncbi.nlm.nih.gov/pubmed/26568649.
6. HHS. Medication-assisted treatment models of care for opioid use disorder in primary care settings. Heal Hum Serv [Internet]. 2016;(28). Available from: http://effectivehealthcare.ahrq.gov/ehc/products/636/2225/opioid-use-disorder-draft-report-160513.pdf.
7. Korthuis PT, McCarty D, Weimer M, Bougatsos C, Blazina I, Zakher B, et al. Primary care-based models for the treatment of opioid use disorder: a scoping review. Ann Intern Med. 2017;166(4):268–78.
8. Lagisetty P, Klasa K, Bush C, Heisler M, Chopra V, Bohnert A. Primary care models for treating opioid use disorders: what actually works? A systematic review. PLoS One. 2017;12:1–40.
9. Wakeman SE, Rigotti NA, Chang Y, Herman GE, Erwin A, Regan S, et al. Effect of integrating substance use disorder treatment into primary care on inpatient and emergency department utilization. J Gen Intern Med [Internet]. 2019;34(6):871–7. Available from: http://link.springer.com/10.1007/s11606-018-4807-x.
10. Green TC, Clarke J, Brinkley-Rubinstein L, BDL M, Alexander-Scott N, Boss R, et al. Postincarceration fatal overdoses after implementing medications for addiction treatment in a statewide correctional system. JAMA Psychiatry. 2018;75:405–7.
11. Tanum L, Solli KK, Latif Z-H, Benth JŠ, Opheim A, Sharma-Haase K, et al. Effectiveness of injectable extended-release naltrexone vs Daily buprenorphine-naloxone for opioid dependence. JAMA Psychiatry [Internet]. 2017;74(12):1197. Available from: http://archpsyc.jama-network.com/article.aspx?doi=10.1001/jamapsychiatry.2017.3206.
12. Lee JD, Nunes EV, Novo P, Bachrach K, Bailey GL, Bhatt S, et al. Comparative effectiveness of extended-release naltrexone versus buprenorphine-naloxone for opioid relapse prevention (X:BOT): a multicentre, open-label, randomised controlled trial. Lancet [Internet]. 2018;391(10118):309–18. Available from: https://linkinghub.elsevier.com/retrieve/pii/S014067361732812X.
13. New York State Department of Health AIDS Institute. Clinical guidelines program – treatment of opioid use disorder [Internet]. 2019. Available from: https://www.hivguidelines.org/substance-use/oud/.

14. Larochelle MR, Bernson D, Land T, Stopka TJ, Wang N, Xuan Z, et al. Medication for opioid use disorder after nonfatal opioid overdose and association with mortality. Ann Intern Med [Internet]. 2018;1–10. Available from: http://annals.org/article.aspx?doi=10.7326/M17-3107.

15. Wakeman SE, Larochelle MR, Ameli O, Chaisson CE, McPheeters JT, Crown WH, et al. Comparative effectiveness of different treatment pathways for opioid use disorder. JAMA Netw Open. 2020;3(2):e1920622.

16. Fiellin DA, Moore BA, Sullivan LE, Becker WC, Pantalon MV, Chawarski MC, et al. Long-term treatment with buprenorphine/naloxone in primary care: results at 2–5 years. Am J Addict. 2008;17:116–20.

17. Soeffing JM, Martin LD, Fingerhood MI, Jasinski DR, Rastegar DA. Buprenorphine maintenance treatment in a primary care setting: outcomes at 1 year. J Subst Abuse Treat [Internet]. 2009;37(4):426–30. Available from: https://doi.org/10.1016/j.jsat.2009.05.003.

18. Mintzer IL, Eisenberg M, Terra M, MacVane C, Himmelstein DU, Woolhandler S. Treating opioid addiction with buprenorphine-naloxone in community-based primary care settings. Ann Fam Med [Internet]. 2007;5(2):146–50. Available from: http://www.annfammed.org/cgi/doi/10.1370/afm.665.

19. Tannous BA, Teng J. Secreted blood reporters: insights and applications. Biotechnol Adv [Internet]. 2011;29(6):997–1003. Available from: http://www.pubmedcentral.nih.gov/articlerender.fcgi?artid=2840630&tool=pmcentrez&rendertype=abstract.

20. Stein MD, Cloe P, Friedmann PD. Brief report: buprenorphine retention in primary care. J Gen Intern Med. 2005;20(11):1038–41.

21. Kunins HV, Sohler NL, Giovanniello A, Thompson D, Cunningham CO. A buprenorphine education and training program for primary care residents: implementation and evaluation. Subst Abus. 2013;34(3):242–7.

22. Holt SR, Segar N, Cavallo DA, Tetrault JM. The addiction recovery clinic: a novel, primary-care-based approach to teaching addiction medicine. Acad Med. 2017;92(5):680–3.

23. Pytell JD, Buresh ME, Graddy R. Outcomes of a novel office-based opioid treatment program in an internal medicine resident continuity practice. Addict Sci Clin Pract [Internet]. 2019;14(1):1–7. Available from: https://doi.org/10.1186/s13722-019-0175-z.

24. Andrilla CHA, Moore TE, Patterson DG. Overcoming barriers to prescribing buprenorphine for the treatment of opioid use disorder: recommendations from rural physicians. J Rural Heal [Internet]. 2019;35(1):113–21. Available from: http://doi.wiley.com/10.1111/jrh.12328.

25. Molfenter T, Knudsen HK, Brown R, Jacobson N, Horst J, Van Etten M, et al. Test of a workforce development intervention to expand opioid use disorder treatment pharmacotherapy prescribers: protocol for a cluster randomized trial. Implement Sci. 2017;12(1):1–9.

26. LaBelle CT, Han SC, Bergeron A, Samet JH. Office-Based Opioid Treatment with buprenorphine (OBOT-B): statewide implementation of the Massachusetts collaborative care model in community health centers. J Subst Abuse Treat [Internet]. 2016;60:6–13. Available from: https://linkinghub.elsevier.com/retrieve/pii/S0740547215001464.

27. Alford DP, LaBelle CT, Kretsch N, Bergeron A, Winter M, Botticelli M, et al. Collaborative care of opioid-addicted patients in primary care using buprenorphine: five-year experience. Arch Intern Med [Internet]. 2011;171(5):425–31. Available from: http://archinte.jamanetwork.com/article.aspx?doi=10.1001/archinternmed.2010.541.

28. DiPaula BA, Menachery E. Physician-pharmacist collaborative care model for buprenorphine-maintained opioid-dependent patients. J Am Pharm Assoc. 2015;55:187–92.

29. Watkins KE, Ober AJ, Lamp K, Lind M, Setodji C, Osilla KC, et al. Collaborative care for opioid and alcohol use disorders in primary care. JAMA Intern Med [Internet]. 2017;177(10):1480. Available from: http://archinte.jamanetwork.com/article.aspx?doi=10.1001/jamainternmed.2017.3947.

30. Haddad MS, Zelenev A, Altice FL. Integrating buprenorphine maintenance therapy into federally qualified health centers: real-world substance abuse treatment outcomes. Drug Alcohol Depend. 2013;131:127–35.

31. Oldfield BJ, Muñoz N, McGovern MP, Funaro M, Villanueva M, Tetrault JM, et al. Integration of care for HIV and opioid use disorder. AIDS [Internet]. 2019;33(5):873–84. Available from: http://journals.lww.com/00002030-201904010-00012.

32. Brunet N, Moore DT, Lendvai Wischik D, Mattocks KM, Rosen MI. Increasing buprenorphine access for veterans with opioid use disorder in rural clinics using telemedicine. Subst Abus. 2020:1–8.
33. Fiellin DA, Pantalon MV, Pakes JP, O'Connor PG, Chawarski M, Schottenfeld RS. Treatment of heroin dependence with buprenorphine in primary care. Am J Drug Alcohol Abuse [Internet]. 2002;28(2):231–41. Available from: http://www.ncbi.nlm.nih.gov/pubmed/12014814.
34. Fiellin DA, Pantalon MV, Chawarski MC, Moore BA, Sullivan LE, O'Connor PG, et al. Counseling plus buprenorphine–naloxone maintenance therapy for opioid dependence. N Engl J Med [Internet]. 2006;355(4):365–74. Available from: http://www.nejm.org/doi/abs/10.1056/NEJMoa055255.
35. Fiellin DA, Barry DT, Sullivan LE, Cutter CJ, Moore BA, O'Connor PG, et al. A randomized trial of cognitive behavioral therapy in primary care-based buprenorphine. Am J Med [Internet]. 2013;126(1):74.e11–7. Available from: http://www.pubmedcentral.nih.gov/articlerender.fcgi?artid=3621718&tool=pmcentrez&rendertype=abstract.
36. Bassuk EL, Hanson J, Greene RN, Richard M, Laudet A. Peer-delivered recovery support services for addictions in the United States: a systematic review. J Subst Abuse Treat [Internet]. 2016;63:1–9. Available from: https://doi.org/10.1016/j.jsat.2016.01.003.
37. McNicholas L, Consensus Panel Chair. Clinical guidelines for the use of buprenorphine in the treatment of opioid addiction. Treat Improv Protoc [Internet]. 2004;40(04–3939):1–172. Available from: http://www.buprenorphine.samhsa.gov/Bup_Guidelines.pdf.
38. Kraus ML, Alford DP, Kotz MM, Levounis P, Mandell TW, Meyer M, et al. Statement of the American Society of Addiction Medicine Consensus Panel on the use of buprenorphine in office-based treatment of opioid addiction. J Addict Med [Internet]. 2011;5(4):254–63. Available from: http://content.wkhealth.com/linkback/openurl?sid=WKPTLP:landingpage&an=01271255-201112000-00003.
39. Sokol R, Albanese M, Chew A, Early J, Grossman E, Roll D, et al. Building a Group-Based Opioid Treatment (GBOT) blueprint: a qualitative study delineating GBOT implementation. Addict Sci Clin Pract [Internet]. 2019;14(1):1–17. Available from: https://doi.org/10.1186/s13722-019-0176-y.
40. Sokol R, LaVertu AE, Morrill D, Albanese C, Schuman-Olivier Z. Group-based treatment of opioid use disorder with buprenorphine: a systematic review. J Subst Abuse Treat [Internet]. 2018;84:78–87. Available from: https://doi.org/10.1016/j.jsat.2017.11.003.
41. Roll D, Spottswood M, Huang H. Using shared medical appointments to increase access to buprenorphine treatment. J Am Board Fam Med. 2015;28(5):676–7.
42. Doorley SL, Ho CJ, Echeverria E, Preston C, Ngo H, Kamal A, et al. Buprenorphine shared medical appointments for the treatment of opioid dependence in a homeless clinic. Subst Abus. 2017;38(1):26–30.
43. Fox AD, Cunningham CO. Abstracts from the 2020 annual meeting of the Society of General Internal Medicine. J Gen Intern Med [Internet]. 2020; Available from: http://link.springer.com/10.1007/s11606-020-05890-3.
44. Uscher-Pines L, Raja P, Mehrotra A, Huskamp HA. Health center implementation of telemedicine for opioid use disorders: a qualitative assessment of adopters and nonadopters. J Subst Abuse Treat [Internet]. 2020;115(April):108037. Available from: https://doi.org/10.1016/j.jsat.2020.108037.
45. Uscher-Pines L, Sousa J, Raja P, Mehrotra A, Barnett M, Huskamp HA. Treatment of opioid use disorder during COVID-19: experiences of clinicians transitioning to telemedicine. J Subst Abuse Treat [Internet]. 2020;118(January):108124. Available from: https://linkinghub.elsevier.com/retrieve/pii/S0740547220303809.
46. Drake C, Yu J, Lurie N, Kraemer K, Polsky D, Chaiyachati KH. Policies to improve substance use disorder treatment with telehealth during the COVID-19 pandemic and beyond. J Addict Med. 2020;14(5):e139–41.
47. Wang L, Weiss J, Ryan EB, Waldman J, Rubin S, Griffin JL. Telemedicine increases access to buprenorphine initiation during the COVID-19 pandemic. J Subst Abuse Treat [Internet]. 2021;124(December 2020):108272. Available from: https://doi.org/10.1016/j.jsat.2020.108272.

48. Harris M, Johnson S, Mackin S, Saitz R, Walley AY, Taylor JL. Low barrier tele-buprenorphine in the time of COVID-19. J Addict Med [Internet]. 2020;Publish Ah(00):12–4. Available from: https://journals.lww.com/10.1097/ADM.0000000000000682.
49. Tofighi B, Grazioli F, Bereket S, Grossman E, Aphinyanaphongs Y, Lee JD. Text message reminders for improving patient appointment adherence in an office-based buprenorphine program: a feasibility study. Am J Addict. 2017;26(6):581–6.
50. Cunningham CO, Giovanniello A, Sacajiu G, Li X, Brisbane M, Sohler NL. Inquiries about and initiation of buprenorphine treatment in an inner-city clinic. Subst Abus [Internet]. 2009;30(3):261–2. Available from: http://www.pubmedcentral.nih.gov/articlerender.fcgi?artid=2746741&tool=pmcentrez&rendertype=abstract.
51. Rawson R, Cousins SJ, McCann M, Pearce R, Van Donsel A. Assessment of medication for opioid use disorder as delivered within the Vermont hub and spoke system. J Subst Abuse Treat [Internet]. 2019;97(August 2018):84–90. Available from: https://doi.org/10.1016/j.jsat.2018.11.003.
52. Brooklyn JR, Sigmon SC. Vermont hub-and-spoke model of care for opioid use disorder. J Addict Med [Internet]. 2017;11(4):286–92. Available from: http://insights.ovid.com/crossref?an=01271255-201708000-00009.
53. D'Onofrio G, Chawarski MC, O'Connor PG, Pantalon MV, Busch SH, Owens PH, et al. Emergency department-initiated buprenorphine for opioid dependence with continuation in primary care: outcomes during and after intervention. J Gen Intern Med [Internet]. 2017;32(6):660–6. Available from: http://link.springer.com/10.1007/s11606-017-3993-2.
54. D'Onofrio G, O'Connor PG, Pantalon MV, Chawarski MC, Busch SH, Owens PH, et al. Emergency department-initiated buprenorphine/naloxone treatment for opioid dependence: a randomized clinical trial. JAMA – J Am Med Assoc. 2015;313(16):1636–44.
55. Naeger S, Mutter R, Ali MM, Mark T, Hughey L. Post-discharge treatment engagement among patients with an opioid-use disorder. J Subst Abuse Treat [Internet]. 2016;69:64–71. Available from: https://doi.org/10.1016/j.jsat.2016.07.004.
56. Englander H, Weimer M, Solotaroff R, Nicolaidis C, Chan B, Velez C, et al. Planning and designing the improving addiction care team (IMPACT) for hospitalized adults with substance use disorder. J Hosp Med [Internet]. 2017;12(5):339–42. Available from: http://www.journalofhospitalmedicine.com/jhospmed/article/136504/hospital-medicine/planning-and-designing-improving-addiction-care-team.
57. Trowbridge P, Weinstein ZM, Kerensky T, Roy P, Regan D, Samet JH, et al. Addiction consultation services – linking hospitalized patients to outpatient addiction treatment. J Subst Abuse Treat [Internet]. 2017;79:1–5. Available from: https://doi.org/10.1016/j.jsat.2017.05.007.
58. Watkins KE, Ober AJ, Lamp K, Lind M, Diamant A, Osilla KC, et al. Implementing the chronic care model for opioid and alcohol use disorders in primary care. Prog Community Heal Partnerships Res Educ Action [Internet]. 2017;11(4):397–407. Available from: https://muse.jhu.edu/article/683610.
59. Hunter SB, Ober AJ, McCullough CM, Storholm ED, Iyiewuare PO, Pham C, et al. Sustaining alcohol and opioid use disorder treatment in primary care: a mixed methods study. Implement Sci [Internet]. 2018;13(1):83. Available from: https://implementationscience.biomedcentral.com/articles/10.1186/s13012-018-0777-y.
60. Cunningham CO, Lum PJ. Integrating buprenorphine treatment for opioid use disorder in primary care settings [Internet]. 2015. Available from: https://ciswh.org/bupmanual.
61. American Society of Addiction Medicine. National practice guidelines for the use of medications in the treatment of addiction involving opioid use [Internet]. 2015. Available from: http://www.asam.org/docs/default-source/practice-support/guidelines-and-consensus-docs/national-practice-guideline.pdf.
62. American Society of Addiction Medicine. National practice guideline for the treatment of opioid use disorder: 2020 focused update. J Addict Med [Internet]. 2020;14(2S):1–91. Available from: https://journals.lww.com/10.1097/ADM.0000000000000633.
63. Simon CB, Tsui JI, Merrill JO, Adwell A, Tamru E, Klein JW. Linking patients with buprenorphine treatment in primary care: predictors of engagement. Drug Alcohol Depend [Internet]. 2017;181(September):58–62. Available from: https://doi.org/10.1016/j.drugalcdep.2017.09.017.

64. McElrath K. Medication-assisted treatment for opioid addiction in the United States: critique and commentary. Subst Use Misuse [Internet]. 2018;53(2):334–43. Available from: https://www.tandfonline.com/doi/full/10.1080/10826084.2017.1342662.

65. Bhatraju EP, Grossman E, Tofighi B, McNeely J, DiRocco D, Flannery M, et al. Public sector low threshold office-based buprenorphine treatment: outcomes at year 7. Addict Sci Clin Pract [Internet]. 2017;12(1):7. Available from: http://ascpjournal.biomedcentral.com/articles/10.1186/s13722-017-0072-2.

66. Payne BE, Klein JW, Simon CB, James JR, Jackson SL, Merrill JO, et al. Effect of lowering initiation thresholds in a primary care-based buprenorphine treatment program. Drug Alcohol Depend [Internet]. 2019;200(May):71–7. Available from: https://doi.org/10.1016/j.drugalcdep.2019.03.009.

67. Cunningham CO, Giovanniello A, Kunins HV, Roose RJ, Fox AD, Sohler NL. Buprenorphine treatment outcomes among opioid-dependent cocaine users and non-users. Am J Addict [Internet]. 2013;22(4):352–7. Available from: http://www.ncbi.nlm.nih.gov/pubmed/23795874.

68. Fox AD, Sohler NL, Starrels JL, Ning Y, Giovanniello A, Cunningham CO. Pain is not associated with worse office-based buprenorphine treatment outcomes. Subst Abus [Internet]. 2012;33(4):361–5. Available from: http://www.ncbi.nlm.nih.gov/pubmed/22989279.

69. Weinstein ZM, Cheng DM, Quinn E, Hui D, Kim H, Gryczynski G, et al. Psychoactive medications and disengagement from office based opioid treatment (obot) with buprenorphine. Drug Alcohol Depend [Internet]. 2017;170:9–16. Available from: https://doi.org/10.1016/j.drugalcdep.2016.10.039.

70. Lee JD, Grossman E, DiRocco D, Gourevitch MN. Home buprenorphine/naloxone induction in primary care. J Gen Intern Med [Internet]. 2009;24(2):226–32. Available from: http://www.ncbi.nlm.nih.gov/pubmed/19089508.

71. Cunningham CO, Giovanniello A, Li X, Kunins HV, Roose RJ, Sohler NL. A comparison of buprenorphine induction strategies: patient-centered home-based inductions versus standard-of-care office-based inductions. J Subst Abuse Treat [Internet]. 2011;40(4):349–56. Available from: http://www.ncbi.nlm.nih.gov/pubmed/21310583.

72. Gunderson EW, Wang X-Q, Fiellin DA, Bryan B, Levin FR. Unobserved versus observed office buprenorphine/naloxone induction: a pilot randomized clinical trial. Addict Behav [Internet]. 2010;35(5):537–40. Available from: http://www.nature.com/articles/nrm2621.

73. Walley AY, Alperen JK, Cheng DM, Botticelli M, Castro-Donlan C, Samet JH, et al. Office-based management of opioid dependence with buprenorphine: clinical practices and barriers. J Gen Intern Med [Internet]. 2008;23(9):1393–8. Available from: http://link.springer.com/10.1007/s11606-008-0686-x.

74. Boston Medical Center, Office-Based Addiction Treatment Training and Assistance. buprenorphine community induction guide for patients [Internet]. Available from: https://www.bmcobat.org/resources/?category=4.

75. Sohler NL, Li X, Kunins HV, Sacajiu G, Giovanniello A, Whitley S, et al. Home- versus office-based buprenorphine inductions for opioid-dependent patients. J Subst Abuse Treat [Internet]. 2010;38(2):153–9. Available from: https://doi.org/10.1016/j.jsat.2009.08.001.

76. Becker WC, Frank JW, Edens EL. Switching from high-dose, long-term opioids to buprenorphine: a case series. Ann Intern Med. 2020;173(1):70–1.

77. Ghosh SM, Klaire S, Tanguay R, Manek M, Azar P. A review of novel methods to support the transition from methadone and other full agonist opioids to buprenorphine/naloxone sublingual in both community and acute care settings. Can J Addict. 2019;10(4):41–50.

78. Brar R, Fairbairn N, Sutherland C, Nolan S. Use of a novel prescribing approach for the treatment of opioid use disorder: buprenorphine/naloxone micro-dosing – a case series. Drug Alcohol Rev. 2020;39(5):588–94.

79. Sordo L, Barrio G, Bravo MJ, Indave BI, Degenhardt L, Wiessing L, et al. Mortality risk during and after opioid substitution treatment: systematic review and meta-analysis of cohort studies. BMJ [Internet]. 2017;357:j1550. Available from: https://www.bmj.com/lookup/doi/10.1136/bmj.j1550.

80. Weinstein LC, Iqbal Q, Cunningham A, Debates R, Landistratis G, Doggett P, et al. Retention of patients with multiple vulnerabilities in a federally qualified health center buprenorphine program: Pennsylvania, 2017–2018. Am J Public Health [Internet]. 2020;110(4):580–6. Available from: https://doi.org/10.2105/AJPH.2019.305525.

81. Haddad MS, Zelenev A, Altice FL. Integrating buprenorphine maintenance therapy into federally qualified health centers: real-world substance abuse treatment outcomes. Drug Alcohol Depend [Internet]. 2013;131(1–2):127–35. Available from: http://www.ncbi.nlm.nih.gov/pubmed/23332439.

82. Bart G. Maintenance medication for opiate addiction: the foundation of recovery. J Addict Dis [Internet]. 2012;31(3):207–25. Available from: http://www.tandfonline.com/doi/abs/10.1080/10550887.2012.694598.

83. Hser YI, Saxon AJ, Huang D, Hasson A, Thomas C, Hillhouse M, et al. Treatment retention among patients randomized to buprenorphine/naloxone compared to methadone in a multisite trial. Addiction. 2014;109(1):79–87.

84. Bozinoff N, Anderson BJ, Bailey GL, Stein MD. Correlates of stigma severity among persons seeking opioid detoxification. J Addict Med. 2018;12:19–23.

85. Fox AD, Masyukova M, Cunningham CO. Optimizing psychosocial support during office-based buprenorphine treatment in primary care: patients' experiences and preferences. Subst Abus [Internet]. 2016;37(1):70–5. Available from: https://www.ncbi.nlm.nih.gov/pmc/articles/PMC4801741/pdf/nihms-747268.pdf.

86. Tetrault JM, Moore BA, Barry DT, O'Connor PG, Schottenfeld R, Fiellin DA, et al. Brief versus extended counseling along with buprenorphine/naloxone for HIV-infected opioid dependent patients. J Subst Abuse Treat [Internet]. 2012;43(4):433–9. Available from: https://doi.org/10.1016/j.jsat.2012.07.011.

87. Dugosh K, Abraham A, Seymour B, McLoyd K, Chalk M, Festinger D. A systematic review on the use of psychosocial interventions in conjunction with medications for the treatment of opioid addiction. J Addict Med [Internet]. 2016;10(2):93–103. Available from: http://www.ncbi.nlm.nih.gov/pubmed/26808307.

88. Donroe JH, Holt SR, O'Connor PG, Sukumar N, Tetrault JM. Interpreting quantitative urine buprenorphine and norbuprenorphine levels in office-based clinical practice. Drug Alcohol Depend [Internet]. 2017;180(August):46–51. Available from: https://doi.org/10.1016/j.drugalcdep.2017.07.040.

89. Starrels JL, Fox AD, Kunins HV, Cunningham CO. They don't know what they don't know: internal medicine residents' knowledge and confidence in urine drug test interpretation for patients with chronic pain. J Gen Intern Med. 2012;27(11):1521–7.

90. Gaither JR, Gordon K, Crystal S, Edelman EJ, Kerns RD, Justice AC, et al. Racial disparities in discontinuation of long-term opioid therapy following illicit drug use among black and white patients. Drug Alcohol Depend [Internet]. 2018;(May):0–1. Available from: https://linkinghub.elsevier.com/retrieve/pii/S0376871618303855.

91. Tenore PL. Advanced urine toxicology testing. J Addict Dis [Internet]. 2010;29(4):436–48. Available from: http://www.tandfonline.com/doi/abs/10.1080/10550887.2010.509277.

92. Starrels JL, Wu B. Urine drug testing: a reference guide for clinicians. Bronx; 2013. https://ciswh.org/bupmanual.

93. Accurso AJ, Lee JD, Mcneely J. High prevalence of urine tampering in an office-based opioid treatment practice detected by evaluating the norbuprenorphine to buprenorphine ratio. J Subst Abuse Treat [Internet]. 2017;83:62–7. Available from: https://doi.org/10.1016/j.jsat.2017.10.002.

94. Holt SR, Donroe JH, Cavallo DA, Tetrault JM. Addressing discordant quantitative urine buprenorphine and norbuprenorphine levels: Case examples in opioid use disorder. Drug Alcohol Depend [Internet]. 2018;186(October 2017):171–4. Available from: https://doi.org/10.1016/j.drugalcdep.2017.12.040.

95. Netherland J, Botsko M, Egan JE, Saxon AJ, Cunningham CO, Finkelstein R, et al. Factors affecting willingness to provide buprenorphine treatment. J Subst Abuse Treat [Internet]. 2009;36(3):244–51. Available from: http://www.ncbi.nlm.nih.gov/pubmed/18715741.

96. Cunningham CO, Kunins H V., Roose RJ, Elam RT, Sohler NL. Barriers to obtaining waivers to prescribe buprenorphine for opioid addiction treatment among HIV physicians. J Gen Intern Med [Internet]. 2007;22(9):1325–9. Available from: http://www.ncbi.nlm.nih.gov/pubmed/17619934.

97. Caviness CM, Anderson BJ, de Dios MA, Kurth M, Stein M. Prescription medication exchange patterns among methadone maintenance patients. Drug Alcohol Depend. 2013;127(1–3):232–8.

98. Lofwall MR, Walsh SL. A review of buprenorphine diversion and misuse: the current evidence base and experiences from around the world. J Addict Med [Internet]. 2014;8(5):315–26. Available from: http://content.wkhealth.com/linkback/openurl?sid=WKPTLP:landingpage&an=01271255-201409000-00004.

99. Goldsworthy RC, Schwartz NC, Mayhorn CB. Beyond abuse and exposure: framing the impact of prescription-medication sharing. Am J Public Health. 2008;98(6):1115–21.

100. Cicero TJ, Surratt HL, Inciardi J. Use and misuse of buprenorphine in the management of opioid addiction. J Opioid Manag. 2007;3(1551–7489 (Print)):302–8.

101. Paone D, Tuazon E, Stajic M, Sampson B, Allen B, Mantha S, et al. Buprenorphine infrequently found in fatal overdose in New York City. Drug Alcohol Depend [Internet]. 2015;155:298–301. Available from: https://linkinghub.elsevier.com/retrieve/pii/S0376871615015987.

102. Fox AD, Chamberlain A, Sohler NL, Frost T, Cunningham CO. Illicit buprenorphine use, interest in and access to buprenorphine treatment among syringe exchange participants. J Subst Abus Treat. 2015;48(1):112–6.

103. Mitchell SG, Kelly S, Brown B, Reisinger HS, Peterson J, Ruhf A, et al. Uses of diverted methadone and buprenorphine by opioid-addicted individuals in Baltimore, Maryland. Am J Addict [Internet]. 2009;18(5):346–55. Available from: http://doi.wiley.com/10.1080/10550490903077820.

104. Godersky ME, Saxon AJ, Merrill JO, Samet JH, Simoni JM, Tsui JI. Provider and patient perspectives on barriers to buprenorphine adherence and the acceptability of video directly observed therapy to enhance adherence. Addict Sci Clin Pract [Internet]. 2019;14(1):11. Available from: https://doi.org/10.1186/s13722-019-0139-3.

105. Godersky ME, Klein JW, Merrill JO, Blalock KL, Saxon AJ, Samet JH, et al. Acceptability and feasibility of a mobile health application for video directly observed therapy of buprenorphine for opioid use disorders in an office-based setting. J Addict Med. 2020:14(4):319–25.

106. Tofighi B, Grossman E, Bereket S, Lee JD. Text message content preferences to improve buprenorphine maintenance treatment in primary care. J Addict Dis [Internet]. 2016;35(2):92–100. Available from: https://doi.org/10.1080/10550887.2015.1127716.

Reachable Moment: Hospital-Based Interventions

4

Zoe M. Weinstein and Honora Englander

Introduction

The opioid use disorder and overdose crisis is hitting hospitals hard. There were over 500,000 hospital admissions for opioid use disorder (OUD) in 2012, costing $15 billion in health care costs and representing nearly a doubling from the prior decade [1]. OUD-related admissions continues to rise, [2, 3] as do morbidity and mortality associated with these admissions [1, 4–7]. Despite this, hospital providers generally feel unprepared to manage OUD, [8] and OUD remains neglected during hospitalization, [9, 10] with over two-thirds of patients not even referred to any follow-up services [11]. Providers are missing this critical touchpoint. Even after hospital encounters for a nonfatal opioid overdose or injection-related infection, where there is evidence of increased 12-month mortality (111 times mortality risk after overdose and 54 times with serious infection) and clear evidence that starting MOUD saves lives, providers continue to neglect to provide treatment [12, 13]. In one study of Veterans Affairs hospitals, only 15% of people with OUD were provided with methadone or buprenorphine during admission. For patients on MOUD before admission, over one-third had MOUD discontinued during admission, and 23% were not restarted after discharge. And only a small fraction (only 11% of those receiving any MOUD) were newly initiated with linkage to care after hospital discharge [14]. Polysubstance use among people with OUD is common, if not the norm – in one study, 70% of hospitalized adults with OUD also used other substances, including methamphetamines, alcohol, and cocaine [15].

Z. M. Weinstein (✉)
General Internal Medicine, Boston University, Boston, MA, USA
e-mail: Zoe.weinstein@bmc.org

H. Englander
Division of Hospital Medicine, Department of Medicine, Oregon Health & Science University, Portland, OR, USA
e-mail: englandh@ohsu.edu

© Springer Nature Switzerland AG 2021
S. E. Wakeman, J. D. Rich (eds.), *Treating Opioid Use Disorder in General Medical Settings*, https://doi.org/10.1007/978-3-030-80818-1_4

A Reachable Moment

Treating addiction during hospitalization is associated with increased post-hospital SUD treatment engagement after discharge [16], reduced SUD severity [17], reduced substance use [15], lower rates of hospital readmission, and reduced against medical advice discharges [17]. In-hospital SUD treatment is also associated with improved patient [18, 19] and provider experience [20].

Specific to OUD, the Substance Abuse and Mental Health Services Administration (SAMHSA) recommends screening for OUD in all general medical settings [21]; however, screening is rarely done in hospitals, which may contribute to the under-identification of OUD among hospitalized patients [22]. Most hospitalized patients with SUD, including those with OUD, want to stop use and want medications to treat addiction [23, 24]. MOUD is the gold standard of care, and all hospitals should be prepared to initiate methadone or buprenorphine for all interested patients with OUD, as recommended by the Institute for Healthcare Improvement [25] to meet the Healthcare Effectiveness Data and Information Set (HEDIS) measure on initiation and engagement in addiction treatment [26].

Medications for Opioid Use Disorder (MOUD) in the Hospital Setting

Appropriate and proactive withdrawal management is essential to support patients to complete other medical care; otherwise, they are at high risk of leaving the hospital prematurely ("against medical advice"), only to be readmitted with more severe disease or die of overdose [27, 28]. Methadone and buprenorphine are the first line medications for opioid withdrawal and should be aggressively titrated, along with adjuvant medications, if needed. Structured assessments such as the Clinical Opiate Withdrawal Scale (COWS) can be used to guide withdrawal management and buprenorphine induction (Fig. 4.1).

Medical management of withdrawal ("detoxification") alone has been shown to be inferior to maintenance MOUD, so hospital providers should always offer patients maintenance instead of merely withdrawal management with opioid agonist therapy [29]. Some hospital leadership, pharmacists, or clinicians may inappropriately believe that methadone and buprenorphine cannot be started or titrated in the hospital; however, these medications can be legally used to manage symptoms while patients are being treated for other medical issues [30–32].

Methadone is a long-acting medication, and in an outpatient setting is often slowly titrated over many weeks to reach a therapeutic dose, by starting at 30 mg and increasing the dose by 5–10 mg typically every 3 days [33]. In the hospital, more aggressive titration may be possible due to 24-hour monitoring, especially if patients have experience at higher doses of methadone, are pregnant, or are at high risk for leaving against medical advice [34]. However, more rapid titration must be balanced with acute medical issues, such as cardiac risk associated with prolonged QTc and medication interactions. While the dose is titrated, patients may struggle with withdrawal symptoms and cravings, making remaining in the hospital a

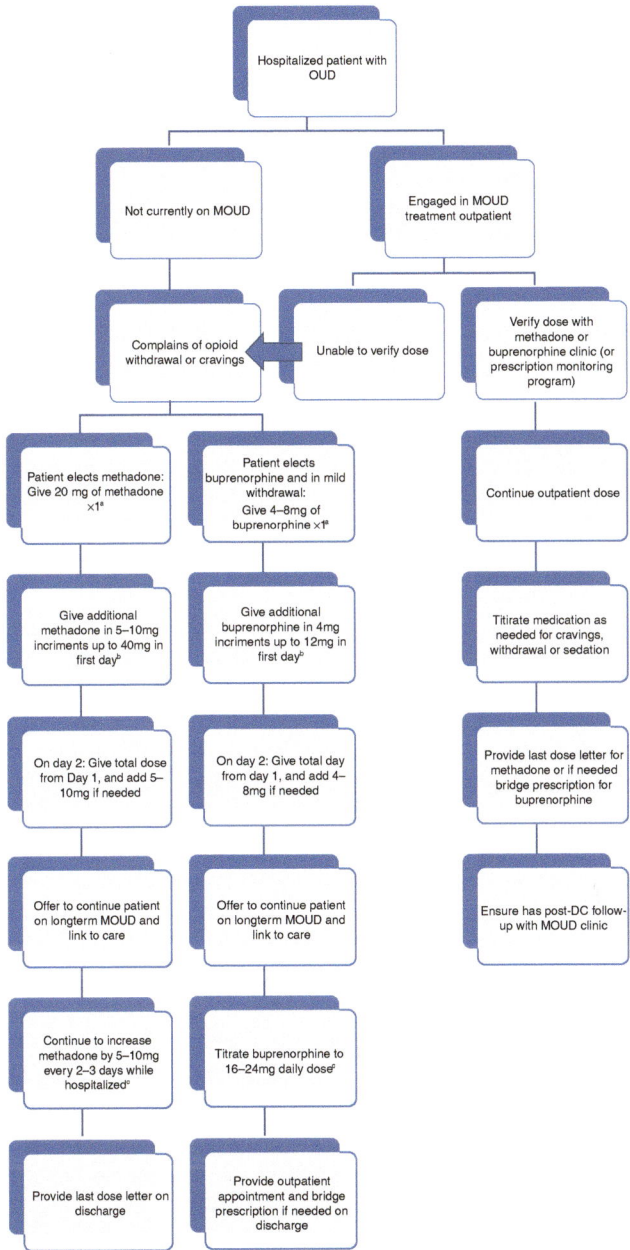

Fig. 4.1 Inpatient opioid withdrawal management. *Abbreviation*: OUD Opioid use disorder, MOUD Medication for opioid use disorder; [a]Consider lower starting dose in patients who are elderly, have impaired liver function and/or severe pulmonary disease, or those with multiple concurrent synergetic and medications; [b]If needed may use additional medications for symptom management including non-steroidal anti-inflammatories, sedative-hypnotics, anti-diarrheals and alpha agonists; [c]If patient refuses maintenance treatment, may offer to taper methadone or bupernorphine during hospitalization by 5 mg or 4 mg per day respectively. Adapted with permission from Boston Medical Center

challenge. Providers should proactively manage these symptoms with additional comfort medications [35]. Direct linkage to community-based opioid treatment programs is crucial to ensure patients can continue to receive methadone immediately following discharge.

Buprenorphine has been shown to be effective in managing acute opioid withdrawal and for long-term treatment initiation both in randomized control trials as well as in real-world hospital settings [29, 36]. Due to its high affinity for the opioid receptor and its partial agonist activity, traditional buprenorphine induction requires stopping all full agonist opioids to avoid the risk of precipitated withdrawal and managing a period of abstinence from all opioids. This may be especially challenging in the hospital, where patients may require high-dose opioids for analgesia due to trauma or other painful conditions, or for patients already on high doses of methadone who require rapid taper off and transition to buprenorphine due to medical complications such as risk for torsade de pointes. While traditional inductions remain a common practice, increasingly, hospital providers are offering low-dose buprenorphine initiations as a cross taper with a full agonit opioid. This apporach is sometimes called a "microdosing" induction, and may be prefereable in certain clinical scenarios in order to avoid painful extended tapers and periods of abstinence from methadone or pain medications required for traditional buprenorphine induction [37–41]. "Microdosing" involves initiating low-dose buprenorphine (typical starting dose of 0.5 mg/day) using sublingual, patch, or buccal formulation of buprenorphine and gradually increasing the buprenorphine dose over 1–7 days while continuing or tapering the full agonist opioids. The specific protocols described in the several case reports and case studies published to date vary. If patients are transitioned from high-dose or long-term methadone, they may require the patch to be placed for 48–72 hours prior to start of the sublingual buprenorphine and some protocols suggest checking urine toxicology for the presence of buprenorphine before initiating the standard sublingual doses [41, 42].

Given buprenorphine's high affinity for the opioid receptor and it's partial agonist activity, historically there has been concern about continuing buprenorphine in the setting of acute pain, especially in the perioperative period, as theoretically the buprenorphine could block the activity of the full agonist opioid pain medication [43]. However, multiple studies now demonstrate that is it both feasible and advisable to continue buprenorphine perioperatively, as analgesia can be achieved, albeit with at times requiring higher doses of opioids [44, 45]. In addition, continuing buprenorphine means that the patient's treatment for OUD remains uninterrupted, minimizing the risk of return to use associated with stopping MOUD [46]. Numerous factors, including patient preferences and post-hospital care transitions, are important when deciding which MOUD to use (Table 4.1).

Naltrexone is an opioid antagonist that can be used to treat OUD. It comes both in a once daily pill and a long-acting injectable form. Antagonist properties make induction difficult, especially in the hospital setting where patients commonly experience pain and have recently used opioids, as naltrexone initiation requires a 7-day period of abstinence from opioid agonists (including methadone, buprenorphine and opioid pain medications) [47]. In addition, the injectable formulation is expensive and is thus not typically available on hospital

Table 4.1 Methadone versus buprenorphine considerations in a hospital setting

	Methadone	Buprenorphine
Acute pain	No problem	May complicate induction[a]
Withdrawal needed prior to initiation	No	Yes[a]
Induction duration	Weeks	Days
Rural geography	Often challenging	Often accessible
Outpatient treatment options	Daily OTP only	Office-based or OTP
Dispensing at SNF	Often challenging	Straightforward

Legend:
OTP Opioid treatment program or methadone clinic, *SNF* Skilled nursing facility
[a]Microdosing may allow initiation of buprenorphine without abstinence from other opioids or withdrawal

formularies (and many outpatient formularies). Evidence for naltrexone is less compelling – studies even in outpatient settings show low rates of treatment initiation [47] and in contrast to methadone and buprenorphine, naltrexone does not decrease risk of HIV, hepatitis, or overdose [33, 48]. For hospital providers, naltrexone utility is likely highest for motivated patients who are currently abstinent but at risk of return to use, and without painful conditions or in patients with co-occurring alcohol use disorder.

Hospital Policies Regarding MOUD: Myths and Truths

Overly restrictive policies and widespread misconceptions about legal barriers to delivering methadone and buprenorphine during hospitalization are common, yet remediable [49]. Methadone for OUD in the hospital is legal, so long as patients are hospitalized for a medical, surgical, obstetric, or psychiatric condition other than withdrawal management alone [30]. Further, providers do not need a DEA-X waiver to prescribe buprenorphine during hospitalization. Outside of hospitals, regulations are different. Current laws require a waiver to prescribe buprenorphine at the time of discharge and prohibit hospital providers (or anyone outside of an opioid treatment program (OTP)) from prescribing methadone for OUD at hospital discharge [50]. While methadone prescribing after discharge should be arranged at an OTP, there is a "72-hour exception" that permits emergency methadone dosing in nonhospital settings, for example, in an emergency department or non-OTP ambulatory setting, 1 day at a time and for 3 day or less [51]. Hospital policies should reflect national guidelines and evidence, and should support first-line methadone, buprenorphine, to treat acute opioid withdrawal. Despite this, many hospitals policies are not guideline adherent [49].

Patients with SUD experience widespread feelings of stigma and discrimination in healthcare settings and may avoid hospital settings or avoid disclosing substance use [52]. Hospitals are no exception [24]. Hospital policies such as restrictive visitor policies, search policies, or those restricting patients' ability to leave the hospital unit or smoke cigarettes may disproportionately harm patients with SUD [53]. Hospital providers can mitigate these potential harms by reviewing and revising policies to integrate principles of harm reduction and trauma-informed care [54–56].

Transitions of Care Considerations

Timely, streamlined access to post-hospital treatment is important to support all patients wishing to continue MOUD after discharge, and hospitals can develop pathways with community SUD treatment partners. Further, there are unique considerations for patients who discharge to skilled nursing facilities (SNF), are at-risk for incarceration (which can interrupt MOUD), who live in rural areas, or who have limited transportation (Table 4.1). Outpatient buprenorphine can be prescribed in office settings by any waivered provider. Outpatient methadone must be prescribed through a federally licensed opioid treatment program (OTP) or "methadone clinic," which are typically located in urban areas and require daily transportation. Direct linkage to methadone clinics is essential, as patients typically need to begin dosing the day after hospital discharge for uninterrupted treatment. Hospital providers should familiarize themselves with local methadone clinics' contact information and admission requirements and initiate the process of direct linkage as early as possible during the hospitalization.

Currently, coordinating methadone at SNF is complicated and there is widespread regional and national practice variation, complicating discharge to SNF [31]. Typically SNF must either transport patients to the clinic daily for dosing, or collaborate with the methadone clinic to obtain a medical exception waiver so that take home doses can be given to SNF staff to be transported to the SNF and dispensed on site. Though stigma and misinterpretation of buprenorphine prescribing restrictions can complicate care coordination of buprenorphine at SNF, generally it is straightforward and should be readily accessible. If SNFs do not have a provider with a DEA-X waiver, then hospital or community providers can prescribe and SNFs can administer buprenorphine. Finally, discrimination toward people with OUD who need post-acute care is pervasive, despite state and federal protections under the American with Disabilities Act [57, 58]. Hospital providers can support more equitable care by knowing and advocating for patients' rights, and by prioritizing relationships with SNFs that commit to providing nondiscriminatory care for people with SUD.

Incarceration may interrupt medication treatment as many prisons and jails do not offer treatment, despite the strong evidence that it reduces post-incarceration overdose deaths [59]. Given risk for forced withdrawal, many patients who fear incarceration decline MOUD initiation. Options to address this include offering extended release buprenorphine, which can be administered every 28 days to maintain treatment, and which has a long half-life, which mitigates typical sublingual buprenorphine withdrawal symptoms [60].

Finally, it is important to consider medical and psychiatric treatment comorbidities when planning post-hospital community SUD treatment. For example, residential addiction treatment settings are typically not equipped to support people who need help with mobility or activities of daily living, most lack capacity to provide wound care or antibiotic infusions [61], and many do not permit patients to leave the premise in the first 30 days of treatment. These factors introduce significant challenges for medically complex patients and are an important opportunity for systems improvement and policy change.

Integrating Harm Reduction into Hospital Care

Patients with OUD may feel stigmatized in hospitals, as many have had past negative experiences with medical providers and institutions [27, 62, 63]. Thus, it is important to proactively engage patients around OUD, especially given that many may struggle to access OUD care in traditional outpatient settings [16]. Further, providers must embrace principles of trauma-informed care [55], avoid stigmatizing language [64], and familiarize themselves with harm reduction strategies to genuinely meet patients where they are at and prevent further morbidity and mortality [65]. Harm reduction may at times contrast with traditional medical models, especially in the hierarchical physician-centered inpatient setting [66]; however, a harm-reduction approach, where the patient is centered as the expert in their own experience and the decision maker in their health, is more likely to engage patients in care [67, 68] (Table 4.2). (See Chap. 10).

Table 4.2 Hospital-based harm reduction strategies

Proactive management of pain and withdrawal	Provide methadone or buprenorphine to treat withdrawal, even if patients do not want to continue long term
	Ensure adequate pain control, including high-dose opioids if needed
Overdose response plan	Prescribe naloxone and provide patient and family education for its use
	Counsel patients for safer use, which includes using with others nearby, avoid mixing substances, employing safer consumption techniques
	Avoid in-hospital use/overdose by ensuring adequate symptom control of pain and withdrawal
Safer use techniques	Review safer injection practices, including preferred injection sites and site rotation, sterile equipment and water use, skin prep, and hand washing
	Provide information on local syringe service programs
	Consider creating a novel hospital-based partnership with a syringe service program [69]
	Consider distributing sterile injection equipment and safer smoking equipment or prescribing syringes and alcohol wipes
Testing and treatment for infectious diseases	Test for HIV, Hepatitis A, B, and C
	Vaccinate for Hepatitis A and B
	Provide testing and treatment for STIs
	Offer HIV Post-exposure (PEP) and Pre-exposure (PrEP) prophylaxis
	Offer curative treatment for Hepatitis C
Linkage to low-barrier care	Offer treatment referrals to MOUD providers who will work with patients whose current goal is not complete abstinence
Tailor medical recommendations to best practices and patient preferences	Offer guideline adherent treatment for conditions (e.g., valve surgery and antibiotics for endocarditis)
	Tailor medical recommendations to patient preferences, honoring patient autonomy and expertise in their own experience [66]
Structure hospital environment to optimize care for people with OUD	Avoid overly restrictive or paternalistic policies when possible (e.g., allow patients to leave the unit if needed to tolerate hospitalization, support patient autonomy and self-determination regarding medical treatment plans)
	Implement trauma-informed hospital practices [55]

Hospital-Based Treatment Models

Addiction consult services (ACS) are one organizational intervention to address needs of hospitalized adults with SUD. Consult services generally include three main activities, including delivering medical and behavioral services, supporting SUD education and culture change [23, 58], and supporting hospital policies and guidance documents [70]. ACS are associated with important patient and provider-level outcomes [8, 16, 19]. Given the siloed nature of SUD care, especially methadone, the many logistical access barriers [67, 71, 72] and patients' medical and socioeconomic complexity, [73] a comprehensive multidisciplinary approach is ideal especially the use of an interprofessional team that includes peers [21, 57]. ACS can also offer expert support for challenging cases such as comanaging pain and OUD, or simultaneous withdrawal from multiple substances.

Currently not all hospitals have the resources or need for formal ACS. However, just as all hospitals prescribe insulin and manage diabetes regardless of whether they have an endocrinology consult service, all hospitals should provide basic OUD care, including withdrawal management, medication initiation, and linkage to post-hospital community OUD treatment. There are numerous national examples of hospitalists, residents, and other interprofessional providers providing targeted SUD interventions including buprenorphine initiation during hospitalization and referral to treatment after discharge [70, 74–76].

The Business Case for Hospital-Based OUD Treatment

Regardless of the treatment model, broad-scale MOUD education and financing are important considerations. Program funding often depends on institutional or payer support, billing-generated revenue, or grant funding. Arguments describing the population health effects of untreated OUD, increased rates of OUD-related hospitalizations, the negative financial impacts associated with poor patient outcomes and high utilization, and gaps in care quality support that hospitals have a stake in the problem [23, 77]. Further arguments favoring support for hospital-based addiction care include research that shows that ACS likely decrease costly inpatient care utilization by decreasing readmissions [17, 78] and that MOUD, which can be initiated by ACS, have been shown to decrease readmissions [79, 80]. Hospital leaders and policymakers should incentivize integration of OUD care as part of hospitalization [81].

Inpatient Addiction Providers as Partners in Quality Care

Addiction specialists and hospitalists can partner with hospital leadership to identify opportunities for systems improvement [82], particularly around training medical staff to prescribe and offer MOUD and naloxone [10], assuring policies are evidence based and trauma informed [55], and supporting patients who have frequent hospitalizations [83]. For example, addiction specialists can partner with multidisciplinary teams to optimize care for patients with endocarditis [84] or evaluate patients for appropriateness for outpatient parenteral antibiotic therapy(OPAT) [61].

Conclusions

Hospitals are at the frontlines of the opioid use disorder and overdose epidemic, caring for patients in times of severe illness, psychiatric crisis, or after overdose. Hospitalization presents a reachable moment to engage patients in harm reduction services and initiate treatment, including MOUD. Addressing OUD in hospitals must become the standard of care. To achieve that end, we must invest in education for providers and create supportive hospital policies that optimize health and safety for patients with OUD. We must push for incentivized metrics to standardize and improve addiction care with the full engagement of hospital leadership. In addition, as hospital-based providers we must continue to challenge ourselves to expand the services we provide to best meet the needs of our patients. For example, providing sterile injection and safer smoking equipment or creating safe consumption sites within our hospitals [69, 85].

References

1. Ronan MV, Herzig SJ. Hospitalizations related to opioid abuse/dependence and associated serious infections increased sharply, 2002–12. Health Aff (Millwood). 2016;35(5):832–7.
2. Agency for Healthcare Research and Quality. Statistical Brief #249. Healthcare Cost and Utilization Project (HCUP). [Internet]. 2019 [cited 2019 Jul 8]. Available from: www.hcup-us.ahrq.gov/reports/statbriefs/sb249-Mental-Substance-Use-Disorder-Hospital-Stays-2016.jsp?utm_source=ahrq&utm_medium=en1&utm_term=Stats&utm_content=1&utm_campaign=ahrq_en6_11_2019.
3. U.S. Census Bureau, Population Division. Annual estimates of the resident population by sex, age, race, and Hispanic origin for the United States and States: April 1, 2010, to July 1, 2018 [Internet]. 2019 [cited 2019 Nov 25]. Available from: https://factfinder.census.gov/faces/tableservices/jsf/pages/productview.xhtml?src=bkmk.
4. Ciccarone D, Unick GJ, Cohen JK, Mars SG, Rosenblum D. Nationwide increase in hospitalizations for heroin-related soft tissue infections: associations with structural market conditions. Drug Alcohol Depend. 2016;163:126–33.
5. Gray ME, Rogawski McQuade ET, Scheld WM, Dillingham RA. Rising rates of injection drug use associated infective endocarditis in Virginia with missed opportunities for addiction treatment referral: a retrospective cohort study. BMC Infect Dis [Internet]. 2018 [cited 2018 Dec 17];18. Available from: https://www.ncbi.nlm.nih.gov/pmc/articles/PMC6201507/.
6. Wurcel AG, Anderson JE, Chui KKH, Skinner S, Knox TA, Snydman DR, et al. Increasing infectious endocarditis admissions among young people who inject drugs. Open Forum Infect Dis. 2016;3(3):ofw157.
7. Song Z. Mortality quadrupled among opioid-driven hospitalizations, notably within lower-income and disabled white populations. Health Aff (Millwood). 2017;36(12):2054–61.
8. Wakeman SE, Pham-Kanter G, Donelan K. Attitudes, practices, and preparedness to care for patients with substance use disorder: results from a survey of general internists. Subst Abuse. 2016;37(4):635–41.

9. Jicha C, Saxon D, Lofwall MR, Fanucchi LC. Substance use disorder assessment, diagnosis, and management for patients hospitalized with severe infections due to injection drug use. J Addict Med. 2019;13(1):69.

10. Rosenthal ES, Karchmer AW, Theisen-Toupal J, Castillo RA, Rowley CF. Suboptimal addiction interventions for patients hospitalized with injection drug use-associated infective endocarditis. Am J Med. 2016;129(5):481–5.

11. Reif S, Acevedo A, Garnick DW, Fullerton C. Reducing behavioral inpatient readmissions for people with substance use disorders: do follow-up services matter? Psychiatr Serv (Washington, DC). 2017;68(8):810–8.

12. Larochelle MR, Bernstein R, Bernson D, Land T, Stopka TJ, Rose AJ, et al. Touchpoints – opportunities to predict and prevent opioid overdose: a cohort study. Drug Alcohol Depend. 2019;204:107537.

13. Larochelle MR, Bernson D, Land T, Stopka TJ, Wang N, Xuan Z, et al. Medication for opioid use disorder after nonfatal opioid overdose and association with mortality: a cohort study. Ann Intern Med. 2018;169(3):137.

14. Priest KC, Lovejoy TI, Englander H, Shull S, McCarty D. Opioid agonist therapy during hospitalization within the Veterans Health Administration: a pragmatic retrospective cohort analysis. J Gen Intern Med. 2020;35:2365–74.

15. King C, Nicolaidis C, Korthuis PT, Priest KC, Englander H. Patterns of substance use before and after hospitalization among patients seen by an inpatient addiction consult service: a latent transition analysis. J Subst Abus Treat. 2020;118:108121.

16. Englander H, Dobbertin K, Lind BK, Nicolaidis C, Graven P, Dorfman C, et al. Inpatient addiction medicine consultation and post-hospital substance use disorder treatment engagement: a propensity-matched analysis. J Gen Intern Med. 2019;34(12):2796–803.

17. Wakeman SE, Metlay JP, Chang Y, Herman GE, Rigotti NA. Inpatient addiction consultation for hospitalized patients increases post-discharge abstinence and reduces addiction severity. J Gen Intern Med. 2017;19:1–8.

18. Collins D, Alla J, Nicolaidis C, Gregg J, Gullickson DJ, Patten A, et al. "If it wasn't for him, I wouldn't have talked to them": qualitative study of addiction peer mentorship in the hospital. J Gen Intern Med [Internet]. 2019 [cited 2019 Nov 21]; Available from: https://doi.org/10.1007/s11606-019-05311-0.

19. Hyshka E, Morris H, Anderson-Baron J, Nixon L, Dong K, Salvalaggio G. Patient perspectives on a harm reduction-oriented addiction medicine consultation team implemented in a large acute care hospital. Drug Alcohol Depend. 2019;204:107523.

20. Englander H, Collins D, Perry SP, Rabinowitz M, Phoutrides E, Nicolaidis C. "We've learned it's a medical illness, not a moral choice": qualitative study of the effects of a multicomponent addiction intervention on hospital providers' attitudes and experiences. J Hosp Med. 2018;13:752–8.

21. Substance Abuse and Mental Health Services Administration. TIP 63: medications for opioid use disorder [internet]. Rockville: Substance Abuse and Mental Health Services Administration; 2018 [cited 2019 Nov 30]. Available from: https://store.samhsa.gov/product/TIP-63-Medications-for-Opioid-Use-Disorder-Full-Document-Including-Executive-Summary-and-Parts-1-5-/SMA19-5063FULLDOC.

22. Wakeman SE, Herman G, Wilens TE, Regan S. The prevalence of unhealthy alcohol and drug use among inpatients in a general hospital. Subst Abuse. 2019;1:1–9.

23. Englander H, Weimer M, Solotaroff R, Nicolaidis C, Chan B, Velez C, et al. Planning and designing the Improving Addiction Care Team (IMPACT) for hospitalized adults with substance use disorder. J Hosp Med. 2017;12(5):339–42.

24. Velez CM, Nicolaidis C, Korthuis PT, Englander H. "It's been an experience, a life learning experience": a qualitative study of hospitalized patients with substance use disorders. J Gen Intern Med. 2017;32(3):296–303.

25. Botticelli M, Gottlieb M, Laderman M. Institute for healthcare improvement: effective strategies for hospitals responding to the opioid crisis [Internet]. Institute for Healthcare Improvement and the Grayken Center for Addiction at Boston Medical Center; 2019 [cited

2019 Nov 25]. Available from: http://www.ihi.org:80/resources/Pages/Publications/Effective-Strategies-for-Hospitals-Responding-to-Opioid-Crisis.aspx.

26. National Committee for Quality Assurance. Initiation and engagement of alcohol and other drug abuse or dependence treatment [Internet]. NCQA. 2019 [cited 2019 Nov 25]. Available from: https://www.ncqa.org/hedis/measures/initiation-and-engagement-of-alcohol-and-other-drug-abuse-or-dependence-treatment/.

27. McNeil R, Small W, Wood E, Kerr T. Hospitals as a 'risk environment': an ethno-epidemiological study of voluntary and involuntary discharge from hospital against medical advice among people who inject drugs. Soc Sci Med. 2014;105:59–66.

28. Zhu H, Wu L-T. Discharge against medical advice from hospitalizations for substance use disorders: the potential impact of the Affordable Care Act. Drug Alcohol Depend. 2019;197:115–9.

29. Liebschutz JM, Crooks D, Herman D, et al. Buprenorphine treatment for hospitalized, opioid-dependent patients: a randomized clinical trial. JAMA Intern Med. 2014;174(8):1369–76.

30. Noska A, Mohan A, Wakeman S, Rich J, Boutwell A. Managing opioid use disorder during and after acute hospitalization: a case-based review clarifying methadone regulation for acute care settings. J Addict Behav Ther Rehabil. 2015;4(2).

31. Pytell JD, Sharfstein JM, Olsen Y. Facilitating methadone use in hospitals and skilled nursing facilities. JAMA Intern Med [Internet]. 2019 [cited 2019 Nov 20]; Available from: https://jamanetwork-com.ezproxy.bu.edu/journals/jamainternalmedicine/fullarticle/2754811.

32. Substance Abuse and Mental Health Services Administration. Special circumstances for providing buprenorphine [Internet]. 2016 [cited 2019 Dec 2]. Available from: https://www.samhsa.gov/medication-assisted-treatment/legislation-regulations-guidelines/special.

33. Joseph H, Stancliff S, Langrod J. Methadone maintenance treatment (MMT): a review of historical and clinical issues. Mt Sinai J Med. 2000;67:18.

34. Hemmons P, Bach P, Colizza K, Nolan S. Initiation and rapid titration of methadone in an acute care setting for the treatment of opioid use disorder: a case report. J Addict Med. 2019;13(5):408.

35. Kleber HD. Pharmacologic treatments for opioid dependence: detoxification and maintenance options. Dialogues Clin Neurosci. 2007;9(4):455–70.

36. Trowbridge P, Weinstein ZM, Kerensky T, Roy P, Regan D, Samet JH, et al. Addiction consultation services – linking hospitalized patients to outpatient addiction treatment. J Subst Abus Treat. 2017;79:1–5.

37. Hämmig R, Kemter A, Strasser J, von Bardeleben U, Gugger B, Walter M, et al. Use of microdoses for induction of buprenorphine treatment with overlapping full opioid agonist use: the Bernese method. Subst Abus Rehabil. 2016;7:99–105.

38. Terasaki D, Smith C, Calcaterra SL. Transitioning hospitalized patients with opioid use disorder from methadone to buprenorphine without a period of opioid abstinence using a microdosing protocol. Pharmacotherapy. 2019;39(10):1023–9.

39. Tang VM, Lam-Shang-Leen J, Brothers TD, Hansen K, Caudarella A, Lamba W, et al. Case series: limited opioid withdrawal with use of transdermal buprenorphine to bridge to sublingual buprenorphine in hospitalized patients. Am J Addict. 2020;29(1):73–6.

40. Raheemullah A, Lembke A. Initiating opioid agonist treatment for opioid use disorder in the inpatient setting: a teachable moment. JAMA Intern Med. 2019;179(3):427–8.

41. Ghosh SM, Klaire S, Tanguay R, Manek M, Azar P. A review of novel methods to support the transition from methadone and other full agonist opioids to buprenorphine/naloxone sublingual in both community and acute care settings. Can J Addict. 2019;10(4):41–50.

42. Hess M, Boesch L, Leisinger R, Stohler R. Transdermal buprenorphine to switch patients from higher dose methadone to buprenorphine without severe withdrawal symptoms. Am J Addict. 2011;20(5):480–1.

43. Alford DP, Compton P, Samet JH. Acute pain management for patients receiving maintenance methadone or buprenorphine therapy. Ann Intern Med. 2006;144(2):127–34.

44. Hansen LE, Stone GL, Matson CA, Tybor DJ, Pevear ME, Smith EL. Total joint arthroplasty in patients taking methadone or buprenorphine/naloxone preoperatively for prior heroin

addiction: a prospective matched cohort study. J Arthroplasty [Internet]. [cited 2016 May 4]; Available from: http://www.sciencedirect.com/science/article/pii/S0883540316000942.

45. Vilkins AL, Bagley SM, Hahn KA, Rojas-Miguez F, Wachman EM, Saia K, et al. Comparison of post-cesarean section opioid analgesic requirements in women with opioid use disorder treated with methadone or buprenorphine. J Addict Med. 2017;11(5):397–401.

46. Lembke A, Ottestad E, Schmiesing C. Patients maintained on buprenorphine for opioid use disorder should continue buprenorphine through the perioperative period. Pain Med [Internet]. [cited 2018 Feb 21]; Available from: https://academic-oup-com.ezproxy.bu.edu/painmedicine/advance-article/doi/10.1093/pm/pny019/4858540.

47. Lee JD, Nunes EV, Novo P, Bachrach K, Bailey GL, Bhatt S, et al. Comparative effectiveness of extended-release naltrexone versus buprenorphine-naloxone for opioid relapse prevention (X:BOT): a multicentre, open-label, randomised controlled trial. Lancet. 2018;391(10118):309–18.

48. Morgan JR, Schackman BR, Weinstein ZM, Walley AY, Linas BP. Overdose following initiation of naltrexone and buprenorphine medication treatment for opioid use disorder in a United States commercially insured cohort. Drug Alcohol Depend. 2019;200:34–9.

49. Priest KC, Englander H, McCarty D. "Now hospital leaders are paying attention": a qualitative study of internal and external factors influencing addiction consult services. J Subst Abus Treat. 2020;110:59–65.

50. U.S. Government. Code of federal regulations. Title 21, Part 1306 [Internet]. Electronic code of federal regulations June 23, 2005. Available from: https://www.ecfr.gov/cgi-bin/text-idx?SID=dd3324c93ad659b4a55e8cca8156a65c&node=se21.9.1306_107&rgn=div8.

51. U.S. Department of Justice. Emergency narcotic addiction treatment [Internet]. [cited 2020 Oct 15]. Available from: https://www.deadiversion.usdoj.gov/pubs/advisories/emerg_treat.htm.

52. Biancarelli DL, Biello KB, Childs E, Drainoni M, Salhaney P, Edeza A, et al. Strategies used by people who inject drugs to avoid stigma in healthcare settings. Drug Alcohol Depend. 2019;198:80–6.

53. McNeil R, Kerr T, Pauly B, Wood E, Small W. Advancing patient-centered care for structurally vulnerable drug-using populations: a qualitative study of the perspectives of people who use drugs regarding the potential integration of harm reduction interventions into hospitals. Addiction. 2016;111(4):685–94.

54. Principles of Harm Reduction [Internet]. Harm reduction coalition. Available from: https://harmreduction.org/about-us/principles-of-harm-reduction/.

55. Substance Abuse and Mental Health Services Administration. Trauma-informed care in behavioral health services. Treatment improvement protocol (TIP) series 57. HHS Publication No. (SMA) 13-4801. [Internet]. Substance Abuse and Mental Health Services Administration; 2014 [cited 2019 Dec 31]. Available from: https://store.samhsa.gov/product/TIP-57-Trauma-Informed-Care-in-Behavioral-Health-Services/SMA14-4816.

56. Trauma Informed Oregon [Internet]. Trauma informed oregon. [cited 2020 Oct 15]. Available from: https://traumainformedoregon.org/.

57. Kimmel SD, Rosenmoss S, Bearnot B, Larochelle M, Walley AY. Rejection of patients with opioid use disorder referred for post-acute medical care before and after an anti-discrimination settlement in Massachusetts. J Addict Med. 2020;15:20–6.

58. Wakeman SE, Rich JD. Barriers to post-acute care for patients on opioid agonist therapy: an example of systematic stigmatization of addiction. J Gen Intern Med. 2017;32(1):17–9.

59. Green TC, Clarke J, Brinkley-Rubinstein L, Marshall BDL, Alexander-Scott N, Boss R, et al. Postincarceration fatal overdoses after implementing medications for addiction treatment in a statewide correctional system. JAMA Psychiat. 2018;75(4):405–7.

60. Ritvo AD, Calcaterra SL, Ritvo JI. Using extended release buprenorphine injection to discontinue sublingual buprenorphine: a case series. J Addict Med. 2020;15:252–4.

61. Englander H, Wilson T, Collins D, Phoutrides E, Weimer M, Korthuis PT, et al. Lessons learned from the implementation of a medically enhanced residential treatment (MERT) model integrating intravenous antibiotics and residential addiction treatment. Subst Abuse. 2018 Mar 29;0(ja):1–25.

62. Appel PW, Oldak R. A preliminary comparison of major kinds of obstacles to enrolling in substance abuse treatment (AOD) reported by injecting street outreach clients and other stakeholders. Am J Drug Alcohol Abuse. 2007;33(5):699–705.

63. Merrill JO, Rhodes LA, Deyo RA, Marlatt GA, Bradley KA. Mutual mistrust in the medical care of drug users. J Gen Intern Med. 2002;17(5):327–33.

64. Kelly JF, Wakeman SE, Saitz R. Stop talking 'dirty': clinicians, language, and quality of care for the leading cause of preventable death in the United States. Am J Med. 2015;128(1):8–9.

65. Thakarar K, Weinstein ZM, Walley AY. Optimising health and safety of people who inject drugs during transition from acute to outpatient care: narrative review with clinical checklist. Postgrad Med J. 2016;postgradmedj-2015-133720.

66. Heller D, McCoy K, Cunningham C. An invisible barrier to integrating HIV primary care with harm reduction services: philosophical clashes between the harm reduction and medical models. Public Health Rep. 2004;119(1):32–9.

67. Appel PW, Ellison AA, Jansky HK, Oldak R. Barriers to enrollment in drug abuse treatment and suggestions for reducing them: opinions of drug injecting street outreach clients and other system stakeholders. Am J Drug Alcohol Abuse. 2004;30(1):129–53.

68. Korthuis PT, Gregg J, Rogers WE, McCarty D, Nicolaidis C, Boverman J. Patients' reasons for choosing office-based buprenorphine: preference for patient-centered care. J Addict Med. 2010;4(4):204–10.

69. Masson CL, Sorensen JL, Grossman N, Sporer KA, Des Jarlais DC, Perlman DC. Organizational issues in the implementation of a hospital-based syringe exchange program. Subst Use Misuse. 2010;45(6):901–15.

70. Priest K, McCarty D. The role of hospitalists in treating opioid use disorder. J Addict Med [Internet]. 2019 [cited 2019 Nov 21];Publish Ahead of Print. Available from: insights. ovid.com.

71. Gryczynski J, Schwartz RP, Salkever DS, Mitchell SG, Jaffe JH. Patterns in admission delays to outpatient methadone treatment in the United States. J Subst Abus Treat. 2011;41(4):431–9.

72. Fisher DG, Reynolds GL, D'Anna LH, Hosmer DW, Hardan-Khalil K. Failure to get into substance abuse treatment. J Subst Abus Treat. 2017;73:55–62.

73. D'Amico MJ, Walley AY, Cheng DM, Forman LS, Regan D, Yurkovic A, et al. Which patients receive an addiction consult? A preliminary analysis of the INREACH (INpatient REadmission post-Addiction Consult Help) study. J Subst Abus Treat. 2019;106:35–42.

74. Englander H. A call to action: hospitalists' role in addressing substance use disorder. J Hosp Med [Internet]. 2019 [cited 2019 Nov 21]; Available from: https://www.journalofhospitalmedicine.com/jhospmed/article/210071/hospital-medicine/call-action-hospitalists-role-addressing-substance-use.

75. Wei J, Defries T, Lozada M, Young N, Huen W, Tulsky J. An inpatient treatment and discharge planning protocol for alcohol dependence: efficacy in reducing 30-day readmissions and emergency department visits. J Gen Intern Med. 2015;30(3):365–70.

76. Bottner R, Moriates C, Tirado C. The role of hospitalists in treating opioid use disorder. J Addict Med [Internet]. 2019 [cited 2020 Jan 27];Publish Ahead of Print. Available from: https://journals.lww.com/journaladdictionmedicine/Citation/publishahead/The_Role_of_Hospitalists_in_Treating_Opioid_Use.99349.aspx.

77. Priest KC, McCarty D. Making the business case for an addiction medicine consult service: a qualitative analysis. BMC Health Serv Res [Internet]. 2019 [cited 2019 Nov 21];19. Available from: https://www.ncbi.nlm.nih.gov/pmc/articles/PMC6842195/.

78. Thompson HM, Hill K, Jadhav R, Webb TA, Pollack M, Karnik N. The substance use intervention team: a preliminary analysis of a population-level strategy to address the opioid crisis at an academic health center. J Addict Med. 2019;13(6):460.

79. Mohlman MK, Tanzman B, Finison K, Pinette M, Jones C. Impact of medication-assisted treatment for opioid addiction on Medicaid expenditures and health services utilization rates in Vermont. J Subst Abus Treat. 2016;67:9–14.

80. Ronquest NA, Willson TM, Montejano LB, Nadipelli VR, Wollschlaeger BA. Relationship between buprenorphine adherence and relapse, health care utilization and costs in privately and publicly insured patients with opioid use disorder. Subst Abus Rehabil. 2018;9:59–78.
81. Kilaru AS, Perrone J, Kelley D, Siegel S, Lubitz SF, Mitra N, et al. Participation in a hospital incentive program for follow-up treatment for opioid use disorder. JAMA Netw Open. 2020;3(1):e1918511.
82. Institute of Medicine (US) Committee on Crossing the Quality Chasm: Adaptation to Mental Health and Addictive Disorders. Improving the quality of health care for mental and substance-use conditions: Quality chasm series [Internet]. Washington (DC): National Academies Press (US); 2006 [cited 2016 Feb 29]. (The National Academies Collection: Reports funded by National Institutes of Health). Available from: http://www.ncbi.nlm.nih.gov/books/NBK19830/.
83. Rico F, Liu Y, Martinez DA, Huang S, Zayas-Castro JL, Fabri PJ. Preventable readmission risk factors for patients with chronic conditions. J Healthc Qual. 2016;38(3):127–42.
84. Yanagawa B, Bahji A, Lamba W, Tan D, Cheema A, Syed I, et al. Endocarditis in the setting of IDU: multidisciplinary management. Curr Opin Cardiol. 2018;33(2):140–7.
85. Burris S, Vernick JS, Ditzler A, Strathdee S. The legality of selling or giving syringes to injection drug users. J Am Pharm Assoc (Washington, DC, 1996). 2002;42(6 Suppl 2):S13–18.

Emergency Department Treatment of Opioid Use Disorder

5

Elizabeth A. Samuels, Edouard Coupet Jr, and Gail D'Onofrio

Introduction

On the frontlines of the opioid overdose epidemic, the ED is caring for increasing numbers of people with substance use disorders (SUDs) overall, and opioid use disorder (OUD) in particular and a key location for linkage to medical and behavioral healthcare. Beyond caring for patients after an opioid overdose, EDs can initiate OUD treatment with medications for opioid use disorder (MOUD), specifically buprenorphine, and provide linkage to treatment and overdose preventing and harm reduction services.

From 1999 to 2020, US drug overdoses more than quadrupled, resulting in the death of over 800,000 people [1–3]. During COVID-19, deaths have continued to escalate [3]. The 12 months ending in May 2020 was the deadliest year period to date, with 81,230 people dying from an opioid overdose [3]. Most of these opioid-related overdose deaths involved potent synthetic opioids, specifically fentanyl [4, 5]. Along with rising overdoses, drug-related visits to the US EDs have also increased. Drug-related ED visits doubled from 2005 to 2014 [6] and from 2016 to 2017; national ED visits for opioid overdose increased by nearly 30% [7]. Individuals treated in the ED for an opioid overdose are at increased risk of repeat overdose and overdose death. After an ED visit for opioid overdose, nearly 20% will have a repeat ED visit for overdose [8]. People treated for an overdose or SUD have a six times higher fatality rate compared to adult ED patients overall [9]. Recent studies from Massachusetts found that among people treated for an opioid overdose, 1% died

E. A. Samuels (✉)
Department of Emergency Medicine, Alpert Medical School of Brown University, Providence, RI, USA
e-mail: elizabeth_samuels@brown.edu

E. Coupet Jr · G. D'Onofrio
Department of Emergency Medicine, Yale School of Medicine, New Haven, CT, USA
e-mail: edouard.coupet@yale.edu; gail.donofrio@yale.edu

© Springer Nature Switzerland AG 2021
S. E. Wakeman, J. D. Rich (eds.), *Treating Opioid Use Disorder in General Medical Settings*, https://doi.org/10.1007/978-3-030-80818-1_5

within 1 month and overall mortality within 12 months is 5.5%. Fewer than 30% received opioid agonist therapy during that time, and if they did their odds of survival were significantly improved [10, 11].

Despite increasing overdose deaths, the availability of evidence-based treatment to reduce morbidity and mortality related to opioid use, engagement in formal addiction treatment and access to harm reduction services remain low [6, 12–14]. Some studies have estimated that nearly 80% of people who needed treatment for OUD were not receiving it [15]. In 2018, there were an estimated 10.3 million people with opioid misuse (3.7% of total population), 2.0 million people with OUD, and 1.17 million people on MOUD [16, 17]. Although ED buprenorphine prescribing has increased from 12.3 per 100,000 ED visits in 2002–2003 to 42.8 per 100,000 ED visits in 2016–2017 (odds ratio for linear trend: 3.31; 95% CI: 1.04–10.5), widespread adoption has not occurred [18].

Harm reduction interventions, such as naloxone distribution and syringe services programs, have proven efficacy to reduce overdose deaths and prevent HIV, HCV, and soft tissue infections. However, limited availability of syringe services programs has been associated with recent outbreaks of HIV as well as national increases in the incidence of endocarditis [19–27]. Although ED physicians have been able to obtain a DATA 2000 waiver since 2002, a recent study in four geographically diverse urban teaching hospitals found that only 3% of physicians (9/683) had completed the waiver training and only 20% indicated a high readiness to initiate buprenorphine [28].

The gaps in treatment engagement and availability of harm reduction services are due to multiple factors. Principle among these are stigma and discrimination, treatment gaps and prescribing restrictions, costs, un- and under-insurance, paraphernalia laws which restrict syringe services availability, and unmet health-related social needs. Emergency medicine clinicians have an important opportunity to help close these gaps and reduce opioid use–related morbidity and mortality. We can do this by identifying patients with OUD, starting treatment for OUD with referral to outpatient providers, providing harm reduction services, and using a multimodal approach to pain control. In this chapter, we will review the identification and assessment of OUD in the ED, treatment initiation and referral, ED harm reduction, and the treatment of pain for patients on MOUD.

Identifying OUD

EDs are increasingly recognized as an ideal setting to identify individuals with untreated OUD, begin treatment, and link them to outpatient care for ongoing management. Still, the ED poses a unique set of challenges in identifying untreated OUD including high staff turnover, limited time, and various competing clinical care duties. In addition to being accurate, an OUD identification tool must be efficient and integrate into any busy ED workflow. There are several tools used to identify OUD that have been validated for the outpatient setting, but few have been evaluated in the ED [29].

Many patients with moderate to severe OUD can be identified by their reason for seeking emergency care, such as overdose, withdrawal, seeking treatment, or injection-related complications, such as soft tissue infections. Simple, short screening tools are best suited for the emergency care setting. The OUD identification tool best suited for the ED is the abbreviated National Institute on Drug Abuse (NIDA) Quick Screen Single Drug Use question: "How many times in the past year have you used an illegal drug or used a prescription medication for nonmedical reasons?" (see Fig. 5.1). Evaluated in a primary care setting, this question was determined to be 100% sensitive and 73.5% specific for SUD, including OUD [30]. If a patient answers yes, ED staff should proceed to assess for presence of OUD with the *Diagnostic and Statistical Manual of Mental Disorders*, 5th Edition (DSM-5) criteria.

Professional organizations and policymakers, including the American College of Emergency Physicians (ACEP), also support use of statewide prescription drug monitoring programs (PDMPs). PMDPs may serve as useful tools that can help identify patients with or at risk for developing OUD. Statewide, they have been shown to reduce opioid-related overdose deaths [31]. Yet use of the PMDP alone has not been shown to be effective in identifying ED patients with OUD [32]. Ultimately, PMDPs are best used in conjunction with clinical history and any other identification tools.

Assessing OUD: DSM-5

Once a patient has been identified as having OUD, ED clinicians should assess the severity of their disease prior to initiating treatment. Patients with moderate to severe OUD, as defined by criteria in the DSM-5, are eligible for treatment with MOUD. The DSM-5 criteria include questions that highlight craving, loss of control, and consequences (see Fig. 5.2). Patients must meet at least two criteria within a 12-month period to be diagnosed with OUD. However, a diagnosis of OUD cannot be made if the individual is only positive for the questions pertaining to tolerance and withdrawal, as these will be positive for all people with opioid dependence without OUD, including individuals on long-term opioids for problems such as sickle cell disease, chronic pain, or those undergoing oncologic treatment.

NIDA Quick Screen Single Question
"How many times in the past year have you used an illegal drug or used a prescription medication for non-medical reasons?"

	Never	Once or Twice	Monthly	Weekly	Daily or Almost Daily
Prescription Opioid Drugs for Non-Medical Reasons?					
Illegal Drugs					

If the patient answers "No" to use of illegal drugs or prescription drugs for non-medical reasons, reinforce abstinence. If the patient answers "Yes", continue to the NIDA-Modified ASSIST
NIDA Quick Screen: https://www.drugabuse.gov/sites/default/files/pdf/nmassist.pdf

Fig. 5.1 NIDA Quick Screen single question

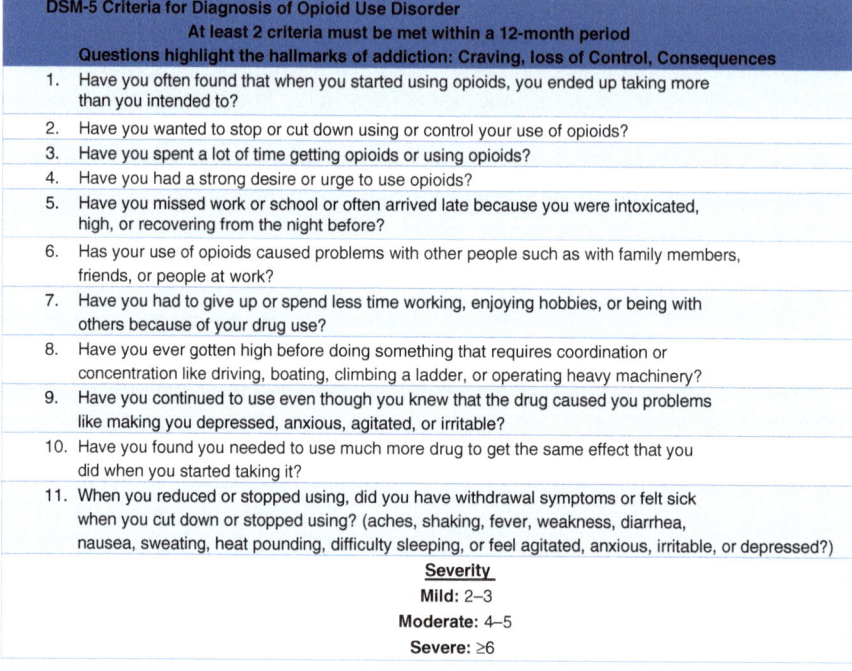

DSM-5 Criteria for Diagnosis of Opioid Use Disorder
At least 2 criteria must be met within a 12-month period
Questions highlight the hallmarks of addiction: Craving, loss of Control, Consequences
1. Have you often found that when you started using opioids, you ended up taking more than you intended to?
2. Have you wanted to stop or cut down using or control your use of opioids?
3. Have you spent a lot of time getting opioids or using opioids?
4. Have you had a strong desire or urge to use opioids?
5. Have you missed work or school or often arrived late because you were intoxicated, high, or recovering from the night before?
6. Has your use of opioids caused problems with other people such as with family members, friends, or people at work?
7. Have you had to give up or spend less time working, enjoying hobbies, or being with others because of your drug use?
8. Have you ever gotten high before doing something that requires coordination or concentration like driving, boating, climbing a ladder, or operating heavy machinery?
9. Have you continued to use even though you knew that the drug caused you problems like making you depressed, anxious, agitated, or irritable?
10. Have you found you needed to use much more drug to get the same effect that you did when you started taking it?
11. When you reduced or stopped using, did you have withdrawal symptoms or felt sick when you cut down or stopped using? (aches, shaking, fever, weakness, diarrhea, nausea, sweating, heat pounding, difficulty sleeping, or feel agitated, anxious, irritable, or depressed?)
Severity
Mild: 2–3
Moderate: 4–5
Severe: ≥6

Fig. 5.2 DSM-5 criteria for diagnosis of opioid use disorder [33]

Engaging Patients

Engaging patients with untreated OUD in the ED to initiate and engage in treatment is potentially challenging and also incredibly rewarding. Having an approach to guide a motivating conversation with patients can help ED clinicians successfully navigate this process. There are a host of strategies clinicians may use to engage with patients, most notable is the Brief Negotiation Interview (BNI). The BNI was derived from motivational interviewing and is ideal for the busy ED setting. Originally, it was studied in patients with alcohol use disorders [34–36]. It is a short counseling session, lasting no more than 10 minutes, that relies on a patient's motivational preparedness to engage in treatment. Motivational interviewing can be conducted by any trained ED clinician, nurse, social worker, substance use counselor, community health worker, or peer recovery specialist. There have been several studies that have demonstrated its effectiveness in enhancing motivation of ED patients with OUD to pursue treatment [34, 37].

The Brief Negotiation Interview

The Brief Negotiation Interview (BNI) consists of four major steps: raise the subject, provide feedback, enhance motivation, and negotiate and advise. In the first step, the ED clinician should ask the patient for permission to discuss their opioid use and its consequences. This should be done in a nonjudgmental, nonconfrontational, and constructive manner. Next, the ED clinician should review the patient's opioid use patterns and provide feedback. The clinician may seek to establish a connection between the patient's opioid use and their ED visit and any other negative consequences surrounding it, including injuries or illnesses. This also serves as an opportunity to provide patient education which may help the patient establish a connection between their opioid use and their presenting ED injury/illness. If the patient does not see this connection, the ED clinician should not force the issue and may instead choose to "agree to disagree."

In the following step, the ED clinician should seek to understand and reinforce the patient's motivation to engage in treatment. To determine the patient's motivation, the ED clinician may start by asking, "On a scale of 1 to 10, how ready are you to accept treatment for your opioid use, with 1 being not ready at all and 10 being very ready?" The patient may select a number and the clinician can respond by exploring why the patient did not select a lower number. For example, if the patient chooses a 3, the clinician may respond with "Great, you are 30% ready; tell me why you did not choose a 2 or a 1?" This provides the patient with an opportunity to identify and explore their reasons for change. If the patient happens to choose a 1, the clinician may ask the patient, "What would have to happen for you to want to make a change?" This allows the patient to generate potentially motivational statements that may invoke change.

The goal of the final step of the BNI is to negotiate a realistic goal with regard to the patient's opioid use. The clinician should start by summarizing the patient's motivations to change and provide any advice. It is important that clinicians understand that some patients may not accept treatment. Instead, clinicians can offer options for referral should the patient change their mind. The interview should conclude with offering harm reduction services, outline plans for next steps, and thank the patient for their time.

Treatment Initiation and Referral

Opioid agonist medications are effective, safe, and evidence-based treatments for opioid withdrawal and OUD that can be provided in any ED by any licensed prescriber. While outpatient methadone maintenance treatment can only be dispensed at licensed opioid treatment programs (OTP), methadone can be administered in the ED setting for opioid withdrawal for up to 72 hours while arranging linkage to an OTP. Unlike methadone, buprenorphine can be prescribed in office-based and clinical settings, previously by any prescribers who had completed the required training and received their Drug Addiction and Treatment Act of 2000 (DATA 2000) waiver or submitted a notice of intent to treat up to 30 patients under the new practice guidelines [38]. Since 2002, ED physicians have been able to administer a buprenorphine dose to treat withdrawal and either obtain a DATA 2000 waiver to prescribe buprenorphine to patients as a bridge to outpatient treatment or provide care at repeat ED visits for up to 3 consecutive days. Currently, only 30% of ED providers report feeling confident in their ability to prescribe buprenorphine and link patients to outpatient care [39]. Barriers to the use of MOUD described in the National Academies of Sciences, Engineering, and Medicine's report *Medications for Opioid Use Disorder Save Lives* [40] include misunderstanding and stigma toward drug addiction, patients with OUD, the medications to treat it, inadequate education of treating clinicians, and current regulations around MOUD. The potential influence of stigma on clinician's ability to provide treatment and erroneous ideas about addiction being a "moral failing" or a choice and not a disease with a neurobiological basis have been reported [40]. Similar attitudes exist with ED clinicians, however; they note that ED-initiated buprenorphine would be feasible with institutional and electronic health record support, training, protocol development, and a referral system for outpatient follow-up [41].

Untreated OUD ranks among the most potentially life-threatening conditions that require treatment in otherwise young and healthy patients. Receipt of MOUD in the year following an ED visit for an opioid overdose is associated with reductions in all-cause and opioid-related mortality [42]. A recent comparative effectiveness study [43] of 40,885 individuals with OUD revealed that while only 15.8% received treatment with opioid agonist therapy, medication was the only treatment associated that reduced risk of an overdose during 3-month (AHR 0.24; 95% CI, 0.14–0.41) and 12-month (AHR, 0.41; 95% CI, 0.31–0.55) follow-up. Treatment initiation with buprenorphine in the ED setting is an effective and feasible intervention. A foundational study examining the effectiveness of ED buprenorphine for initiation of OUD treatment among ED patients with moderate or severe OUD demonstrated that patients who were provided ED buprenorphine with a brief intervention and primary care follow-up were significantly more likely to be engaged in formal OUD treatment at 30 days (78% [95% CI 70–85%]), compared with referral alone (37% [95% CI 28–47%]) and brief intervention with a facilitated, direct referral (45% [95% CI: 36–54%]; $p < 0.001$) [37]. Participants in the buprenorphine group also significantly reduced the number of days per week they used illicit opioids compared to the other study arms ($p < .001$ for both time and intervention effects; $p = .02$ for the interaction effect). Use declined from 5.4 days (95% CI, 5.1–5.7) to 0.9 days (95% CI, 0.5–1.3) among those getting buprenorphine. Individuals in the referral group reduced use from 5.4 days a week (95% CI, 5.1–5.7) to 2.3 days (95% CI, 1.7–3.0). Participants in the brief intervention group reduced use from 5.6 days a week (95% CI, 5.3–5.9) to 2.4 days (95% CI, 1.8–3.0) [37].

This seminal study demonstrated not only feasibility of beginning buprenorphine in ED, but also that ED OUD treatment with buprenorphine could be a key strategy to address gaps in treatment access. ED buprenorphine initiation was also found to be cost effective [44]. Expansion of use of buprenorphine for treatment of opioid withdrawal and OUD has been supported and promoted by ACEP through the Emergency Quality (E-QUAL) Network Opioid Initiative [45], an ACEP point-of-care online buprenorphine prescribing support tool and phone application [46], and the development of emergency medicine tailored waiver courses. EDs are increasingly implementing protocols to start patients on buprenorphine for treatment of OUD. Some link patients to hospital-based ED bridge programs or low-barrier access clinics that stabilize patients on medication for OUD and subsequently link patients to outpatient office-based or OTPs for ongoing treatment. Other EDs provide referral directly to community-based OTPs or office-based treatment clinicians [47, 48].

Patients with moderate to severe OUD administered buprenorphine in the ED should have symptoms of opioid withdrawal according to the Clinical Opioid Withdrawal Scale (COWS) [49, 50] of 8 or greater should not have taken any long-acting opioids within the past 24 hours to 72 hours depending on type (Table 5.1) or short-acting opioids within the past 6–12 hours, and should be medically stable. Buprenorphine should be started as either a buprenorphine monoproduct or combination buprenorphine–naloxone formulation, starting with 4–8 mg buprenorphine if in moderate withdrawal (Fig. 5.3). Patients with more severe withdrawal will need a higher dosage. Peak plasma level should be reached within 30 minutes to one hour. Patients can be reassessed within 30–60 minutes. If withdrawal symptoms are improved, but not fully resolved, another 4–8 mg buprenorphine can be given depending on repeat COWS.

Most individuals will do well with a dose of 12–16 mg on the first day, however higher doses may be needed. If there is no improvement in symptoms, then other causes of the patient's symptoms should be considered. It is important that the individual feels in control of their withdrawal symptoms and withdrawal symptoms should be resolved or significantly improved prior to discharge. Patients can be safely started on buprenorphine if they are pregnant. Opioid agonist treatment during pregnancy can improve maternal and neonatal outcomes and is recommended by the American College of Obstetricians and Gynecologists [51]. Historically, it was recommended to use buprenorphine monoproduct rather than buprenorphine–naloxone combination formulations to avoid possible prenatal exposure to naloxone [52]; however, the naloxone in buprenorphine–naloxone is not bioavailable when taken orally/sublingually [53] and recent research has found it to be safe and with similar outcomes as buprenorphine monoproduct [54, 55].

Buprenorphine can be given to patients treated after an opioid overdose. Several case studies have reported buprenorphine administration to patients in withdrawal after naloxone reversal of an opioid overdose or precipitated withdrawal resulting from administration of an opioid antagonist (naloxone or naltrexone) [56–60].

Patients can be discharged with a prescription for 16 mg buprenorphine/4 mg naloxone once a day until a follow-up appointment can be made ideally within 7 days of the ED visit. Having an established referral mechanism is key to ensure

Table 5.1 Time course of opioid withdrawal following last use for common opioids

Drug	Onset, hours	Peak	Resolution, days
Buprenorphine	4–48	96 h	14–21
Fentanyl (intravenous)	2–5	8–12 h	4–5
Heroin	6–12	24–72 h	7–10
Short acting prescription opioids	6–12	24–72 h	7–10
Long acting opioids (i.e. Oxycontin)	24–36	2–5 days	10–14
Methadone	24–72+	4–6 days	14–21

Reference: Herring et al. [61]

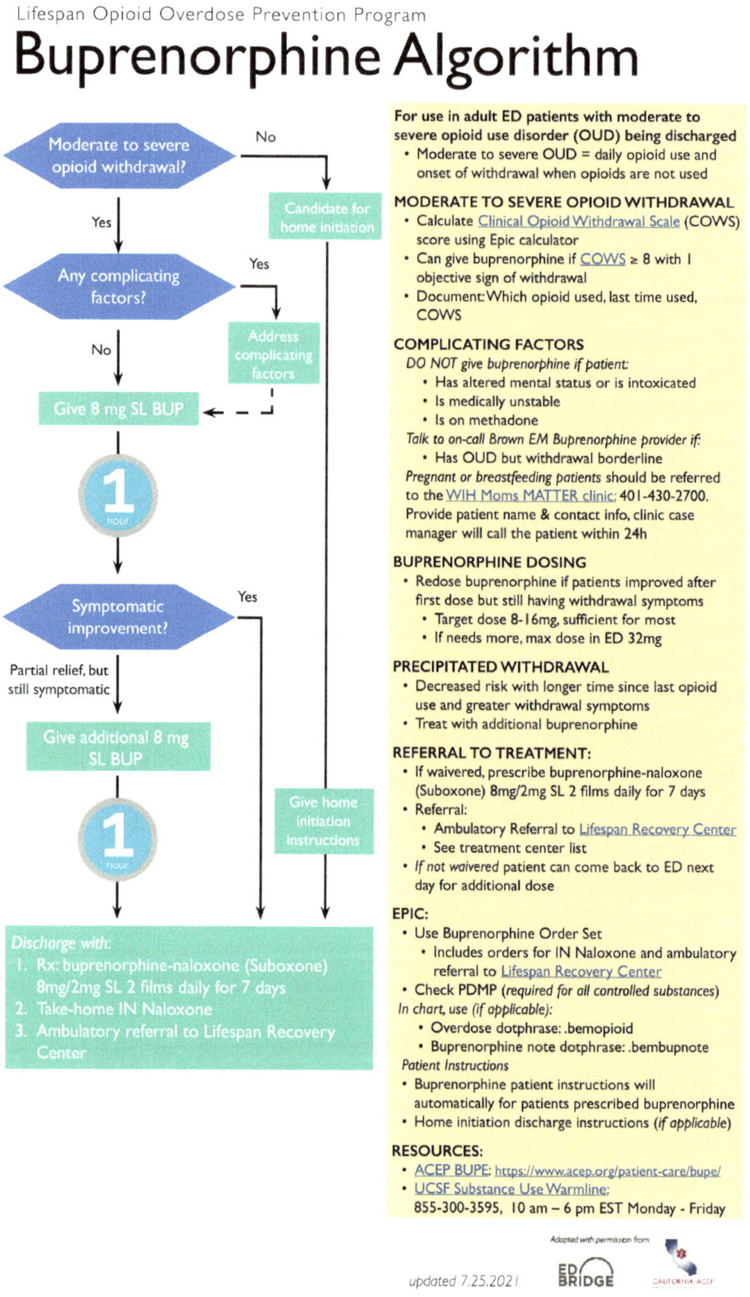

Lifespan Opioid Overdose Prevention Program

Buprenorphine Algorithm

Moderate to severe opioid withdrawal? — No

Yes

Candidate for home initiation

Any complicating factors? — Yes

No

Address complicating factors

Give 8 mg SL BUP

1 hour

Symptomatic improvement? — Yes

Partial relief, but still symptomatic

Give additional 8 mg SL BUP

1 hour

Give home initiation instructions

Discharge with:
1. Rx: buprenorphine-naloxone (Suboxone) 8mg/2mg SL 2 films daily for 7 days
2. Take-home IN Naloxone
3. Ambulatory referral to Lifespan Recovery Center

For use in adult ED patients with moderate to severe opioid use disorder (OUD) being discharged
- Moderate to severe OUD = daily opioid use and onset of withdrawal when opioids are not used

MODERATE TO SEVERE OPIOID WITHDRAWAL
- Calculate Clinical Opioid Withdrawal Scale (COWS) score using Epic calculator
- Can give buprenorphine if COWS ≥ 8 with 1 objective sign of withdrawal
- Document: Which opioid used, last time used, COWS

COMPLICATING FACTORS
DO NOT give buprenorphine if patient:
- Has altered mental status or is intoxicated
- Is medically unstable
- Is on methadone
Talk to on-call Brown EM Buprenorphine provider if:
- Has OUD but withdrawal borderline
Pregnant or breastfeeding patients should be referred to the WIH Moms MATTER clinic: 401-430-2700. Provide patient name & contact info, clinic case manager will call the patient within 24h

BUPRENORPHINE DOSING
- Redose buprenorphine if patients improved after first dose but still having withdrawal symptoms
  - Target dose 8-16mg, sufficient for most
  - If needs more, max dose in ED 32mg

PRECIPITATED WITHDRAWAL
- Decreased risk with longer time since last opioid use and greater withdrawal symptoms
- Treat with additional buprenorphine

REFERRAL TO TREATMENT:
- If waivered, prescribe buprenorphine-naloxone (Suboxone) 8mg/2mg SL 2 films daily for 7 days
- Referral:
  - Ambulatory Referral to Lifespan Recovery Center
  - See treatment center list
- *If not waivered* patient can come back to ED next day for additional dose

EPIC:
- Use Buprenorphine Order Set
  - Includes orders for IN Naloxone and ambulatory referral to Lifespan Recovery Center
- Check PDMP *(required for all controlled substances)*
In chart, use (if applicable):
  - Overdose dotphrase: .bemopioid
  - Buprenorphine note dotphrase: .bembupnote
Patient Instructions
- Buprenorphine patient instructions will automatically for patients prescribed buprenorphine
- Home initiation discharge instructions *(if applicable)*

RESOURCES:
- ACEP BUPE: https://www.acep.org/patient-care/bupe/
- UCSF Substance Use Warmline: 855-300-3595, 10 am – 6 pm EST Monday - Friday

Adapted with permission from

updated 7.25.2021   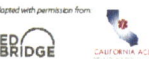 ED BRIDGE   CALIFORNIA ACEP

Fig. 5.3 Example ED buprenorphine algorithm. (Image Courtesy of the Lifespan Opioid Overdose Prevention Program, Brown Emergency Medicine)

timely follow-up and successful treatment engagement and maintenance. This can be through pre-established clinic walk-in hours, providing an appointment time and location, or navigation from a health promotion advocate, community health worker, or peer recovery coach. All patients started on buprenorphine should be discharged with take-home naloxone and a prescription for buprenorphine whether or not they have an appointment for the following day.

Buprenorphine Side Effects

The primary risk of provision of buprenorphine in the ED is precipitated withdrawal. It is important to reassess patients between doses of buprenorphine. As buprenorphine is a partial agonist, there is a ceiling effect which reduces risk of respiratory depression. Prior to giving someone buprenorphine, one should be aware of other toxidromes or conditions and be particularly careful that the patient is not febrile or septic, which will make the COWS score inaccurate.

Precipitated withdrawal is caused when buprenorphine is administered in the setting of recent opioid use or use of a long-acting opioid, such as methadone, and the patient is not in sufficient withdrawal. To prevent this, standard buprenorphine induction should be avoided in patients currently taking long-acting opioids, particularly methadone. Table 5.1 details the recommended durations of time patients should have not taken a long-acting opioid, by opioid type. If patients do experience precipitated withdrawal, which is very uncommon, the most effective treatments are additional doses of buprenorphine [61]. To sufficiently treat withdrawal, enough buprenorphine needs to be given to saturate the opioid receptors, which can require doses up to and surpassing 24 mg. Adjunct medications may be given for comfort, but these have limited effectiveness [61, 62]. These medications include ibuprofen, antiemetics, antidiarrheals, clonidine, and lorazepam.

Unobserved "Home" Initiation

If patients are not in withdrawal at the time of their ED visit, they can be given a prescription for buprenorphine/naloxone with instructions for an unobserved initiation. After an overdose reversed with naloxone, buprenorphine can be administered if the withdrawal symptoms are significant; however these may resolve after the naloxone is metabolized, so patients who are no longer experiencing withdrawal symptoms can be provided a prescription for buprenorphine with home initiation instructions as well. Patients should be provided clear instructions (Fig. 5.4) about how to take buprenorphine [63]. Phone applications and online resources are available to help support and guide patients [64]. Just as with patients started on buprenorphine in the ED, all patients undergoing home initiation should be discharged with take-home naloxone.

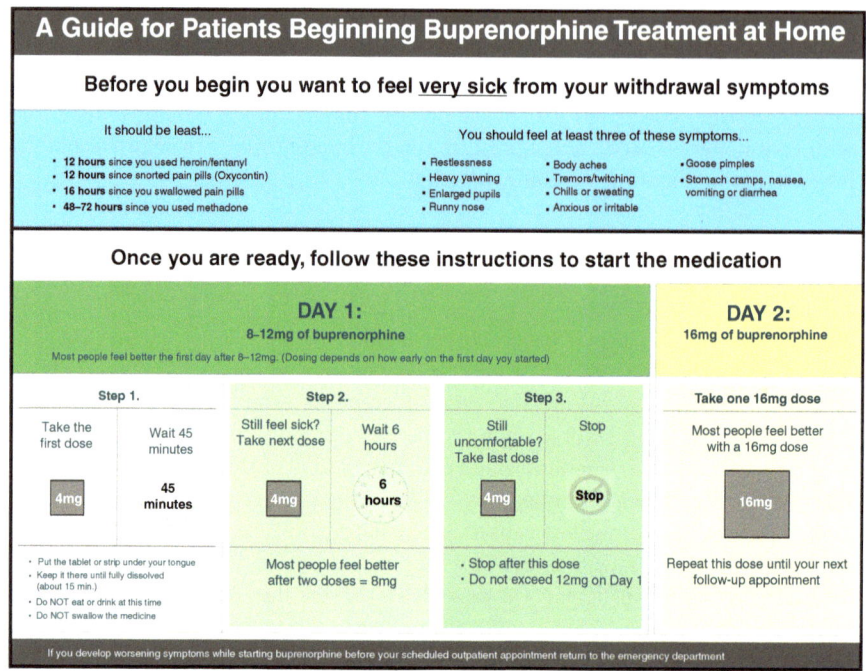

Fig. 5.4 Unobserved buprenrophine initiation patient instructions. (Image Courtesy of the Yale Department of Emergency Medicine)

Harm Reduction

In addition to provision of treatment, harm reduction strategies to reduce substance-use related morbidity and mortality are central to a comprehensive ED approach to OUD. Harm reduction is an approach which seeks to reduce drug-related harm while respecting individuals' autonomy. Community harm reduction strategies include naloxone distribution, syringe services programs, and supervised consumption/injection facilities.

Naloxone is an opioid antagonist that reverses the effects of an opioid overdose. Community naloxone distribution programs have demonstrated that lay people, particularly people who inject drugs, can reliably administer naloxone in the event of a witnessed overdose [65–69]. Community distribution of naloxone began in the 1990s and has been shown to reduce population-level overdose deaths [70], reduce deaths among people released from prison [71], and to be cost-effective when provided to people who use heroin [72]. It is also associated with a reduction in opioid-related ED visits when co-prescribed with opioids for chronic pain by a primary care provider [65, 66, 70, 73, 74]. Since 2014, naloxone distribution has substantially increased through community-based harm reduction organizations, public health departments, pharmacies, and other medical settings. People at increased risk for overdose include people who inject opioids, people who use opioids and have been recently released from prison [75, 76], concurrent opioid use with other sedating medications (i.e., benzodiazepines) or substances (i.e. alcohol) [77], and people taking opioids with significant comorbidities such as liver disease, renal impairment, COPD, and obstructive sleep apnea [78].

Naloxone can be prescribed by any ED prescriber and picked up at an outpatient pharmacy, but to improve access, many EDs distribute naloxone directly to patients at risk of opioid overdose [79–82]. In states allowing for provider-to-patient distribution of naloxone, EDs can provide patients at risk of overdose with take-home naloxone in a pre-assembled "kit" that includes administration instructions, a mouth barrier for rescue breathing, and two doses of naloxone. In states that allow for third-party prescribing, providers can prescribe naloxone to individuals who are concerned for overdose risk among a family member or friend.

Naloxone can be given intramuscularly (IM) or intranasally (IN). IM naloxone can be prescribed as two single-dose vials, 0.4 mg/ML with a 3 cc syringe and 1-inch 23G needle (Table 5.2). This formulation requires drawing up the medication into a syringe prior to administration and is the cheapest type of naloxone available. Evzio™ is an FDA approved prefilled IM naloxone autoinjector. It has a single dose of naloxone 2 mg/0.4 mL, and comes in packs of two. While it is easy to use, it is significantly more expensive and requires prior insurance authorization, limiting its utility in the ED setting.

Intranasal (IN) naloxone is available in generic and FDA-approved formulations. Generic IN naloxone is prescribed as two 2 mg/2 mL prefilled luer-lock needle-less syringes to be dispensed with a mucosal atomization device. This formulation requires assembly before use. FDA-approved IN naloxone, Narcan®, contains 4 mg of naloxone and requires no assembly. It is very easy to use, but more expensive than the generic formulation.

Table 5.2 Naloxone formulations and characteristics

	Generic intramuscular	Evzio™ auto-injector	Generic intranasal	Narcan® nasal spray
Dose	0.4 mg/mL or 4 mg/10 mL	2 mg/0.4 mL	1 mg/ mL	4 mg/0.1 mL
Titratable dose	x		x	
Assembly required	x		x	
Cost	$10–15	$4100 (brand) $178 (generic)	$40–70	$130–150
Prescription & quantity	#2 single-use 1 mL vials OR 10 mL multidose vial PLUS #2 3 mL syringe w/23–25 gauge 1–1.5 inch IM needles; 2 refills	#1 two-pack of two 2 mg/0.4 mL prefilled auto- injector devices; 2 refills	#2 2 mL Luer-Jet™ Luer-Lock needleless syringe plus #2 mucosal atomizer devices (MAD-300); 2 refills	#1 two-pack of two 4 mg/0.1 mL intranasal devices; 2 refills

Primary considerations for ED naloxone distribution include state regulatory barriers, which can limit direct patient naloxone distribution and third-party prescribing, cost, and patient education. Naloxone is covered by most insurance plans. Any trained staff member can provide overdose prevention, response, and naloxone administration education. Narcan® includes patient use instructions in the box, but patient education is best done in person in combination with facilitation of treatment referral. Education can also be done with a video [81].

Syringe services programs [83, 84] and supervised consumption facilities (also known as overdose prevention centers or supervised injection facilities) have demonstrated lower HIV/HCV transmission rates, injection drug risk behaviors, decreased overdose incidents, and more rapid entry into treatment programs [85–87]. Recommended by the WHO and CDC, syringe services programs teach safe injection practices and provide sterile injection supplies to individuals who inject drugs. These programs have been shown to reduce HIV and HCV transmission without increasing substance use [83, 88–92]. Syringe services programs provide additional services that benefit patients including HIV and HCV testing, naloxone distribution, personalized support, and linkage to care. If available, patients who inject drugs should be referred to syringe services programs for continued access to harm reduction and support. In many states, syringes can also be purchased at a pharmacy. Despite their public health utility, many states severely restrict syringe access at pharmacies or community-based syringe services programs, especially in southeast and midwest US and rural communities [93]. Despite the evidence supporting the positive public health impact of supervised consumption sites, as of the date of publication, there has yet to be a publicly sanctioned supervised consumption site operating in the US. Several states and cities are seeking to open such facilities.

Treating Acute Pain in Patients on Medications for Addiction Treatment

Treatment of acute pain in patients on MOUD requires a multimodal approach. Patients with OUD are at significant risk for having their pain undertreated, as they will have increased opioid tolerance, hyperalgesia, and often face significant stigma in healthcare settings. Understanding the importance of effective pain management and discrimination patients may have experienced in healthcare settings related to pain management because of their OUD history is crucial. Some patients may also have concerns about exposure to opioids for pain and potentially resuming use of opioids. The most important first step in pain management is for clinicians to have an honest, open, and patient-centered discussion with patients about the use of non-opioids as well as opioids for pain control [94, 95].

MOUD should be continued in all patients taking MOUD; however, a patient's basal buprenorphine or methadone dose should not be thought of as providing any pain management [96]. Pain control should be added onto a patient's regular MOUD regimen, recognizing that patients who are opioid tolerant will require higher doses at shorter intervals of opioid analgesics than an opioid naïve patient. Splitting the dosing of buprenorphine to every 4, 8, or 12 hours or increasing the dose can maximize the analgesic properties of buprenorphine. Methadone dosing should be kept in a single dose after confirmed with a patient's OTP. The emergency clinician should make contact with the outpatient provider to discuss any changes made to buprenorphine dosing for improved pain control. Barring contraindications, acetaminophen and NSAIDs should be utilized at regular intervals and appropriate dosing. In the acute setting, regional anesthesia using peripheral nerve blocks may also provide relief [94, 95].

Intravenous nonopioid analgesics for severe pain include low-dose ketamine and intravenous lidocaine. Ketamine is a NMDAR antagonist, and at low, sub-dissociative dosages it has been shown to have good analgesic and opioid-sparing effects [94, 95, 97]. There are a range of ED protocols. Initial infusions range from 0.1 to 0.3 mg/kg IV over 15 minutes [97–100]. Lidocaine is a sodium channel antagonist and, like ketamine, is an opioid-sparing analgesic. It is less studied in the ED setting compared to ketamine and should not be used in patients with cardiac dysrhythmias [101, 102]. It is started with an initial bolus of 1–1.5 mg/kg followed by an infusion of 1.5–3 mg/kg/h [94, 95, 97, 101, 102]. Cardiac dysrhythmias are contraindications for use of IV lidocaine.

Opioid agonists with a high affinity for the opioid receptor can also be utilized for severe pain not relieved by nonopioid medications [94, 96]. Buprenorphine can be given intravenously for severe pain or in patients who cannot take sublingual or oral medications. Intravenous buprenorphine can be given as 0.3 mg diluted in volume of 10 mL over 3–5 minutes IV. It can be re-dosed within 30 minutes. There is no clinical ceiling on the analgesic effects of buprenorphine, but patients should be monitored closely as respiratory depression can occur at high doses of buprenorphine [94, 96]. While buprenorphine binds to most of the mu opioid receptors, there will be some unbound receptors that high-affinity opioid agonists, such a hydromorphone, fentanyl, or oxycodone, can bind to [103]. To be effective, patients will need much higher than usual doses [104]. Patients should be monitored closely with additional opioid administration, as there is an increased risk of respiratory depression. For patients being discharged in whom split dosing sublingual buprenorphine is not effective, oxycodone can be added. All adjustments to a patient's buprenorphine or addition of other opioid agonists should be done in consultation with a patient's outpatient provider. For severe pain in patients that are going to be admitted to the hospital, intravenous opioids such as fentanyl or hydromorphone in addition to low-dose ketamine are all options.

Conclusion

Untreated OUD results in high rates of overdose and death. The ED provides an important opportunity to provide lifesaving care to people with untreated OUD, including initiation of evidence-based treatment with buprenorphine and provision of harm reduction services. ED-initiated buprenorphine is safe and highly effective. Expanding its use will require not only education and training for all ED clinicians, but also addressing gaps in emergency clinician education, regulatory restrictions, and clinician stigma toward people with OUD and MOUD. The success of starting OUD treatment in the ED with buprenorphine depends on successful linkage to outpatient treatment providers. As the capacity for ED buprenorphine expands, outpatient buprenorphine treatment must also expand to ensure access to timely and longitudinal care.

References

1. Centers for Disease Control and Prevention. Multiple cause of death 1999–2017 on CDC WONDER online database: National Center for Health Statistics.; December 2018. Available from: https://wonder.cdc.gov/mcd.html.
2. NIDA. Overdose death rates 2019 [updated January 2019]. Available from: https://www.drugabuse.gov/related-topics/trends-statistics/overdose-death-rates.
3. CDC Health Alert Network. Increase in fatal drug overdoses across the United States driven by synthetic opioids before and during the COVID-19 pandemic. Atlanta: Centers for Disease Control and Prevention; 2020 [updated December 17]. Available from: https://www.cdc.gov/media/releases/2020/p1218-overdose-deaths-covid-19.html.
4. Rudd RA, Seth P, David F, Scholl L. Increases in drug and opioid-involved overdose deaths – United States, 2010–2015. MMWR Morb Mortal Wkly Rep. 2016;65(5051):1445–52.
5. Scholl L, Seth P, Kariisa M, Wilson N, Baldwin G. Drug and opioid-involved overdose deaths – United States, 2013–2017. MMWR Morb Mortal Wkly Rep. 2018;67(5152):1419–27.
6. Weiss A, Bailey M, O'Malley L, Barrett M, Elixhauser A, Steiner C. Patient characteristics of opioid-related inpatient stays and emergency department visits nationally and by state, 2014. Agency for Healthcare Research and Quality: Rockville; 2017.
7. Vivolo-Kantor AM, Seth P, Gladden RM, Mattson CL, Baldwin GT, Kite-Powell A, et al. Vital signs: trends in emergency department visits for suspected opioid overdoses – United States, July 2016-September 2017. MMWR Morb Mortal Wkly Rep. 2018;67(9):279–85.
8. Olfson M, Wall M, Wang S, Crystal S, Blanco C. Risks of fatal opioid overdose during the first year following nonfatal overdose. Drug Alcohol Depend. 2018;190:112–9.
9. Krawczyk N, Eisenberg M, Schneider KE, Richards TM, Lyons BC, Jackson K, et al. Predictors of overdose death among high-risk emergency department patients with substance-related encounters: a data linkage cohort study. Ann Emerg Med. 2020;75(1):1–2.
10. Larochelle M, Liebschutz J, Zhang F, Ross-Degnan D, Wharam J. Opioid prescribing after nonfatal overdose and association with repeated overdose. Ann Intern Med. 2016;165(5):376–7.
11. Weiner SG, Baker O, Bernson D, Schuur JD. One-year mortality of patients after emergency department treatment for nonfatal opioid overdose. Ann Emerg Med. 2020;75(1):13–7.
12. NIDA. Nationwide Trends. June 25, 2015. Available from: https://www.drugabuse.gov/publications/drugfacts/nationwide-trends.
13. White AM, Slater ME, Ng G, Hingson R, Breslow R. Trends in alcohol-related emergency department visits in the United States: results from the nationwide emergency department sample, 2006 to 2014. Alcohol Clin Exp Res. 2018;42(2):352–9.
14. Mack KA, Jones CM, Ballesteros MF. Illicit drug use, illicit drug use disorders, and drug overdose deaths in metropolitan and nonmetropolitan areas – United States. MMWR Surveill Summ. 2017;66(19):1–12.
15. Park-Lee E, Lipari RN, Hedden SL, Kroutil LA, Porter JD. Receipt of services for substance use and mental health issues among adults: Results FROM the 2016 National Survey on Drug Use and Health: Substance Abuse and Mental Health Services Administration; 2017.
16. Substance Abuse and Mental Health Services Administration. Key substance use and mental health indicators in the United States: Results from the 2018 National Survey on Drug Use and Health (HHS Publication No. PEP19-5068, NSDUH Series H-54). Rockville: Center

for Behavioral Health Statistics and Quality, Substance Abuse and Mental Health Services Administration; 2019.

17. Substance Abuse and Mental Health Services Administration. Key substance use and mental health indicators in the United States: results from the 2018 National Survey on Drug Use and Health. Center for Behavioral Health Statistics and Quality, Substance Abuse and Mental Health Services Administration: Rockville; 2019.

18. Rhee TG, D'Onofrio G, Fiellin DA. Trends in the use of buprenorphine in US emergency departments, 2002–2017. JAMA Netw Open. 2020;3(10):e2021209.

19. Fleischauer AT, Ruhl L, Rhea S, Barnes E. Hospitalizations for endocarditis and associated Health care costs among persons with diagnosed drug dependence – North Carolina, 2010–2015. MMWR Morb Mortal Wkly Rep. 2017;66(22):569–73.

20. Gray ME, Rogawski McQuade ET, Scheld WM, Dillingham RA. Rising rates of injection drug use associated infective endocarditis in Virginia with missed opportunities for addiction treatment referral: a retrospective cohort study. BMC Infect Dis. 2018;18(1):532.

21. Hartman L, Barnes E, Bachmann L, Schafer K, Lovato J, Files DC. Opiate injection-associated infective endocarditis in the Southeastern United States. Am J Med Sci. 2016;352(6):603–8.

22. Keeshin SW, Feinberg J. Endocarditis as a marker for new epidemics of injection drug use. Am J Med Sci. 2016;352(6):609–14.

23. Schranz AJ, Fleischauer A, Chu VH, Wu LT, Rosen DL. Trends in drug use-associated infective endocarditis and heart valve surgery, 2007 to 2017: a study of statewide discharge data. Ann Intern Med. 2019;170(1):31–40.

24. Wurcel AG, Anderson JE, Chui KKH, Skinner S, Knox TA, Snydman DR, et al. Increasing infectious endocarditis admissions among young people who inject drugs. Open Forum Infect Di. 2016;3(3).

25. Goedel WC, King MRF, Lurie MN, Galea S, Townsend JP, Galvani AP, et al. Implementation of syringe services programs to prevent rapid human immunodeficiency virus transmission in rural counties in the United States: a modeling study. Clin Infect Dis 2020;70(6):1096–102.

26. Gonsalves GS, Crawford FW. Dynamics of the HIV outbreak and response in Scott County, IN, USA, 2011–15: a modelling study. Lancet HIV. 2018;5(10):e569–e77.

27. Davis CS, Carr DH, Samuels EA. Paraphernalia laws, criminalizing possession and distribution of items used to consume illicit drugs, and injection-related harm. Am J Public Health. 2019:e1–4.

28. Hawk K, D'Onofrio G, Chawarski M, O'Connor P, Cowan E, Lyons M, et al. Barriers and facilitators to clinician readiness to provide emergency department-initiated buprenorphine: results of a survey and qualitative analysis. JAMA Netw Open. 2020;3:e204561.

29. Duber HC, Barata IA, Cioe-Pena E, Liang SY, Ketcham E, Macias-Konstantopoulos W, et al. Identification, management, and transition of care for patients with opioid use disorder in the emergency department. Ann Emerg Med. 2018;72(4):420–31.

30. Smith PC, Schmidt SM, Allensworth-Davies D, Saitz R. A single-question screening test for drug use in primary care. Arch Intern Med. 2010;170(13):1155–60.

31. Patrick SW, Fry CE, Jones TF, Buntin MB. Implementation of prescription drug monitoring programs associated with reductions in opioid-related death rates. Health Aff. 2016;35(7):1324–32.

32. Hawk K, D'Onofrio G, Fiellin DA, Chawarski MC, O'Connor PG, Owens PH, et al. Past-year prescription drug monitoring program opioid prescriptions and self-reported opioid use in an emergency department population with opioid use disorder. Acad Emerg Med. 2018;25(5):508–16.

33. American Psychiatric Association. Diagnostic and statistical manual of mental disorders. 5th ed; 2013. p. 541. https://doi.org/10.1176/appi.books.9780890425596.

34. Pantalon MV, Dziura J, Li F-Y, Owens PH, O'Connor PG, D'Onofrio G. An interventionist adherence scale for a specialized brief negotiation interview focused on treatment engagement for opioid use disorders. Subst Abus. 2017;38(2):191–9.

35. D'Onofrio G, Pantalon MV, Degutis LC, Fiellin DA, O'Connor PG. Development and implementation of an emergency practitioner–performed brief intervention for hazardous and harmful drinkers in the emergency department. Acad Emerg Med. 2005;12(3):249–56.

36. D'Onofrio G, Fiellin DA, Pantalon MV, Chawarski MC, Owens PH, Degutis LC, et al. A brief intervention reduces hazardous and harmful drinking in emergency department patients. Ann Emerg Med. 2012;60(2):181–92.

37. D'Onofrio G, O'Connor PG, Pantalon MV, Chawarski MC, Busch SH, Owens PH, et al. Emergency department-initiated buprenorphine/naloxone treatment for opioid dependence: a randomized clinical trial. JAMA. 2015;313(16):1636–44.

38. Kampman K, Jarvis M. American Society of Addiction Medicine (ASAM) national practice guideline for the use of medications in the treatment of addiction involving opioid use. J Addict Med. 2015;9(5):358–67.

39. Lowenstein M, Kilaru A, Perrone J, Hemmons J, Abdel-Rahman D, Meisel ZF, et al. Barriers and facilitators for emergency department initiation of buprenorphine: a physician survey. Am J Emerg Med. 2019;37(9):1787–90.

40. National Academies of Sciences, Engineering, and Medicine. Medications for opioid use disorder save lives. Washington, DC: The National Academies Press; 2019.

41. Im DD, Chary A, Condella A, Vongsachang H, Carlson L, Vogel L, et al. 121 emergency providers' attitudes towards opioid use disorder and emergency department-initiated buprenorphine treatment: a mixed-methods study. Ann Emerg Med. 2018;72(4):S52.

42. Larochelle MR, Bernson D, Land T, Stopka TJ, Wang N, Xuan Z, et al. Medication for opioid use disorder after nonfatal opioid overdose and association with mortality: a cohort study. Ann Intern Med. 2018;169(3):137–45.

43. Wakeman SE, Larochelle MR, Ameli O, Chaisson CE, McPheeters JT, Crown WH, et al. Comparative effectiveness of different treatment pathways for opioid use disorder. JAMA Netw Open. 2020;3(2):e1920622.

44. Busch SH, Fiellin DA, Chawarski MC, Owens PH, Pantalon MV, Hawk K, et al. Cost-effectiveness of emergency department-initiated treatment for opioid dependence. Addiction. 2017;112(11):2002–10.

45. American College of Emergency Physicians. E-QUAL network opioid initiative. 2019. Available from: https://www.acep.org/administration/quality/equal/emergency-quality-network-e-qual/e-qual-opioid-initiative/.

46. Ketcham E, Ryan S. Buprenorphine use in the emergency department tool. Dallas: American College of Emergency Physicians; 2018. Available from: https://www.acep.org/patient-care/bupe/.

47. D'Onofrio G, McCormack RP, Hawk K. Emergency departments – a 24/7/365 option for combating the opioid crisis. N Engl J Med. 2018;379(26):2487–90.

48. Substance Abuse and Mental Health Services Administration. Use of medications for opioid use disorder in emergency departments. Rockville: National Mental Health and Substance Use Policy Laboratory; 2019. Contract No.: HHS Publication No. XXXXXX.

49. Ries R, Fiellin D, Miller S, Saitz R. Principles of addiction medicine. 5th ed. Philadelphia: Wolters Kluwer Publishers; 2014.

50. Schuckit MA. Treatment of opioid-use disorders. N Engl J Med. 2016;375(4):357–68.

51. American College of Obstetricians and Gynecologists. Opioid use and opioid use disorder in pregnancy Committee Opinion No. 711. Obstet Gynecol. 2017(130):e81–94.

52. Johnson RE, Jones HE, Fischer G. Use of buprenorphine in pregnancy: patient management and effects on the neonate. Drug Alcohol Depend. 2003;70:S87–101.

53. Fudala PJ, Bridge TP, Herbert S, Williford WO, Chiang CN, Jones K, et al. Office-based treatment of opiate addiction with a sublingual-tablet formulation of buprenorphine and naloxone. N Engl J Med. 2003;349(10):949–58.

54. Debelak K, Morrone WR, O'Grady KE, Jones HE. Buprenorphine + naloxone in the treatment of opioid dependence during pregnancy-initial patient care and outcome data. Am J Addict. 2013;22(3):252–4.

55. Wiegand SL, Stringer EM, Stuebe AM, Jones H, Seashore C, Thorp J. Buprenorphine and naloxone compared with methadone treatment in pregnancy. Obstet Gynecol. 2015;125(2):363–8.

56. Herring AA, Schultz CW, Yang E, Greenwald MK. Rapid induction onto sublingual buprenorphine after opioid overdose and successful linkage to treatment for opioid use disorder. Am J Emerg Med. 2019;37(12):2259–62.
57. Carroll GG, Wasserman DD, Shah AA, Salzman MS, Baston KE, Rohrbach RA, et al. Buprenorphine field initiation of ReScue treatment by emergency medical services (Bupe FIRST EMS): a case series. Prehosp Emerg Care. 2020:1–5.
58. Phillips RH, Salzman M, Haroz R, Rafeq R, Mazzarelli AJ, Pelletier-Bui A. Elective naloxone-induced opioid withdrawal for rapid initiation of medication-assisted treatment of opioid use disorder. Ann Emerg Med. 2019;74(3):430–2.
59. Chhabra N, Aks SE. Treatment of acute naloxone-precipitated opioid withdrawal with buprenorphine. Am J Emerg Med. 2020;38(3):691 e3–4.
60. Szczesniak LM, Calleo VJ, Sullivan RW. Buprenorphine therapy in the setting of induced opioid withdrawal from oral naltrexone: a case report. Harm Reduct J. 2020;17(1):71.
61. Herring AA, Perrone J, Nelson LS. Managing opioid withdrawal in the emergency department with buprenorphine. Ann Emerg Med. 2019;73(5):481–7.
62. Love JS, Perrone J, Nelson LS. Should buprenorphine be administered to patients with opioid withdrawal in the emergency department? Ann Emerg Med. 2018;72(1):26–8.
63. Lee JD, Vocci F, Fiellin DA. Unobserved "home" induction onto buprenorphine. J Addict Med. 2014;8(5):299–308.
64. Amston Studio LLC. Buprenorphine home induction. New Haven. Available from: https://apps.apple.com/us/app/buprenorphine-home-induction/id1449302173.
65. Piper TM, Stancliff S, Rudenstine S, Sherman S, Nandi V, Clear A, et al. Evaluation of a naloxone distribution and administration program in New York City. Subst Use Misuse. 2008;43(7):858–70.
66. Doe-Simkins M, Walley AY, Epstein A, Moyer P. Saved by the nose: bystander-administered intranasal naloxone hydrochloride for opioid overdose. Am J Public Health. 2009;99(5):788–91.
67. Enteen L, Bauer J, McLean R, Wheeler E, Huriaux E, Kral AH, et al. Overdose prevention and naloxone prescription for opioid users in San Francisco. J Urban Health. 2010;87(6):931–41.
68. Bennett A, Bell A, Tomedi L, Hulsey E, Kral A. Characteristics of an overdose prevention, response, and naloxone distribution program in Pittsburgh and Allegheny County, Pennsylvania. J Urban Health. 2011;88:1020–30.
69. Strang J, Manning V, Mayet S, Best D, Titherington E, Santana L, et al. Overdose training and take-home naloxone for opiate users: prospective cohort study of impact on knowledge and attitudes and subsequent management of overdoses. Addiction. 2008;103(10):1648–57.
70. Walley AY, Xuan Z, Hackman HH, Quinn E, Doe-Simkins M, Sorensen-Alawad A, et al. Opioid overdose rates and implementation of overdose education and nasal naloxone distribution in Massachusetts: interrupted time series analysis. BMJ. 2013;346:f174.
71. Bird SM, McAuley A, Perry S, Hunter C. Effectiveness of Scotland's National Naloxone Programme for reducing opioid-related deaths: a before (2006-10) versus after (2011-13) comparison. Addiction. 2016;111(5):883–91.
72. Coffin PO, Sullivan SD. Cost-effectiveness of distributing naloxone to heroin users for lay overdose reversal. Ann Intern Med. 2013;158:1–9.
73. Coffin PO, Behar E, Rowe C, Santos GM, Coffa D, Bald M, et al. Nonrandomized intervention study of naloxone coprescription for primary care patients receiving Long-term opioid therapy for pain. Ann Intern Med. 2016;165(4):245–52.
74. Maxwell S, Bigg D, Stanczykiewicz K, Carlberg-Racich S. Prescribing naloxone to actively injecting heroin users: a program to reduce heroin overdose deaths. J Addict Dis. 2006;25(3):89–96.
75. Binswanger IA, Blatchford PJ, Mueller SR, Stern MF. Mortality after prison release: opioid overdose and other causes of death, risk factors, and time trends from 1999 to 2009. Ann Intern Med. 2013;159(9):592–600.

76. Bukten A, Stavseth MR, Skurtveit S, Tverdal A, Strang J, Clausen T. High risk of overdose death following release from prison: variations in mortality during a 15-year observation period. Addiction. 2017;112(8):1432–9.
77. Garg RK, Fulton-Kehoe D, Franklin GM. Patterns of opioid use and risk of opioid overdose death among Medicaid patients. Med Care. 2017;55(7):661–8.
78. Nadpara PA, Joyce AR, Murrelle EL, Carroll NW, Carroll NV, Barnard M, et al. Risk factors for serious prescription opioid-induced respiratory depression or overdose: comparison of commercially insured and veterans health affairs populations. Pain Med. 2018;19(1):79–96.
79. Samuels E. Emergency department naloxone distribution: a Rhode Island department of health, recovery community, and emergency department partnership to reduce opioid overdose deaths. R I Med J (2013). 2014;97(10):38–9.
80. Samuels EA, Baird J, Yang ES, Mello MJ. Adoption and utilization of an emergency department naloxone distribution and peer recovery coach consultation program. Acad Emerg Med. 2019;26(2):160–73.
81. Samuels EA, Hoppe J, Papp J, Whiteside L, Raja AS, Bernstein E. Emergency department naloxone distribution: key considerations and implementation strategies. American College of Emergency Physicians: Irving; 2015.
82. Dwyer K, Walley AY, Langlois BK, Mitchell PM, Nelson KP, Cromwell J, et al. Opioid education and nasal naloxone rescue kits in the emergency department. West J Emerg Med. 2015;16(3):381–4.
83. Platt L, Minozzi S, Reed J, Vickerman P, Hagan H, French C, et al. Needle and syringe programmes and opioid substitution therapy for preventing HCV transmission among people who inject drugs: findings from a Cochrane Review and meta-analysis. Addiction. 2018;113(3):545–63.
84. Sawangjit R, Khan TM, Chaiyakunapruk N. Effectiveness of pharmacy-based needle/syringe exchange programme for people who inject drugs: a systematic review and meta-analysis. Addiction. 2017;112(2):236–47.
85. Potier C, Laprevote V, Dubois-Arber F, Cottencin O, Rolland B. Supervised injection services: what has been demonstrated? A systematic literature review. Drug Alcohol Depend. 2014;145:48–68.
86. Wood E, Tyndall MW, Zhang R, Stoltz JA, Lai C, Montaner JS, et al. Attendance at supervised injecting facilities and use of detoxification services. N Engl J Med. 2006;354(23):2512–4.
87. Marshall B, Milloy M, Wood E, Montaner J, Kerr T. Reduction in overdose mortality after the opening of North America's first medically supervised safer injecting facility: a retrospective population-based study. Lancet. 2011;377(9775):1429–37.
88. Palmateer N, Kimber J, Hickman M, Hutchinson S, Rhodes T, Goldberg D. Evidence for the effectiveness of sterile injecting equipment provision in preventing hepatitis C and human immunodeficiency virus transmission among injecting drug users: a review of reviews. Addiction. 2010;105(5):844–59.
89. MacArthur GJ, van Velzen E, Palmateer N, Kimber J, Pharris A, Hope V, et al. Interventions to prevent HIV and Hepatitis C in people who inject drugs: a review of reviews to assess evidence of effectiveness. Int J Drug Policy. 2014;25(1):34–52.
90. Aspinall EJ, Nambiar D, Goldberg DJ, Hickman M, Weir A, Van Velzen E, et al. Are needle and syringe programmes associated with a reduction in HIV transmission among people who inject drugs: a systematic review and meta-analysis. Int J Epidemiol. 2014;43(1):235–48.
91. Des Jarlais D, Perlis T, Arasteh K, Torian L, Hagan H, Beatrice S, et al. Reductions in hepatitis C virus and HIV infections among injecting drug users in New York City, 1990–2001. AIDS. 2005:S20–5.
92. Nguyen TQ, Weir BW, Des Jarlais DC, Pinkerton SD, Holtgrave DR. Syringe exchange in the United States: a national level economic evaluation of hypothetical increases in investment. AIDS Behav. 2014;18(11):2144–55.
93. Davis CS, Carr DH, Samuels EA. Paraphernalia laws, criminalizing possession and distribution of items used to consume illicit drugs, and injection-related harm. Am J Public Health. 2019;109(11):1564–7.

94. Coffa D, Harter K, Smith B, Snyder H, Windels S. Acute pain and perioperative management in opioid use disorder: pain control in patients on buprenorphine, methadone, or naltrexone. 2018. Available from: https://static1.squarespace.com/static/5acbce828f51302409d8bdcb/t/5acda2 600e2e72484fd5b7e3/1523425889927/SHOUT+GUIDELINE+-+periop+and+acute+pain-+03-28-2018.pdf.
95. Project SHOUT: support for hospital opioid use treatment. Available from: https://sarah--windels-b4j2.squarespace.com/guidelines.
96. Alford DP, Compton P, Samet JH. Acute pain management for patients receiving maintenance methadone or buprenorphine therapy. Ann Intern Med. 2006;144(2):127–34.
97. Lee EN, Lee JH. The effects of low-dose ketamine on acute pain in an emergency setting: a systematic review and meta-analysis. PLoS One. 2016;11(10):e0165461.
98. Beaudoin FL, Lin C, Guan W, Merchant RC. Low-dose ketamine improves pain relief in patients receiving intravenous opioids for acute pain in the emergency department: results of a randomized, double-blind, clinical trial. Acad Emerg Med. 2014;21(11):1193–202.
99. Bowers KJ, McAllister KB, Ray M, Heitz C. Ketamine as an adjunct to opioids for acute pain in the emergency department: a randomized controlled trial. Acad Emerg Med. 2017;24(6):676–85.
100. Karlow N, Schlaepfer CH, Stoll CRT, Doering M, Carpenter CR, Colditz GA, et al. A systematic review and meta-analysis of ketamine as an alternative to opioids for acute pain in the emergency department. Acad Emerg Med. 2018;25(10):1086–97.
101. Masic D, Liang E, Long C, Sterk EJ, Barbas B, Rech MA. Intravenous lidocaine for acute pain: a systematic review. Pharmacotherapy. 2018;38(12):1250–9.
102. Silva L, Scherber K, Cabrera D, Motov S, Erwin PJ, West CP, et al. Safety and efficacy of intravenous lidocaine for pain management in the emergency department: a systematic review. Ann Emerg Med. 2018;72(2):135–44 e3.
103. Huhn AS, Strain EC, Bigelow GE, Smith MT, Edwards RR, Tompkins DA. Analgesic effects of hydromorphone versus buprenorphine in buprenorphine-maintained individuals. Anesthesiology. 2019;130(1):131–41.
104. Kornfeld H, Manfredi L. Effectiveness of full agonist opioids in patients stabilized on buprenorphine undergoing major surgery: a case series. Am J Ther. 2010;17(5):523–8.

Treating Opioid Use Disorder in Correctional Settings

6

Rachel Simon, Josiah D. Rich, and Sarah E. Wakeman

Introduction

In the United States, there are approximately 2.2 million individuals who are currently incarcerated in prison or jail and another 4.6 million who are under correctional supervision through probation or parole [1, 2]. [See Table 6.1 for definitions.] Many more individuals are cycling through the correctional system annually – in 2017, there were over 10 million admissions to county jails and another 606,000 to state and federal prisons [1, 2]. This, however, was not always the case. For the past 40 years, the number of individuals under correctional control in the US has increased exponentially, with a 500% increase in individuals incarcerated in jails and prisons since 1980. The epidemic of mass incarceration overlaps with the epidemic of drug use and addiction, principally as a result of the "War on Drugs," established during the Nixon administration when President Nixon declared that "public enemy number one is drug abuse" and instigated this "war." The "War on Drugs" expanded under President Reagan with the establishment of strict drug sentencing policies, including mandatory minimums, which led to an unprecedented increase in incarceration due to drug-related crimes. In state prisons, the number of people incarcerated for a drug offense has increased tenfold since 1980, and people charged with a drug offense now account for one out of every five individuals behind bars [3]. Half of individuals incarcerated in federal prisons are there for a drug offense. These numbers likely underestimate the true impact of the War on Drugs and incarceration as many more people are detained or imprisoned for charges which are related to drugs and drug policies, for example, acquisitive crimes like low-level property charges or theft.

R. Simon (✉) · S. E. Wakeman
Department of Medicine, Massachusetts General Hospital, Boston, MA, USA
e-mail: rsimon3@partners.org

J. D. Rich
Brown University, The Miriam and Rhode Island Hospitals, Providence, RI, USA

© Springer Nature Switzerland AG 2021
S. E. Wakeman, J. D. Rich (eds.), *Treating Opioid Use Disorder in General Medical Settings*, https://doi.org/10.1007/978-3-030-80818-1_6

Table 6.1 Terminology related to correctional control

Term	Definition
Prison	Facilities that are run by the state or the federal government that typically hold individuals with sentences of more than 1 year
Jail	Facilities that are locally operated and hold individuals awaiting trial or sentencing or both, as well as individuals sentenced to a term of less than 1 year
Probation	Community supervision that is mandated by a court in lieu of incarceration.
Parole	Community supervision where individuals are conditionally released from prison/jail to serve the remaining portion of their sentence in the community.

Minoritized individuals, including Black, Latinx, and Indigenous people, experience the greatest burden of harm from the US drug policies. Despite similar rates of drug use and selling between White and Black individuals, Black people are more likely to be arrested; when arrested, are more likely to be convicted; and when convicted, are more likely to have longer prison sentences than White people [4]. Black people are six times more likely to be incarcerated than White people and Hispanic/Latinx individuals are approximately three times more likely [5]. One out of three Black men can expect to experience incarceration in their lifetime, as compared to one out of every seventeen White men. The mass incarceration of minoritized individuals is no accident; racism is inherent in this nation's drug policy. It has been shown that the "War on Drugs" has operated as a system of social control targeting low-income Black and Latinx communities, resulting in legalized discrimination similar to slavery and the Jim Crow laws [6, 7].

This chapter will provide an overview of the prevalence of OUD in correctional settings and a primer on treatment for OUD during incarceration and during the vulnerable transition period from corrections back to the community.

A Note on Language

Incarceration is one of the most stigmatizing and traumatizing events an individual can experience. While often a tremendously negative experience while incarcerated, the event of incarceration has far-reaching, life-long implications after release. Social resources, including food stamps, housing, and social security, and other economic opportunities such as the ability to apply for educational financial aid and secure different employment opportunities, become severely limited as a result of institutionalized discrimination related to incarceration. Language is a powerful mediator of this stigma and can play an important role in how individuals and society as a whole view the experience of incarceration [8]. Terminology used to describe individuals who have been affected by the criminal legal system often includes derogatory and dehumanizing language, including offender, ex-felon, criminal, and prisoner. Person-first and centered language is a way for healthcare professionals, and society as a whole, to begin to combat this stigma and offer patients a less discriminatory, human-centered experience in healthcare. Examples of less-stigmatizing terminology include person who has experienced incarceration, person who is incarcerated, or a person who has been imprisoned. Similarly, increasingly the term "criminal legal system" is used to replace the term "criminal justice system" as a way to acknowledge the often discriminatory, unjust impact this system has on minoritized communities and people of low socioeconomic status.

Opioid Use Disorder in Corrections

As a consequence of the War on Drugs, a majority of those who have experienced incarceration have a substance use disorder (SUD). In their most recent report on drug use and addiction, the Bureau of Justice Statistics found that 63% of people in jail and 58% of people in state prison met criteria for drug use disorder based on the *Diagnostic and Statistical Manual of Mental Disorders–IV* (DSM-IV, which has since been replaced by the DSM–5 and has reclassified drug abuse or dependence as substance use disorder) [9]. While statistics on the prevalence of opioid use disorder (OUD) specifically were not collected, the report did note that around one-fifth of incarcerated individuals reported regular use of heroin or other nonprescribed opioids in the month prior to incarceration. A meta-analysis on the prevalence of drug use in correctional facilities found significant heterogeneity among studies (between 10–60% of individuals met DSM–IV criteria for drug abuse/dependence) thought to be at least partially due to variable study design and diagnostic definitions [10]. Nonetheless, it has been shown that approximately one-quarter of individuals with OUD are arrested and/or incarcerated each year [11]. As a result, healthcare providers in the community who care for people with OUD are very likely to have patients who have experienced incarceration, and/or are currently under correctional custody.

Healthcare in Corrections

When Medicare and Medicaid were established in 1965 through the Social Security Act, it was prohibited for either agency to pay for healthcare in the country's prisons and jails, an exclusion that is commonly referred to as the "inmate exception" [12]. As a result, correctional institutions are each responsible for providing healthcare to the people who are incarcerated within their facility, which has resulted in a patchwork of systems that typically involves healthcare service provision through an outside contractor or through the department of corrections directly [13, 14]. Because each correctional facility approaches healthcare differently, the quantity and quality of services offered varies greatly. In addition to the high rate of substance use disorder, people who are incarcerated face a high burden of other medical and psychiatric comorbidities. The landmark Supreme Court ruling, *Estelle v Gamble* of 1976, established that to not provide community standard care for an incarcerated person's medical condition is cruel and unusual punishment and thus a violation of the Eighth Amendment [15]. However, numerous medical organizations have expressed concern that the vast majority of people who are incarcerated receive substandard care because correctional healthcare programs are under-resourced, are separated from mainstream medicine, and lack regulatory oversight and quality control mandates [16].

History of Opioid Use Disorder Treatment in Corrections

Most jails and prisons across the country do not provide people who are incarcerated with medication to treat OUD, including methadone, buprenorphine, or naltrexone. A survey of the state and federal prison systems in 2009 found that 28 systems (55%) offer methadone to inmates in some situations, largely for inmates with OUD who are pregnant. Seven state prison systems (14%) offer buprenorphine to some inmates [17]. Naltrexone was not surveyed in this study. In 2017, it was estimated that only 5% of individuals with OUD who are incarcerated receive pharmacotherapy for OUD, which is especially distressing given the evidence that MOUD, specifically opioid agonist therapy (OAT) with methadone or buprenorphine, has been shown to be the most effective treatment [18].

While it is unknown how many correctional facilities offer naltrexone, it is estimated that this medication is offered much more frequently than OAT. Alkermes, the pharmaceutical company that manufactures the extended-release intramuscular naltrexone product Vivitrol, has been marketed heavily to the criminal legal system, specifically to drug court judges. Vivitrol has been advertised as the "safest" way to treat OUD in correctional facilities because it is a pure opioid antagonist. Alkermes has been accused of subtly emphasizing stigma against OAT for its own product's benefit by describing Vivitrol as a "nonaddictive" substance, unable to "get someone high" and much less likely to be diverted [19]. Alkermes has also lobbied intensely in state legislatures to prioritize the incorporation of Vivitrol as OUD treatment in correctional facilities [20]. Extended-release naltrexone has been shown to reduce recurrence of opioid use compared to placebo or no medication; however, it is less effective than buprenorphine at improving retention in treatment and reducing recurrence of opioid use [21–23]. It is also not associated with a reduction in overdose, unlike methadone and buprenorphine which have been consistently shown to reduce both fatal and nonfatal overdose [18, 24]. This is a particularly important distinction given the marked increase in fatal overdose in the immediate period post-release from incarceration [25]. In December 2019, the Federal Drug Administration issued a public warning letter to Alkermes in response to a print advertisement for Vivitrol, stating that this advertisement failed to disclose the risks of this medication in regards to causing a fatal overdose at the end of a treatment period, if the medication were discontinued or if the opioid blockade effect were to be overcome with sufficient opioids [26].

Correctional staff have historically been reluctant to offer MOUD, specifically OAT, because of concerns around cost, diversion, and the mistaken belief that pharmacotherapy is not an appropriate or effective way to treat OUD for those who are incarcerated. The most common reason prison systems cited for not offering MOUD was because they "prefer drug-free detoxification over providing methadone or buprenorphine" [12]. Educational initiatives for correctional staff on addiction, as well as establishing linkages to community supports, have been shown to change these attitudes [27].

The treatment landscape, however, is changing. Over the past 10 years, more correctional facilities are offering MOUD as the result of increased public awareness and concern surrounding the opioid overdose crisis as well as recent court cases that established the imperative of offering this treatment. *Pesce v. Coppinger* was a lawsuit filed on behalf of Geoffrey Pesce, a man with OUD treated with methadone who had been in recovery for many years and was facing incarceration in Middletown House of Corrections, a jail in Essex County, Massachusetts, where his methadone would have been discontinued [28]. In November 2018, a federal court judge issued an injunction requiring the Massachusetts sheriff to provide Pesce with continued access to methadone during his incarceration. A few years later, a similar lawsuit, *DiPierro v Hurwitz*, was filed against the federal Bureau of Prisons by Stephanie DiPierro, a woman with OUD treated with methadone. She similarly won continued access to this medication, marking the first time a nonpregnant woman will be able to receive methadone while in custody of the federal Bureau of Prisons [29]. At the time of this writing, there are similar ongoing lawsuits in Kansas, Missouri, Maine, and Washington.

Aside from pharmacotherapy, psychosocial interventions and recovery supports such as 12-step mutual support groups, substance use education, therapeutic communities, and religious groups have also been employed in the correctional setting. One study estimated that the majority of state prisons offer drug and alcohol education (74%) and some form of substance use counseling (54%), and a minority (20%) offer therapeutic communities [30]. However, there is no evidence to support the efficacy of these programs. A recent Cochrane review found there was no evidence to support psychosocial interventions as providing any additional benefit to pharmacological maintenance treatment [31]. Furthermore, recurrence rates after counseling alone for treatment of OUD are high [32]. There is also little evidence that therapeutic communities are effective for the treatment of OUD, when compared to other outpatient programs or residential treatment programs. Two studies of therapeutic communities for individuals within prisons have shown reduced rates of recidivism when compared to no treatment or mental health counseling; efficacy with regards to OUD was not studied [33, 34].

Consequences of Lack of OUD Treatment in Corrections

Given the limited access to the most effective, evidence-based treatments in correctional facilities, patients with OUD are at high risk of opioid withdrawal when they are incarcerated. A survey of jails found that only 28% offered alcohol or opioid medically supervised withdrawal and estimated that over 1 million individuals go through untreated withdrawal in the jail system annually [35]. This likely underestimates the prevalence of untreated opioid withdrawal as medically supervised withdrawal for alcohol is more common. Even when medically supervised opioid withdrawal is offered, often opioids are not utilized, and when they are, the opioid agonist taper is typically rapid (a few days) and leaves individuals with ongoing untreated withdrawal symptoms [36].

Given this minimal access to care, it is not surprising that patients with OUD have negative experiences of withdrawal management when they are incarcerated

[37]. Untreated opioid withdrawal is extremely distressing and traumatic for patients, and in extreme cases can lead to death [38]. Suffering through untreated withdrawal as a result of being forcibly withdrawn from methadone or buprenorphine in facilities that still don't offer OAT is also a reason people subsequently don't engage in OAT after release [39, 40].

Some patients will use nonprescribed opioids surreptitiously while incarcerated as a means to manage their withdrawal or ongoing cravings, which puts them at risk of complications, most notably overdose and a wide variety of infections given they are using in isolation with fear of retribution, and without access to safe injection supplies. Approximately 30–60 individuals die in prison from a drug overdose each year, with rates increasing with the introduction of fentanyl into the opioid supply [41].

Given lack of access to opioid agonist therapy and less access to drugs like heroin, individuals with OUD use less or no opioids while they are incarcerated, which decreases their opioid tolerance. When released, these individuals are at markedly high risk of opioid overdose as they now have increased access to opioids with a tolerance that has declined. Individuals are over one hundred times more likely to die of drug overdose in the 2 weeks post-release, and 12 times more likely to die of any cause, than their counterparts in the community [42]. A meta-analysis of drug-related deaths after release from prison confirms these findings [43]. In addition to the significant impact on mortality, release from incarceration is associated with high morbidity. A study of over 40,000 patients released from corrections showed that 1 out of 12 people was hospitalized for an acute condition in the first 90 days post-release, a rate much higher than the general population of Medicare beneficiaries [44]. Many of these individuals were hospitalized secondary to mental health conditions and poisoning, which includes accidental and intentional poisoning and drug overdose.

Furthermore, studies have also shown that when opioid agonist therapy is tapered or discontinued during incarceration, individuals are less likely to re-engage in treatment once released and to delay getting care for their OUD as compared to those who are continued on their OAT [45]. In sum, there are adverse medical consequences to restricting access to MOUD in the correctional setting, including opioid withdrawal syndrome, death, risk of fatal overdose and hospitalization post-release, and decreased likelihood of future engagement in treatment. In addition to the increased medical challenges, relapse to opioid use after release from incarceration challenges all other components of successful reentry including housing, transportation nutrition, steady income, and daily structure.

Implementing Medication for OUD Treatment in Corrections

When MOUD is provided to individuals who are incarcerated, the mortality rate post-release plummets. A large, prospective observation study in England compared all cause and drug-related mortality in the month after release from prison between those given OAT in prison and those who were not. They found a significant reduction in all-cause mortality (HR 0.25) and drug-related mortality (HR 0.15).

Preliminary data from implementation of a comprehensive MOUD program initiated in 2016 in the Rhode Island Department of Corrections found a 60% reduction in overdose deaths in the 6 months post release (RR 0.4) [46]. The number needed to treat to prevent a death from overdose was eleven. The mortality benefits are not only seen after release; it has also been shown that provision of OAT in corrections reduces all-cause mortality in prison. One study demonstrated a 75% reduction in mortality among those on OAT in prison as compared to those who were not (adjusted HR 0.26) [47].

Additional benefits have been shown with the provision of MOUD in correctional facilities, notably that patients are more likely to engage in community treatment for their OUD after release and that they are more quickly connected to a prescriber post release [48]. Patients who receive MOUD in corrections are less likely to test positive for nonprescribed opioids [49, 50]. They are also less likely to acquire Hepatitis C and HIV.

Qualitative work has also been done among people with OUD in correctional facilities on their experience with MOUD provision. A study conducted in Rhode Island of 40 individuals who received MOUD found a range of benefits, including decreased prevalence of nonprescribed opioid use inside the facility, improved general environment, and increased post-release intentions to continue MOUD, along with the benefit of not having to go through withdrawal while incarcerated [51].

Overdose Prevention and Naloxone Distribution

Given the high risk of overdose after release from incarceration, overdose education and naloxone distribution (OEND) programs are increasingly being incorporated into jails and prisons prerelease. OEND programs distribute naloxone kits and provide education to individuals on how to identify and reverse overdose as a bystander. These programs typically also include education on Good Samaritan Laws, which protect individuals present at an overdose from prosecution for low-level drug-related offenses when they call for emergency help.

Studies among people who are in correctional custody or who have experienced incarceration show approximately one-third of individuals have experienced an overdose personally, and the majority (70–80%) have witnessed an overdose [52, 53]. These studies demonstrate that most of the time emergency services are not called because of fear of police involvement, particularly for individuals who are under community supervision (probation or parole). Importantly, the vast majority of individuals who have witnessed or experienced an overdose express interest and willingness to participate in OEND training.

OEND programs have been shown to increase knowledge of overdose prevention and management, and importantly have been shown to decrease overdose deaths post release [54, 55]. They have also been shown to increase the use of naloxone in the community, both for the individuals who are provided with the naloxone at release as well as for other individuals [56]. Interestingly, a study at Riker's Island jail in New York City provided OEND to the incarcerated people's visitors and documented that these naloxone kits were distributed to surrounding communities with high levels of opioid overdose [53].

Caring for Patients with OUD Who Have Experienced Incarceration

Clinicians that take care of patients with OUD who have experienced incarceration must be aware of the specific health, socioeconomic, and legal implications that incarceration has on their patients' general health and specifically on their OUD. In addition to the risks of treatment discontinuation, opioid withdrawal, and increased risk of overdose post release, there are other health consequences of incarceration, including trauma, social isolation, and poor control of other medical and psychiatric conditions.

For these reasons, it is important to create a trusting relationship over time and establish an environment where patients feel comfortable sharing their incarceration history with their healthcare providers. These conversations must be done with sensitivity, given the stigma associated with this experience. Ways to create space for people to feel safe sharing their incarceration history may include using trauma-informed approaches to care, using non-stigmatizing, non-threatening language, and incorporating general social determinants of health screening, which may include history-taking related to incarceration among other questions completed by the patient before the visit. For providers exploring this during a patient visit, prefacing a question about prior incarceration with a statement such as follows: "Many of my patients have experienced incarceration, which has impacted their health. Has this ever happened to you or a loved one?" is a phrasing which may help [57]. Of course, a patient may not feel comfortable disclosing this information; the most important thing is for the provider to build trust and to communicate that the clinical setting is a safe space for them to share their concerns and experiences. Lastly, it is important not to ask or document why a patient was incarcerated as this can expose patients to stigma and the harms of conscious and unconscious negative bias from their healthcare team and can impact future clinicians who access their medical record.

While progress is being made to increase access to MOUD within correctional facilities, the vast majority of people with OUD will not have access to first-line pharmacotherapy while incarcerated. Physicians in the community should not assume their patients were able to access medication while incarcerated and should ask their patients if and how their OUD was addressed.

As described above, the first few months post release represent an incredibly high-risk time in an individual's life. During a first post-release visit, in addition to obtaining a comprehensive history of substance use, physicians should ensure that patients have naloxone and know how to use it, initiate MOUD if able, and build trust and rapport. For patients who are currently injecting drugs discussion of safer injection practices, provision of sterile injection equipment, testing for HIV and HCV, confirmation that patients have been vaccinated against HAV and HBV, and discussion of pre-exposure prophylaxis treatment for HIV are important interventions. For female patients, discussion of contraception for women who do not wish to become pregnant is also important. Physicians should also try to elicit any barriers to obtaining ongoing medical care, such as difficulties with transportation or restrictions as a result of parole or probation conditions, and work to minimize these challenges to ensure continuity of care.

For patients who are engaged in treatment for their OUD in the community, the threat of incarceration can create clinical challenges. For those patients who are aware of an impending incarceration, the patient and clinician should discuss the risk of forced opioid withdrawal when incarcerated. If the patient is on opioid agonist therapy, there is a considerable chance their OAT will not be continued while incarcerated, depending upon what jurisdiction they are in. This creates a clinically dangerous situation for patients and it is difficult to find a way to counsel patients, as arguably the criminal legal system is forcing healthcare professionals to consider alternatives that are not in the best medical interest of the patient. Extended-release injectable buprenorphine is a clinical option for individuals who are justice-involved, given the prolonged half-life (4 weeks) and slow taper. Fortunately, the tide has started to shift, and more correctional facilities are offering MOUD. For physicians who care for individuals with OUD who have experienced incarceration, advocating that their state prison and district jails offer OUD is a crucial way to improve their patients' health.

Another important point of advocacy is the decriminalization of drug use. Decriminalization of drug use would encourage individuals with unhealthy substance use and SUD to get the treatment they need, and prevent much of the decompensation of and trauma associated with SUD that occurs as a result of incarceration [58]. Furthermore, resources spent on the war on drugs would be able to be redirected to evidenced-based public health interventions to prevent and treat SUD in the community. Portugal, a country that decriminalized drug use 20 years ago, has seen incredible benefits across the societal spectrum, including decreased rates of drug use, HIV infection, and drug-related overdose [59].

Innovating Around Care for OUD in Correctional Settings

There is increasing recognition of the importance of providing MOUD and other treatment services for people with OUD in the correctional setting. A comprehensive planning and implementation guideline recently published by the National Council for Behavioral Health and Vital Strategies emphasizes that for correctional facilities seeking to implement provision of MOUD, it is strongly recommend to garner the support of both medical and security staff [60]. As described earlier, correctional staff may harbor misconceptions and stigma about the treatment of OUD, which may be a barrier to implementation of evidence-based treatment. The RI Department of Corrections (DOC), the first statewide DOC in the United States to offer all three FDA-approved medications for OUD, offers educational materials for this purpose. Correctional staff may also express concerns about medication diversion; however, anecdotal data from facilities where MOUD is implemented have shown that nonprescribed use of buprenorphine and methadone decreases when it is prescribed to patients with a clinical indication [51]. Regardless, the RI DOC, for example, has been able to decrease the risk of diversion by separating medication lines for MOUD, choosing formulations that are difficult to divert (including using a crushed buprenorphine tablet as opposed to the film) and having patients talk in front of a correctional officer after taking their medication.

There are multiple ways that MOUD can be offered within a correctional facility. While naltrexone can be prescribed and administered by any licensed physician, physician assistant, or nurse practitioner, buprenorphine currently can only be prescribed by a healthcare professional who has obtained a Drug Enforcement Agency (DEA) X-waiver. Methadone can only be dispensed in a federally accredited and certified opioid treatment program (OTP). These medications can be delivered offsite by an external provider, onsite by an external provider, or onsite by the correctional facility, where the correctional facility completes the accreditation to become an OTP. Regardless of the way MOUD is administered, it would be ideal to offer all three medications (methadone, buprenorphine, and naltrexone), just as they should be available in the community. Patients must be able to continue the medication they were on prior to incarceration and also be able to initiate the medication that best fits their individual medical needs, and not be limited by restrictions placed by the correctional facility. However, it is incumbent upon the system that starts a patient on any of these medications to ensure that it is possible to continue the medication after release. To not do so risks creating, perhaps, an even greater risk of post-release overdose. Universal screening for chronic opioid use and OUD should be performed upon arrival to the correctional facility, in order to quickly identify patients who are at risk for opioid withdrawal and/or those who would benefit from MOUD. Treatment for OUD should be offered without administrative or medical barriers, including lengthy pretreatment assessments. Treatment should not be discontinued for any reason besides evidence that it is causing clinical harm to the patient; contingencies based on behavior must not play a role. Furthermore, while psychosocial and behavioral counseling should be offered to patients with OUD, they should not be mandatory for treatment [61].

Additional challenges in the treatment of OUD in corrections include difficulty with accessing patients' medical records from the community, as correctional healthcare systems are typically separate from community healthcare systems and use their own electronic medical record system. This makes it difficult to determine if patients have been previously diagnosed with OUD and if they are on treatment. Furthermore, correctional healthcare providers have described an issue termed "dual loyalty," whereby they are placed in situations in which they are asked, explicitly or implicitly, to consider the interests of the correctional system and staff in their professional duties [62, 63]. An example is being asked to disclose a patient's clinical information for security purposes. Lastly, in jails, it is often unknown when patients will be released, creating difficulty with transitions in medical care. For OUD treatment specifically, the RI DOC has worked to minimize barriers in transition by partnering with an external vendor to provide MOUD on site; at release, patients can continue to get their OUD at this vendor's community sites. Transitions clinics or partnerships with community care providers offer another option for linkage to treatment after release.

Conclusions

Many individuals with opioid use disorder in the United States will experience incarceration as a result of the laws that criminalize substance use. Minoritized populations are disproportionately harmed by incarceration because of inherent racism in US drug policy. Despite the high prevalence of OUD within correctional facilities, access to evidence-based treatment, specifically opioid agonist therapy, remains minimal resulting in serious short- and long-term health consequences for this population, most alarmingly the high risk of fatal overdose in the immediate post-release period. Healthcare providers who care for patients with OUD in the community need to be attuned to the impact of incarceration on a patients' OUD treatment, be able to continue or rapidly initiate MOUD following release, and to advocate for improved care behind bars, linkage to appropriate care post release, as well as the decriminalization of drug use.

References

1. Zeng Z. Jail inmates in 2017. Bureau of Justice Statistics (BJS); 2019 [cited 2020Mar2]. Available from: https://www.bjs.gov/index.cfm?ty=pbdetail&iid=65471.
2. Bronson J, Carson A. Prisoners in 2017. Bureau of Justice Statistics; 2019 [cited 2020Mar2]. Available from: http://www.bjs.gov/index.cfm?ty=pbdetail&iid=6546.
3. Sawyer W, Wagner P. Mass incarceration: the whole pie 2019. Prison Policy Initiative; 2019 [cited 2020Mar2]. Available from: https://www.prisonpolicy.org/reports/pie2019.html.
4. Report to the United Nations on Racial Disparities in the U.S. Criminal Justice System. The sentencing project; 2018 [cited 2020Mar2]. Available from: https://www.sentencingproject.org/publications/un-report-on-racial-disparities/.
5. Carson EA. Prisoners in 2016 [Internet]. Bureau of Justice Statistics; 2018 [cited 2020Mar2]. Available from: http://www.bjs.gov/index.cfm?ty=pbdetail&iid=6187/.
6. Fellner J. Race, drugs, and law enforcement in the United States [Internet]. Human Rights Watch; 2010 [cited 2020Mar2]. Available from: https://www.hrw.org/news/2009/06/19/race-drugs-and-law-enforcement-united-states#.
7. Rosino ML, Hughey MW. The war on drugs, racial meanings, and structural racism: a holistic and reproductive approach. Am J Econ Sociol. 2018;77(3–4):849–92.
8. Tran NT, Baggio S, Dawson A, O'Moore É, Williams B, Bedell P, et al. Words matter: a call for humanizing and respectful language to describe people who experience incarceration. BMC Int Health Human Rights. 2018;18(1):1–6.
9. Bronson J, Stroop J, Zimmer S, Berzofsky M. Drug use, dependence, and abuse among state prisoners and jail inmates, 2007–2009 [Internet]. Bureau of Justice Statistics; 2017 [cited 2020Mar2]. Available from: http://www.bjs.gov/index.cfm?ty=pbdetail&iid=5966.
10. Fazel S, Bains P, Doll H. Substance abuse and dependence in prisoners: a systematic review. Addiction. 2006;101(2):181–91.
11. Boutwell AE, Nijhawan A, Zaller N, Rich JD. Arrested on heroin: A national opportunity. J Opioid Manag. 2007;3(6):328–32.

12. Health coverage options for incarcerated people. HealthCare.gov; [cited 2020Mar2]. Available from: https://www.healthcare.gov/incarcerated-people/.

13. Jails: Inadvertent Health Care Providers. How county correctional facilities are playing a role in the safety net [Internet]. The Pew Charitable Trusts; 2018 [cited 2020Mar2]. Available from: https://www.pewtrusts.org/-/media/assets/2018/01/sfh_jails_inadvertent_health_care_providers.pdf.

14. State prisons and the delivery of hospital care [Internet]. The Pew Charitable Trusts; 2018 [cited 2020Mar2]. Available from: https://www.pewtrusts.org/en/research-and-analysis/reports/2018/07/19/state-prisons-and-the-delivery-of-hospital-care.

15. https://www.law.cornell.edu/supremecourt/text/429/97.

16. Fiscella K, Beletsky L, Wakeman SE. The inmate exception and reform of correctional health care. Am J Public Health. 2017;107(3):384–5.

17. Nunn A, Zaller N, Dickman S, Trimbur C, Nijhawan A, Rich JD. Methadone and buprenorphine prescribing and referral practices in US prison systems: results from a Nationwide Survey. Drug Alcohol Depend. 2009;105(1–2):83–8.

18. Wakeman SE, Larochelle MR, Ameli O, Chaisson CE, Mcpheeters JT, Crown WH, et al. Comparative effectiveness of different treatment pathways for opioid use disorder. JAMA Netw Open. 2020;3(2):e1920622. Published 2020 Feb 5.

19. Harper J. To grow market share, a drugmaker pitches its product to judges [Internet]. NPR; 2017 [cited 2020Mar2]. Available from: https://www.npr.org/sections/health-shots/2017/08/03/540029500/to-grow-market-share-a-drugmaker-pitches-its-product-to-judges.

20. Harper J. A drugmaker tries to cash in on the opioid epidemic, one state law at a time [Internet]. NPR; 2017 [cited 2020Mar2]. Available from: https://www.npr.org/sections/health-shots/2017/06/12/523774660/a-drugmaker-tries-to-cash-in-on-the-opioid-epidemic-one-state-law-at-a-time.

21. Krupitsky E, Zvartau E, Blokhina E, et al. Randomized trial of long-acting sustained-release naltrexone implant vs oral naltrexone or placebo for preventing relapse to opioid dependence. Arch Gen Psychiatry. 2012;69(9):973–81.

22. Lee JD, Friedmann PD, Kinlock TW, et al. Extended-release naltrexone to prevent opioid relapse in criminal justice offenders. N Engl J Med. 2016;374(13):1232–42.

23. Lee JD, Nunes EV Jr, Novo P, et al. Comparative effectiveness of extended-release naltrexone versus buprenorphine-naloxone for opioid relapse prevention (X:BOT): a multicentre, open-label, randomised controlled trial. Lancet. 2018;391(10118):309–18.

24. Larochelle MR, Bernson D, Land T, et al. Medication for opioid use disorder after non-fatal opioid overdose and association with mortality: a cohort study. Ann Intern Med. 2018;169(3):137–45.

25. Binswanger IA, Blatchford PJ, Mueller SR, Stern MF. Mortality after prison release: opioid overdose and other causes of death, risk factors, and time trends from 1999 to 2009. Ann Intern Med. 2013;159(9):592–600.

26. Center for Drug Evaluation and Research. Alkermes, Inc. Warning Letter [Internet]. U.S. Food and Drug Administration; [cited 2020Mar2]. Available from: https://www.fda.gov/inspections-compliance-enforcement-and-criminal-investigations/warning-letters/alkermes-inc-597260-12022019.

27. Friedmann PD, Wilson D, Knudsen HK, Ducharme LJ, Welsh WN, Frisman L, et al. Effect of an organizational linkage intervention on staff perceptions of medication-assisted treatment and referral intentions in community corrections. J Subst Abuse Treat. 2015;50:50–8.

28. Pesce V. Coppinger [Internet]. ACLU Massachusetts; 2019 [cited 2020Mar2]. Available from: https://www.aclum.org/en/cases/pesce-v-coppinger.

29. DiPierro V. Hurwitz [Internet]. ACLU Massachusetts; 2019 [cited 2020Mar2]. Available from: https://www.aclum.org/en/cases/dipierro-v-hurwitz.

30. Taxman FS, Perdoni ML, Harrison LD. Drug treatment services for adult offenders: the state of the state. J Subst Abuse Treat. 2007;32(3):239–54.

31. Amato L, Minozzi S, Davoli M, Vecchi S, Ferri M, Mayet S. Psychosocial combined with agonist maintenance treatments versus agonist maintenance treatments alone for treatment of opioid dependence. Cochrane Database Syst Rev. 2004;(4):CD004147.
32. Mattick RP, Breen C, Kimber J, Davoli M, Breen R. Methadone maintenance therapy versus no opioid replacement therapy for opioid dependence. Cochrane Database Syst Rev. 2003;(4):CD002209.
33. Sacks S, Sacks JY, Mckendrick K, Banks S, Stommel J. Modified TC for MICA offenders: crime outcomes. Behav Sci Law. 2004;22(4):477–501.
34. Wexler HK, Melnick G, Lowe L, Peters J. Three-year reincarceration outcomes for amity in-prison therapeutic community and aftercare in California. Prison J. 1999;79(3):321–36.
35. Fiscella K, Pless N, Meldrum S, Fiscella P. Alcohol and opiate withdrawal in US jails. Am J Public Health. 2004;94(9):1522–4.
36. Jeanmonod R, Harding T, Staub C. Treatment of opiate withdrawal on entry to prison. Addiction. 1991;86(4):457–63.
37. Mitchell SG, Kelly SM, Brown BS, Reisinger HS, Peterson JA, Ruhf A, et al. Incarceration and opioid withdrawal: the experiences of methadone patients and out-of-treatment heroin users. J Psychoactive Drugs. 2009;41(2):145–52.
38. Darke S, Larney S, Farrell M. Yes, people can die from opiate withdrawal. Addiction. 2016;112(2):199–200.
39. Maradiaga JA, Nahvi S, Cunningham CO, Sanchez J, Fox AD. "I kicked the hard way. I got incarcerated". Withdrawal from methadone during incarceration and subsequent aversion to medication assisted treatments. J Subst Abuse Treat. 2016;62:49–54.
40. Fu JJ, Zaller ND, Yokell MA, Bazazi AR, Rich JD. Forced withdrawal from methadone maintenance therapy in criminal justice settings: a critical treatment barrier in the United States. J Subst Abus Treat. 2013;44(5):502–5.
41. Mortality in State Prisons, 2001–2014 – Statistical Tables [Internet]. Bureau of Justice Statistics; 2016 [cited 2020Mar2]. Available from: http://www.bjs.gov/index.cfm?ty=pbdetail&iid=5866.
42. Binswanger IA, Stern MF, Deyo RA, Heagerty PJ, Cheadle A, Elmore JG, et al. Release from prison — a high risk of death for former inmates. N Engl J Med. 2007;356(2):157–65.
43. Merrall ELC, Kariminia A, Binswanger IA, Hobbs MS, Farrell M, Marsden J, et al. Meta-analysis of drug-related deaths soon after release from prison. Addiction. 2010;105(9):1545–54.
44. Wang EA, Wang Y, Krumholz HM. A high risk of hospitalization following release from correctional facilities in Medicare beneficiaries. JAMA Intern Med. 2013;173(17):1621.
45. Rich JD, Mckenzie M, Larney S, Wong JB, Tran L, Clarke J, et al. Methadone continuation versus forced withdrawal on incarceration in a combined US prison and jail: a randomised, open-label trial. Lancet. 2015;386(9991):350–9.
46. Green TC, Clarke J, Brinkley-Rubinstein L, Marshall BDL, Alexander-Scott N, Boss R, et al. Postincarceration Fatal Overdoses After Implementing Medications for Addiction Treatment in a Statewide Correctional System. JAMA Psychiatry. 2018;75(4):405–7.
47. Larney S, Gisev N, Farrell M, Dobbins T, Burns L, Gibson A, et al. Opioid substitution therapy as a strategy to reduce deaths in prison: retrospective cohort study. Drug Alcohol Depend. 2014;146.
48. Zaller N, Mckenzie M, Friedmann PD, Green TC, Mcgowan S, Rich JD. Initiation of buprenorphine during incarceration and retention in treatment upon release. J Subst Abuse Treat. 2013;45(2):222–6.
49. Gordon MS, Kinlock TW, Schwartz RP, O'Grady KE. A randomized clinical trial of methadone maintenance for prisoners: findings at 6 months post-release. Addiction. 2007;103(8):1333–42.
50. Mckenzie M, Zaller N, Dickman SL, Green TC, Parikh A, Friedmann PD, et al. A randomized trial of methadone initiation prior to release from incarceration. Subst Abus. 2012;33(1):19–29.
51. Brinkley-Rubinstein L, Peterson M, Clarke J, Macmadu A, Truong A, Pognon K, et al. The benefits and implementation challenges of the first state-wide comprehensive medication for addictions program in a unified jail and prison setting. Drug Alcohol Depend. 2019;205:107514.

52. Curtis M, Dietze P, Aitken C, Kirwan A, Kinner SA, Butler T, and Stoove M. Acceptability of prison-based take-home naloxone programmes among a cohort of incarcerated men with a history of regular injecting drug use. Harm Reduct J. 2018;15(48):1–9.
53. Wagner KD, Harding RW, Kelley R, Labus B, Verdugo SR, Davidson PJ et al. Post-overdose interventions triggered by calling 911: centering the perspectives of people who use drugs (PWUDs). PLoS One. 2019;14(10):e0223823.
54. Horton M, Mcdonald R, Green TC, Nielsen S, Strang J, Degenhardt L, et al. A mapping review of take-home naloxone for people released from correctional settings. Int J Drug Policy. 2017;46:7–16.
55. Bird SM, Mcauley A, Perry S, Hunter C. Effectiveness of Scotland's National Naloxone Programme for reducing opioid-related deaths: a before (2006–10) versus after (2011–13) comparison. Addiction. 2016;111(5):883–91.
56. Wenger LD, Showalter D, Lambdin B, Leiva D, Wheeler E, Davidson PJ, et al. Overdose education and naloxone distribution in the San Francisco county jail. J Correct Health Care. 2019;25(4):394–404.
57. Sue K. How to talk with patients about incarceration and health. AMA J Ethics. 2017;19(9):885–93.
58. https://drugpolicy.org/resource/its-time-us-decriminalize-drug-use-and-possession#why-is-decriminalization-the-solution.
59. Hughes CE, Stevens A. The effects of the decriminalization of drug use in Portugal. Discussion paper. Oxford: The Beckley Foundation; 2007.
60. https://www.thenationalcouncil.org/wp-content/uploads/2020/01/MAT_in_Jails_Prisons_Toolkit_Final_2020-01-30.pdf.
61. http://nationalacademies.org/hmd/reports/2019/medications-for-opioid-use-disorder-save-lives.
62. Pont J, Stover H, Wolff H. Dual loyalty in prison health care. Am J Public Health. 2012;102(3):475–80.
63. Allen SA, Wakeman SE, Cohen RL, Rich JD. Physicians in US prisons in the era of mass incarceration. Int J Prison Health. 2010;6(3):100–6.

Use of the ECHO Model to Support Treatment of Opioid Use Disorder

7

Miriam Komaromy, Judy Bartlett, and Prabhat Chand

Overview

The Extension for Community Healthcare Outcomes (ECHO) model offers a way for primary care providers (PCPs) to develop expertise in addressing opioid use disorder (OUD) and other substance use disorders (SUDs). ECHO uses videoconferencing to connect multiple primary care teams simultaneously with addiction treatment specialists and builds treatment capacity via mentorship and case-based learning (Fig. 7.1).

This type of applied learning helps to transition medical providers from having only knowledge to having confidence in their skills, an ability to navigate challenges that arise during treatment, and a willingness to treat patients with OUD. ECHO is designed to expand access to care by developing capacity to treat common complex conditions, such as OUD, in underserved areas. Fueled by extensive funding opportunities from the federal government, ECHO has now been widely implemented in the US to train primary care providers to treat OUD, especially in rural and traditionally underserved settings. In addition, the model has been tailored to other settings (e.g., inpatient addiction consult services), to different types of providers (e.g., recovery coaches/community health workers and

M. Komaromy (✉)
Grayken Center for Addiction, General Internal Medicine, Boston Medical Center, Boston University, Boston, MA, USA
e-mail: Miriam.Komaromy@bmc.org

J. Bartlett
Bartlett Evaluation, Albuquerque, NM, USA
e-mail: judy@bartlettevaluation.com

P. Chand
Centre for Addiction Medicine, Department of Psychiatry, National Institute of Mental Health and Neurosciences (NIMHANS), Bangalore, India
e-mail: chand@nimhans.ac.in

© Springer Nature Switzerland AG 2021
S. E. Wakeman, J. D. Rich (eds.), *Treating Opioid Use Disorder in General Medical Settings*, https://doi.org/10.1007/978-3-030-80818-1_7

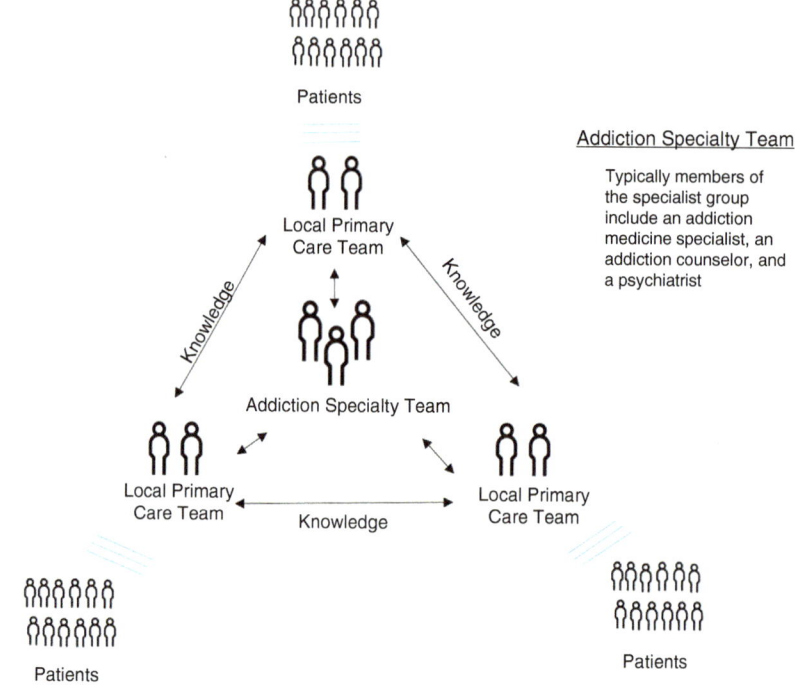

Patients

Addiction Specialty Team

Typically members of
the specialist group
include an addiction
medicine specialist, an
addiction counselor, and
a psychiatrist

Local Primary
Care Team

Knowledge

Knowledge

Addiction Specialty Team

Local Primary
Care Team

Local Primary
Care Team

Knowledge

Patients

Patients

Fig. 7.1 The ECHO Model for addressing OUD

behavioral health providers), and to successful treatment models (e.g., Massachusetts Nurse Care Manager Model, Vermont Hub-and-Spoke model) [1, 2]. ECHO has also been applied to treatment of SUDs in many other countries, including Canada, India, Vietnam, and Australia [3, 4].

What Is the ECHO Model?

The ECHO model is an approach to medical education that is designed to leverage the specialized knowledge of medical experts (typically from academic medical settings) to train PCPs (who typically offer care for common complex diseases in their own communities). Traditional continuing medical education is based on lectures and can convey facts but is not suitable for helping PCPs to develop new skills or become confident and competent in the application of new knowledge. ECHO programs, in contrast, offer ongoing sessions that bring together medical experts and PCPs, who learn by presenting de-identified patient cases to the experts and to colleagues and receiving feedback and guidance on medical management. When PCPs participate in weekly ECHO sessions over a period of months, they develop their knowledge and understanding of disease management and receive ongoing feedback about their patients' care. The medical specialists who lead the sessions are often faculty at academic medical centers, while learners are typically clinicians practicing in community health centers, together with other members of the care team, such as nurses, community health workers, or behavioral health providers.

The ECHO model differs from telemedicine. In telemedicine, a specialist is connected via video with a single patient who is geographically distant from them. In ECHO sessions, the specialist is connected with PCPs (or other learners), rather than with a patient, and provides mentorship and suggestions for patient care rather than providing care directly. In this way, ECHO leverages the scarce and costly resource of a specialist's time and knowledge to train a large number of PCPs, who are then able to provide specialized care to a very large number of patients. In contract, telemedicine allows a specialist to provide care for one remote patient at a time and does not increase overall capacity.

This model, which was developed in New Mexico in 2003, was pioneered by Dr. Sanjeev Arora with the goal of expanding access to treatment for hepatitis C in a large, rural state in an era when the disease was prevalent, treatment was toxic, and access to specialty care was very limited. The model has since spread nationally and internationally and has been applied to training different types of healthcare workers to address a wide variety of diseases. To date, approximately 650 ECHO programs have been implemented in more than 37 countries [5]. One resource for locating ECHO programs is the website of the ECHO Institute, echo.unm.edu.

An ECHO program brings together faculty and learners who wish to focus on a particular disease or group of conditions. Examples include HIV, autism, rheumatology, or women's health. An ECHO program may consist of ongoing ECHO sessions or may be limited to a fixed number of sessions, such as 10 or 12. A typical ECHO session (Table 7.1) lasts 1–2 hours and recurs 1–4 times per month. Sessions are conducted over a secure video platform and typically include 15–30 participants. Fewer participants make it difficult to maintain a rich discussion, while a larger group encourages passive participation and decreases opportunities for participants to present cases.

Sessions usually begin with one of the specialists giving a brief lecture with slides on a topic related to OUD care. This is followed by a primary care provider or team presenting the case of a patient from their practice in de-identified fashion. A facilitator from the specialist team leads a discussion of the case, following a standardized flow that is designed to engage the participants (Table 7.2). Without

Table 7.1 Defining features of ECHO programs

Focus on a common complex disease (e.g., hepatitis C) or group of diseases (e.g., rheumatologic disorders)

Connect a few specialists (often from academic medical centers) with multiple frontline general care providers or teams (often primary care medical providers who are practicing in rural or traditionally-underserved areas)

Utilize a secure, multipoint videoconferencing platform

Focus on case-based learning, with participants presenting actual, de-identified cases from their own practice and receiving feedback/coaching on care management

Offer a brief talk by a specialist on some aspect of care for the disease of interest

Include only healthcare providers/team members; patients do not participate in ECHO sessions

Table 7.2 Standardized flow of a case-based discussion during an ECHO session

1. Participating team or provider presents a de-identified case of one of their current patients, highlighting specific questions.
2. Facilitator summarizes the case and asks the presenter for any corrections or additions.
3. Other participants are invited to ask clarifying questions.
4. Specialist team is invited to ask clarifying questions.
5. Other participants are invited to offer care management recommendations.
6. Specialist team is invited to offer recommendations.
7. Facilitator leads further discussion.
8. Facilitator summarizes key recommendations.
9. After the session, facilitator emails the presenter a brief written summary of recommendations.

this type of formal structure, the specialists tend to dominate the conversation and participants are less likely to offer questions or treatment suggestions [6]. At the end of the discussion, the facilitator summarizes the recommendations for care, which are also emailed to the presenting team.

ECHO programs often find it difficult to attract physician participants, and other primary care team members frequently constitute the majority of program participants, including nurse practitioners, physician assistants, counselors, nurses, medical assistants, and community health workers. Training and supporting these participants is an excellent goal for an ECHO program. If programs wish to attract physicians, they may need to address barriers to physician participation. These include systemic pressures to protect productivity and thus avoid activities that decrease the number of patient visits. Options include providing financial incentives to the physician or clinical organization, offering the ECHO program outside of typical weekday clinic hours, and offering free continuing professional education credits.

History of ECHO for SUDs and OUD

In 2005, shortly after the first ECHO program was launched with a focus on hepatitis C, a second ECHO program was initiated with a focus on coaching PCPs on the treatment of addiction and mental health disorders. This program, called Integrated Addictions and Psychiatry [7], operated continuously in New Mexico for 13 years. Starting in 2006, other academic medical centers began to implement their own ECHO programs while the University of New Mexico continued to add ECHO programs focused on a wide variety of diseases. However, few other institutions [8] attempted to launch programs focused on substance use disorders until the opioid overdose epidemic began to be a national concern. More recently numerous federal agencies included implementation of an Opioid ECHO program as an option in their requests for proposals (RFPs), including Substance Abuse and Mental Health Services Administration (SAMHSA), National Institute on Drug Abuse (NIDA), and Health Resources and Services Administration (HRSA), catalyzing broad adoption of the model [1, 9, 10].

Why Is ECHO Needed for OUD?

For the past 20 years, physicians have been required by federal law to take an 8-hour training course to prescribe medication (buprenorphine/naloxone) for office-based treatment of OUD. More recent legislation requires nonphysician healthcare providers to take an even longer 24-hour training course. More recently, new practice guidelines allow providers who submit a notice of intent to treat up to 30 patients at a time to obtain an x-waiver without completing the previously required training, however providers who want to be able to treat more than 30 patients must still complete the 8-24 hour training. On the surface, these federal requirements seem intended to prepare healthcare providers to treat OUD, making an opioid-focused ECHO program unnecessary. In fact, it is unknown whether these required trainings actually increase knowledge or improve clinical care and many clinicians who participate in the 8- to 24-hour training do not go on to actually prescribe medication for OUD (MOUD). Those who do prescribe typically treat far fewer patients than federal law allows.

Studies have shown that many factors are involved in clinicians' hesitance to treat with MOUD, including lack of confidence, lack of behavioral health support, and resistance to prioritizing this patient population over other patients [11, 12]. Indeed, starting to treat patients who have OUD can be quite challenging; many have co-occurring mental or physical health diagnoses and other substance use disorders. Patients who have OUD may be hesitant to seek care and may anticipate being treated poorly by the medical system. Medical providers may also correctly perceive that the way they have been accustomed to interacting with patients who have SUDs is not likely to result in a favorable outcome. Stigma toward substance use disorders affects patients and also the providers who choose to care for them [13].

For these reasons, it can be helpful for clinicians to engage in ongoing learning about how to work with patients who have SUDs. The technical knowledge about how to prescribe the medications is only a small part of what is needed. Instead, ECHO programs tend to focus on techniques for effective communication, such as motivational interviewing; on how to respond to evidence of recurrence of use without triggering the patient to drop out of lifesaving care; and on how to overcome stigma toward people who use drugs, which is still highly prevalent in the medical system.

During an ECHO session, when medical providers present patients who have OUD, they can describe their tentative plan for treatment and receive feedback. The specialist team often includes counselors or social workers who are experts in addiction treatment and can provide invaluable suggestions about how to communicate with patients and promote their engagement with care. Medical experts from the specialist team can offer advice about managing medication side effects or treating co-occurring medical problems. And, finally, fellow participants—other primary care teams—can offer support and practical suggestions. By presenting patients iteratively over several months, PCPs build their knowledge and skills and begin asking more complex and nuanced questions.

What Is the Impact of ECHO Programs and of Opioid ECHO Programs in Particular?

Participation in ECHO programs increases medical providers' knowledge and satisfaction with treating a wide variety of illnesses [14, 15]. When PCPs participated in a hepatitis C ECHO program, their treatment outcomes were indistinguishable from outcomes achieved by academic liver specialists [16]. Nursing homes supported by a geriatric teleECHO program reduced the use of physical and chemical restraints [17].

ECHO programs focused on pain have produced changes in provider behavior (such as increased referral to physical medicine, increased prescribing of non-opioid pain medications, and decreased opioid prescribing) [8, 18–20].

The perceived value of ECHO programs for supporting treatment of OUD is evidenced by the fact that universities in most US states have implemented ECHO programs focused on training medical providers to treat OUD and other SUDs, including programs offered by 69 academic medical institutions [21].

Participants in ECHO programs focused on SUDs and OUD report that the advice they receive when they present patient cases leads to changes in their treatment plans and that they apply knowledge learned during others' case presentations to the care of patients in their own practices [6]. In Pennsylvania, Opioid ECHO was associated with improvements in provider knowledge and ability to treat OUD [9]. When ECHO was included as a component of California's implementation of the Hub-and-Spoke model, evaluators found marked increases in the number of providers prescribing buprenorphine and the number of patients receiving treatment [1]. A preliminary evaluation of the New York Health and Hospitals' buprenorphine ECHO program found that providers' self-efficacy increased but few providers started prescribing after ECHO participation [10]. A study of the first decade of the addiction-focused ECHO program in New Mexico found that the number of buprenorphine-waivered providers working in traditionally underserved areas increased much faster in New Mexico compared with the rest of the nation [7]. A recent systematic review concluded that Opioid ECHO improves physician preparedness to treat opioid use disorder [22].

However, studies also identified barriers to ECHO participation, including the amount of time required and the related loss of clinical productivity and revenue [23, 24]. Future adaptations of the ECHO model may need to focus on providing more flexible options for participation, such as supplementing ECHO participation with an option for one-to-one learning. An ongoing study in New Mexico, funded by Agency for Healthcare Research and Quality (AHRQ), engages providers in an Opioid ECHO program focused on MOUD, and then offers additional facilitation to participating clinics if they are not making progress in establishing or expanding MOUD treatment programs based on ECHO participation alone. The study is also evaluating the impact of a financial incentive for participants (Julie Griffin Salvador, personal communication, 2/21/2020).

In summary, ECHO has been broadly implemented in the US as a way to address the opioid use disorder and overdose epidemic, and published data demonstrate that engaging in an opioid-focused ECHO program is associated with improvements in opioid prescribing practices among participants. ECHO participation is also associated with increases in providers' knowledge and confidence regarding their ability to treat OUD, in the number of buprenorphine-waivered providers (particularly in traditionally-underserved areas), and in the number of patients treated. However, to date, evidence of the impact of opioid ECHO programs is relatively weak and includes no results from randomized controlled trials [25, 26].

Expansion Beyond a Focus on Outpatient Treatment of OUD and Academic Expertise

In the last few years, the ECHO model has been applied to SUD treatment in a number of innovative ways. This includes the use of ECHO to support the provision of inpatient addiction consultation (see Box 7.1). ECHO is also being expanded beyond the traditional approach of drawing experts from academic medical settings, and in some cases community health center networks have used specialists from their own networks rather than from universities (see Box 7.2). Several ECHO programs also target learners who are not medical providers, but rather community health workers, nurses, or addiction counselors (see Box 7.3). In addition, ECHO programs focused on SUDs have been launched in several other countries outside of the US (including Canada, India, Australia, and Vietnam) [3, 4] (See Box 7.4).

Box 7.1 Expanding the Scope of ECHO to the Hospital Setting
Interview with Honora Englander, MD, Associate Professor of Medicine, Division of Hospital Medicine, Department of Medicine, Oregon Health & Science University

Since Oregon Health Sciences University (OHSU) launched its hospital-based IMPACT program in 2015, Dr. Honora Englander has been inundated with requests from hospital staff and administrators, "How can we improve addiction care at our hospital?" In addition to publishing tools to support hospital-based addiction care, Dr. Englander viewed launching an ECHO as a natural way to support dissemination: There was an obvious need from both the clinician and patient perspectives and OHSU had a mature ECHO infrastructure.

> The faculty [of the *SUD in Hospital Care ECHO*] are providing a master class in how to talk about addiction.—ECHO participant

The ECHO faculty includes two doctors, a social worker, a peer, a pharmacist, and a nurse; the participants were even more diverse, adding hospital administrators, NPs, PAs, and community-based providers who collaborated with hospitals. In January 2020, the Hospital ECHO started its fourth 12-week cohort. When they launched in early 2019, they focused narrowly on OUD care but have evolved based on feedback from participants, who asked for more information about care for methamphetamine and alcohol use and more support around how to interact with patients. The ECHO incorporates role plays and many of the case-based discussions focus on what harm reduction and trauma-informed care should like in the hospital setting.

> Simply acknowledging the distress both between patients and providers as well as within providers themselves really resonated with the ECHO participants.—Dr. Englander

As Dr. Englander explained, a hospital-based harm reduction conversation is very different from a clinic-based conversation. In hospitals, where the default expectation is that the provider rather than the patient holds most of the decision-making power, the clash between medical models and harm reduction is intensified and unique struggles emerge. For example, how does a hospital team best manage a patient with a life-threatening infection who continues to inject substances?

The goals of OHSU's Hospital ECHO do not include replicating the IMPACT model (described more in Chap. 4), which is a fully staffed, inter-professional addiction consult service. "I don't think that is realistic for all hospitals," said Dr. Englander. Instead, OHSU has designed this ECHO with a broader goal in mind: changing the standard of care in hospitals across the country based on four key elements: (1) adopting a framework that SUDs are treatable, chronic diseases; (2) initiating and bridging patients to MOUD; (3) implementing harm reduction practices, including naloxone distribution; and (4) providing pathways to support care after hospitalization.

The next steps for the OHSU team include continuing to support the champions emerging from prior ECHO cohorts (e.g., via shadowing opportunities at OHSU), tailoring an ECHO to hospital-based peers, and expanding the current ECHO beyond Oregon.

Box 7.2 An OUD ECHO Led by a Federally Qualified Health Center
Interview with Abby Letcher, MD, Neighborhood Health Centers of the Lehigh Valley

A relatively new, federally qualified health center (FQHC) in Pennsylvania is paving a remarkable pathway to better serve people with OUD in their community: a pathway that other FQHCs can adopt. ECHO is one of several tools that Neighborhood Health Centers of Lehigh Valley (NHCLV) uses.

In 2016, NHCLV didn't provide OUD treatment and, according to Dr. Abby Letcher, they knew *nothing* about it. Within 3 years, NHCLV has become a high-volume OUD practice. They began in 2017 with funding to expand medication for OUD (MOUD) and an invitation to participate in an Opioid ECHO run out of the University of New Mexico. Dr. Letcher attended the weekly ECHO sessions for 6 months, which she described as "transformative," and took away three lessons: First, harm reduction isn't crazy; it's good medicine. Primary care settings can actively decrease stigma and become welcoming oases. Finally, MOUD is not hard.

But culture and practice change *is* hard. And Dr. Letcher saw ECHO as a critical tool for catalyzing a community-wide transformation. By early 2019, NHCLV had launched its own ECHO program to serve Lehigh Valley, called *Community Response to the Opioid Epidemic*, becoming one of only a handful of ECHO programs designed and implemented by an FQHC rather than an academic medical center.

Although Lehigh Valley had a few methadone programs, the predominant paradigm was abstinence. As NHCLV became the first local primary care practice to provide MOUD, their community partners—treatment and recovery programs, as well as resource organizations focused on housing, food, job readiness, etc.— began asking questions: What's the evidence? How do we do this? How do we partner with you? The NHCLV ECHO was designed to answer these questions.

> We recognized that our partners needed support to unpack their own stigma and start moving forward … there were no platforms for people to learn from each other… [NHCLV] needed to be bold in this activist primary care niche.

The start-up costs to become an ECHO hub are relatively low, and NHCLV received support from the Lehigh Valley Health Network and from the free training offered by the ECHO Institute in New Mexico. NHCLV's experience with ECHO—as both spoke and hub—has played a role in transforming individuals, NHCLV itself, and the overall network in Lehigh Valley serving people with OUD. As one example, the ER is now conducting MOUD inductions. One reason that ECHO catalyzes change, Dr. Letcher believes, is that participants often see themselves or their family members represented in the case presentations. "That turns on a light bulb and allows stigma to fall away: This is the kind of care that I want for my sister."

Box 7.3 Expanding the Scope of ECHO Beyond Office-Based Care
Interview with Danna Gobel MSW LCSW, Education Program Manager, Boston Medical Center's Office-Based Addiction Treatment (OBAT)

Under the leadership of Colleen T. Labelle, MSN, RN-BC, CARN, Director STATE OBAT and, Director Boston Medical Center (BMC) OBAT Training and Technical Assistance, BMC OBAT has developed several successful ECHO programs focused primarily on office-based treatment of Opioid Use Disorder (OUD) in New England. More recently the team has launched an ECHO program called, "SUD Care Continuum," which has completed a very successful 6-month cycle, with a second round preparing to launch. This ECHO has been led by Medical Director, Rachel King, MD, and serves learners who are providing acute SUD treatment, including staff from inpatient detoxification programs, transitional care settings, crisis stabilization programs, and methadone treatment programs. The original aim was to encourage bridging of care with Medication for Addiction Treatment (MAT).

For this program the BMC ECHO team is collaborating with the Massachusetts Bureau of Substance Addiction Services (BSAS). According to program manager, Danna Gobel, the BMC ECHO team "wanted to avoid a message that 'BMC is telling you what to do,' and so most of the recruitment of participants was done by BSAS. The panel did not include a psychiatrist, but a mental health clinician who was well known in the acute treatment community." Most of the participants in this ECHO program have been counselors, social workers, recovery coaches, and nurses.

The initial goal of the program was to promote MAT and encourage more care across the continuum, with the integration of evidence-based treatments for long term. The BMC team anticipated this would be met with substantial resistance from participants. Instead, there has generally been a positive attitude with little pushback, and with the perspective that medication treatment is one of the useful tools in recovery. Going into the second round, the makeup of the panelists and aim has shifted. Understanding that many of the case-based questions were more clinical in nature, the ECHO team has added to its panel a licensed mental health clinician who works in a methadone clinic. The aim will be recognizing and discussing solutions to common gaps in the continuum of care. The curriculum includes the use of medication and also innovative topics such as the harm reduction principles; working with patients who are justice-involved; brain injury and SUD; engaging with parents involved with child protection; and understanding diversity in sexuality and gender. The addition of a licensed mental health clinician will allow for more in-depth and interdisciplinary discussion of how to address complicated patient situations, such as co-occurring mental illness and trauma.

Comments from the program evaluation included:

I can now provide more accurate info and not reinforce stereotypes of MAT.

I continue to provide medication for addiction while aggressively using motivational interviewing and other behavioral techniques to help them stop using other substances.

This course opened my eyes to the inter-professional possibilities of our program.

[I have] a better understanding of what they (patients) are going through, and [this] has had an impact on how clients are treated.

Gobel and the rest of the BMC ECHO team are excited to be able to share their knowledge and also to learn from care providers who work in the SUD treatment continuum outside of traditional office-based care settings.

Box 7.4 Rapid Expansion of ECHO to Support SUD Treatment in India

Interview with Dr. Prabhat Chand, Professor of Psychiatry, National Institute of Mental Health and Neurosciences, Bangalore, India

As a young psychiatrist practicing at the prestigious Indian National Institute of Mental Health and Neurosciences (NIMHANS), Dr. Prabhat Chand worried about the huge number of Indians who have problems with mental health or substance use, but are unable to access treatment—estimated at 75% of this population. Dr. Chand read early publications about the ECHO model and became convinced that he could adapt the model to address mental illness and addiction in India. He spent 4 months in New Mexico learning everything he could about ECHO, and started his first ECHO program in India in 2014.

The NIMHANS ECHO programs target healthcare workers who serve the most marginalized populations, and so in addition to training physicians and other licensed healthcare providers, their programs serve a wide variety of other types of frontline providers. They have adapted the model in various ways to meet the needs of their audience. Many of these providers do not have access to computers or Internet, and so most access ECHO video sessions on their phones. Chand and colleagues identified a need to enhance the ECHO case-based learning sessions with other forms of learning, and have added supplementary web-based teaching modules. Some rural healthcare workers have limited comfort with learning through reading, and so the modules tend to be very simple and brief, and include short quizzes on content. In order to earn a certificate of completion, participants are required to engage in the ECHO sessions and also complete the modules and pass the quizzes, but can make an unlimited number of attempts to do so.

NIMHANS has had to bridge the major challenge of language barriers in India, since so many rural providers speak only or primarily a local dialect, or pronounce Hindi in such differing ways that communication is difficult. NIMHANS ECHO sessions include real-time summaries of the case discussions on a whiteboard in order to assist with communication. Since 2015 the group has also been providing ECHO sessions in many languages to target participants in different states.

Chand and his group have just completed their 29th ECHO cohort, and have engaged more than 6000 participants, including some in India's most remote and impoverished regions.

Conclusion

The ECHO model offers a promising approach to expanding the pool of outpatient healthcare providers who are interested in treating OUD and other SUDs, as well as increasing their confidence and ability to do so. ECHO programs have been widely implemented for these purposes. The model is also being applied in a variety of innovative ways to enhance treatment of OUD using specific models of outpatient care, to improve treatment in the inpatient setting, and to expand treatment of OUD and other SUDs in countries outside of the US. Rigorous evaluation of the clinical impact of the ECHO model for OUD is largely lacking, as is research on how to overcome identified barriers to participation. Finally, since many programs are currently grant funded, sustainable funding sources are needed if the programs are to continue beyond the current liberal availability of funding aimed at addressing the opioid use disorder and overdose epidemic.

References

1. Darfler K, Sandoval J, Antonini VP, Urada D. Preliminary results of the evaluation of the California Hub and Spoke Program. J Subst Abus Treat. 2020;108:26–32. https://doi.org/10.1016/j.jsat.2019.07.014.
2. Miele GM, Caton L, Freese TE, McGovern M, Darfler K, Antonini VP, Perez M, Rawson R. Implementation of the hub and spoke model for opioid use disorders in California: rationale, design and anticipated impact. J Subst Abus Treat. 2020;108:20–5. https://doi.org/10.1016/j.jsat.2019.07.013.
3. Sagi MR, Aurobind G, Chand P, Ashfak A, Karthick C, Kubenthiran N, Murthy P, Komaromy M, Arora S. Innovative telementoring for addiction management for remote primary care physicians: a feasibility study. Indian J Psychiatry. 2018;60(4):461. https://doi.org/10.4103/psychiatry.IndianJPsychiatry_211_18.
4. Dubin RE, Flannery J, Taenzer P, Smith A, Smith K, Fabico R, Zhao J, Cameron L, Chmelnitsky D, Williams R, Carlin L. ECHO Ontario chronic pain & opioid stewardship: providing access and building capacity for primary care providers in underserviced, rural, and remote communities. Stud Health Technol Inform. 2015;209:15–22. https://doi.org/10.3233/978-1-61499-505-0-15.
5. The website of the ECHO Institute at the University of New Mexico (echo.unm.edu). Accessed 2/20/2020
6. Komaromy M, Bartlett J, Manis K, Arora S. Enhanced primary care treatment of behavioral disorders with ECHO case-based learning. Psychiatr Serv. 2017;68(9):873–5. https://doi.org/10.1176/appi.ps.201600471.
7. Komaromy M, Duhigg D, Metcalf A, Carlson C, Kalishman S, Hayes L, Burke T, Thornton K, Arora S. Project ECHO (Extension for Community Healthcare Outcomes): A new model for educating primary care providers about treatment of substance use disorders. Subst Abuse. 2016;37(1):20–4. Available from: http://www.ncbi.nlm.nih.gov/pubmed/26848803.
8. Anderson D, Zlateva I, Davis B, Bifulco L, Giannotti T, Coman E, Spegman D. Improving pain care with project ECHO in community health centers. Pain Med. 2017;18(10):1882–9. Available from: http://www.ncbi.nlm.nih.gov/pubmed/29044409.
9. Kawasaki S, Francis E, Mills S, Buchberger G, Hogentogler R, Kraschnewski J. Multi-model implementation of evidence-based care in the treatment of opioid use disorder in Pennsylvania. J Subst Abus Treat. 2019;106:58–64. https://doi.org/10.1016/j.jsat.2019.08.016.
10. Tofighi B, Isaacs N, Byrnes-Enoch H, Lakew R, Lee JD, Berry C, Schatz D. Expanding treatment for opioid use disorder in publicly funded primary care clinics: exploratory evaluation of the NYC health+ hospitals buprenorphine ECHO program. J Subst Abus Treat. 2019;106:1–3. https://doi.org/10.1016/j.jsat.2019.08.003.
11. Hutchinson E, Catlin M, Andrilla CH, Baldwin LM, Rosenblatt RA. Barriers to primary care physicians prescribing buprenorphine. Ann Family Med. 2014;12(2):128–33. https://doi.org/10.1370/afm.1595.
12. Huhn AS, Dunn KE. Why aren't physicians prescribing more buprenorphine? J Subst Abus Treat. 2017;78:1–7. https://doi.org/10.1016/j.jsat.2017.04.005.

13. Madden EF. Intervention stigma: how medication-assisted treatment marginalizes patients and providers. Soc Sci Med. 2019;232:324–31. https://doi.org/10.1016/j.socscimed.2019.05.027.
14. Bouchonville MF, Hager BW, Kirk JB, Qualls CR, Arora S. Endo echo improves primary care provider and community health worker self-efficacy in complex diabetes management in medically underserved communities. Endocr Pract. 2018;24(1):40–6.
15. Lewiecki EM, Jackson A, Lake AF, Carey JJ, Belaya Z, Melnichenko GA, Rochelle R. Bone health TeleECHO: a force multiplier to improve the care of skeletal diseases in under-served communities. Curr Osteoporos Rep. 2019;17(6):474–82. https://doi.org/10.1007/s11914-019-00543-9.
16. Arora S, Thornton K, Murata G, Deming P, Kalishman S, Dion D, Parish B, Burke T, Pak W, Dunkelberg J, Kistin M. Outcomes of treatment for hepatitis C virus infection by primary care providers. N Engl J Med. 2011;364(23):2199–207. https://doi.org/10.1056/NEJMoa1009370.
17. Gordon SE, Dufour AB, Monti SM, et al. Impact of a videoconference educational intervention on physical restraint and antipsychotic use in nursing homes: results from the ECHO-AGE pilot study. J Am Med Dir Assoc. 2016;17:554–6.
18. Frank JW, Carey EP, Fagan KM, Aron DC, Todd-Stenberg J, Moore BA, Kerns RD, Au DH, Ho PM, Kirsh SR. Evaluation of a telementoring intervention for pain management in the Veterans Health Administration. Pain Med. 2015;16(6):1090–100. Available from: http://www.ncbi.nlm.nih.gov/pubmed/25716075.
19. Katzman JG, Qualls CR, Satterfield WA, Kistin M, Hofmann K, Greenberg N, Swift R, Comerci GD, Fowler R, Arora S. Army and Navy ECHO pain telementoring improves clinician opioid prescribing for military patients: an observational cohort study. J Gen Intern Med. 2019;34(3):387–95. Available from: https://www.ncbi.nlm.nih.gov/pubmed/?term=30382471.
20. Díaz S, Zhao J, Cronin S, Jaglal S, Bombardier C, Furlan AD. Changes in opioid prescribing behaviors among family physicians who participated in a weekly tele-mentoring program. J Clin Med. 2020;9(1):14. https://doi.org/10.3390/jcm9010014.
21. The website of the ECHO Institute at the University of New Mexico (https://echo.unm.edu/locations/global). Accessed 2/20/2020.
22. Puckett HM, Bossaller JS, Sheets LR. The impact of project ECHO on physician preparedness to treat opioid use disorder: a systematic review. Addict Sci Clin Pract. 2021;16:6. https://doi.org/10.1186/s13722-021-00215-z.
23. Salvador J, Bhatt S, Fowler R, Ritz J, James R, Jacobsohn V, Brakey HR, Sussman AL. Engagement with project ECHO to increase medication-assisted treatment in rural primary care. Psychiatr Serv. 2019;70(12):1157–60. https://doi.org/10.1176/appi.ps.201900142.
24. Scott JD, Unruh KT, Catlin MC, et al. Project ECHO: a model for complex, chronic care in the Pacific Northwest region of the United States. J Telemed Telecare. 2012;18(8):481–4.
25. McBain RK, Sousa JL, Rose AJ, Baxi SM, Faherty LJ, Taplin C, Chappel A, Fischer SH. Impact of project ECHO models of medical tele-education: a systematic review. J Gen Intern Med. 2019;1:1–6. https://doi.org/10.1007/s11606-019-05291-1.
26. Zhou C, Crawford A, Serhal E, Kurdyak P, Sockalingam S. The impact of project ECHO on participant and patient outcomes: a systematic review. Acad Med. 2016;91(10):1439–61. https://doi.org/10.1097/ACM.0000000000001328.

The Power of Team: Introduction to Interprofessional Care Teams in Opioid Use Disorder Treatment

8

Christopher J. Shaw, Jacqueline Bango,
Stephen Hayward Keizer, and Madeleine Sedlack

An Example of Interprofessional Care for OUD

The Massachusetts General Hospital Inpatient Addiction Consult Team

The Interprofessional team–based model of care is not a new concept. It has proven to be effective for patients with chronic illnesses such as diabetes, hypertension, and HIV which require frequent monitoring and assessment. It has also been effective in helping manage the unique needs for patients requiring palliative care or hospice services. Interprofessional teams leverage strengths of different disciplines to promote health and wellbeing of patients. The patient is the hub and center for the team and person-centered care is essential. This care concept can also be practiced across general medical settings, from primary care to long-term care and skilled nursing facilities to inpatient hospital settings.

C. J. Shaw (✉)
Addiction Consult Team (ACT), Substance Use Disorder Initiative, Massachusetts General Hospital, Boston, MA, USA
e-mail: cshaw@partners.org

J. Bango
Addiction Consult Team (ACT), Massachusetts General Hospital, Boston, MA, USA
e-mail: jbango@partners.org

S. H. Keizer
Bridge Clinic & Addiction Consult Team (ACT), Massachusetts General Hospital, Boston, MA, USA
e-mail: SKEIZER@mgh.harvard.edu

M. Sedlack
Institute of Health Professions & Addiction Consult Team (ACT), Massachusetts General Hospital, Boston, MA, USA

© Springer Nature Switzerland AG 2021
S. E. Wakeman, J. D. Rich (eds.), *Treating Opioid Use Disorder in General Medical Settings*, https://doi.org/10.1007/978-3-030-80818-1_8

Interprofessional teams are particularly important for patients who are marginalized by the healthcare system. This is true for patients with stigmatizing illnesses as well as populations of people who are treated with disregard. It is important to understand that patients with OUD often don't come to a hospital by choice. People who experience an opioid overdose are brought to the hospital by family, emergency medical services (EMS), or the police. Patients with serious bacterial infections or other medical complications of OUD may delay seeking care and treatment due to the prospects of the emotional pain of being treated poorly by hospital staff or suffering through undertreated opioid withdrawal. Hospital staff blind to their own biases and stigma toward persons with OUD can inflict emotional pain on patients. This combination of physical and emotional distress can result in patients leaving the hospital before completing recommended treatment. They are often labeled as "drug-seekers, addicts, junkies, and abusers." The attitudes of hospital staff can be the greatest deterrents to seeking care, particularly for patients who have previously experienced discrimination in healthcare settings.

An interprofessional team approach can be effective in helping patients navigate challenges encountered in hospital setting and reduce the perception of the hospital as a "risk environment" [2]. The interprofessional team welcomes patients into care, identifies and treats opioid cravings, encourages patients to complete treatment, and advocates for them with hospital staff. Through education and modeling of care the interprofessional team also promotes healing and helps eradicate stigma from hospital staff [2].

An example of interprofessional collaboration in the care of patients hospitalized with OUD is the Massachusetts General Hospital (MGH) inpatient Addiction Consult Team (ACT). Started in 2014, ACT is a unique collaboration between medicine, psychiatry, nursing, and social work. It includes physicians, advanced practice nurses, social workers, pharmacists, and students in each of these disciplines. Perhaps most importantly, ACT employs recovery coaches who are people who have shared lived experience with patients diagnosed with SUD [2]. ACT provides both medication recommendations for opioid use disorder (OUD) and other types of SUD, as well as direct linkage to other therapies including residential treatment, intensive outpatient treatment, outpatient group and individual therapy, psychiatry, recovery coaching, and peer support meetings. In seeking to delivering the highest quality of care for patients and families, ACT meets the WHO's definition of interprofessional collaboration, and its primary focus is on this goal. Now in its eighth year, the ACT provided nearly 10,000 consults to over 6,000 unique patients in its first 6 years alone. ACT's mission is to promote the health and wellness of hospitalized patients with SUD. To elucidate the necessary components of interprofessional care for patients with OUD, this chapter will provide a detailed description of the structure and function of ACT.

Shared Roles and Responsibilities

Each ACT discipline has a role to play in assisting patients. Supporting a patient's goals is the responsibility of the entire team, and so is knowledge of resources. Medical and psychiatric physicians and advanced practice nurses help teams manage and ease a patient's withdrawal and make recommendations for treatment. The role of the medical provider is to ensure that patients receive appropriate medications such as methadone or buprenorphine. ACT providers also ensure all patients with OUD have a prescription for intranasal naloxone in hand when discharged from the hospital and consider other harm reduction interventions such as initiation of pre-exposure prophylaxis medication to prevent HIV, distribution of safer use supplies, and discussion of safer use practices [3].

Fueled by resilience and advocacy, social workers meet with patients at the bedside to help them identify their unique goals and bring forth their own internal resources combined with external supports to help them achieve these [4]. Recovery coaches have lived experiences to share with staff and patients. Their teaching and modeling behavior for patients and staff are invaluable assets to the program. ACT pharmacists and students play an important role in teaching patients and educating staff. Team pharmacists provide medication teaching and education that helps patients appreciate the role and value of sustained medication treatment. There is often overlapping of visits from one discipline to the other, and frequent joint visits are made to a patient so they can see the coordination and collaboration of care on their behalf.

ACT members use every resource at their disposal to help a patient stay in the hospital and receive the care they need. While OUD treatment initiation and direct linkage to ongoing community-based care are the goals for all interested patients, ACT's first goal is relationship building, engagement, and identifying each unique patient's goals.

The interdisciplinary nature of the team helps facilitate this process. Social workers and recovery coaches offer extensive resource information about available outpatient and community-based treatment and all ACT disciplines are aware of a range of resources which are available in the hospital. The social workers and recovery coaches on ACT work collaboratively with the medical/psychiatric providers to provide a multifaceted approach to treatment planning. Since OUD is a condition influenced by many factors that can stem from both genetic and environmental factors, an interdisciplinary team–based approach to treatment that takes into consideration all of these complex factors is critical to help patients achieve the best possible outcomes [5].

Treatment is not one-size-fits-all, particularly for hospitalized patients who are often struggling with significant medical complexity, co-occurring psychiatric illness, and structural barriers to health. Building partnerships with other hospital services that can provide different treatment options of interest to patients can motivate a patient from alternative angles. The interdisciplinary team is invaluable as it recognizes the need to address this complex condition from a variety of different angles and recognizes that one single approach to treatment may not be sufficient for many of the patients we care for.

ACT social workers have expertise in motivational interviewing. Motivational interviewing is an approach that operates under the premise that patients are the experts on their own lives, and the role of the worker is simply to help bring to the surface the wisdom and knowledge that patients already possess to help them work through ambivalence and achieve their goals [6]. Using a strengths-based approach, social workers identify what internal and external barriers may be keeping a patient "stuck" and work with them to challenge and change these barriers. Whether a patient's goal is harm reduction, total cessation, or simply improving their quality of life, the next step lies in collaborating with patients to create a treatment plan that is realistic and feasible given their biological, psychological, and social factors, and one that is in line with a patient's goals and level of readiness [7]. ACT social workers work in partnership with patients to identify what they feel will be most helpful to support their goals, provide psycho-education around available treatment options, and arrange direct linkage to the form of care that is most appropriate to meet their needs.

As one social worker describes in her own words:

My role includes helping patients assess their substance use and to decide if changes would be in their best interest. When patients explore their history of substance use, they reveal an overwhelming array of losses, challenges, and barriers to recovery that would require a team of experts to address adequately. Fortunately, access to an interprofessional team such as ACT affords precisely that. There is an added benefit of being part of a team as a patient will be open to talking to a member of the team after having met another member who started the process of building trust and establishing rapport. Patients who see a team of professionals working closely with each other to ensure they get optimal treatment can recognize that they are not only a member of the team, but they are the most valued member of all.

Team building includes the patient as the central focus of the team and improving patient care as the ultimate goal [9]. Starting with the patient story and the opportunity to improve this person's life is the best way for team members to prioritize the same goals [9]. Team members each bring their unique background and training, and all understand the diverse range of skills, roles, responsibilities, and this valuable feedback loop among the group [10]. For interprofessional care to function successfully, it is vital that team members respect each colleague's autonomy as well as the unique experience and knowledge that they bring to the team. Interprofessional collaboration requires that each team member engages not only with patients but with other team members as well.

Interprofessional Team Communication

Effective communication is a crucial and necessary ingredient for a successful interprofessional team. To facilitate this, ACT gathers as a team for daily hour-long rounds to discuss patient cases and interdisciplinary care needs. A common goal of daily rounds is for all team members to come together and get to know each other better and have an opportunity to offer treatment advice utilizing expertise from their particular lens. This ensures that a patient's care benefits from the multiple perspectives of the interprofessional team, and meeting attendance by all team members is essential and expected. The Robert Wood Johnson Foundation's (RWJF) [8] definition of interprofessional collaboration in healthcare identifies the necessity for cultural change. It emphasizes that each discipline works together to engage with patients and those who support them.

Healthcare providers overall share a common cultural value to improve patient outcomes [9].

Members of a team include multiple cadres of staff who have a variety of professional training and life experiences. This plurality lends itself to the power and creativity of the group. Successful interprofessional teams fully embrace and appreciate the unique viewpoints, contributions, and talents that each discipline and team member possess [8]. One discipline is not more important than another, power balance and fairness to all is the priority. Therefore, having adequate "face time" is vital and every discipline must have equal status in these team meetings. Each team member helps actualize the group by making the ethos of the group his/her ethos and does not indulge in their own private opinions and prejudices. Individualism, arrogance, and power have no place in the interprofessional team model. Brainstorming of options is focused on maximizing benefits for patients, not puffing up positions unique to a particular discipline. Teams are open to the possibility that there is always more than one solution (not either–or, instead, both–and). Assumptions are just that, and finding ways to minimize, lessen, resolve issues is the goal.

A healthy and robust team promotes confidence in each of its members and encourages open sharing. Each individual is empowered to share perspectives in supportive environments safely. This resilience of team members is especially necessary when caring for patients with OUD, as it is necessary for these individuals to have the ongoing hope and grounding to continuously push back against societal beliefs that addiction is not a treatable illness. Resilience is defined as an ability to adapt and bounce back when things don't go as planned and it is best cultivated in collaborative connections with others [9]. Relationships with others reduces isolation and collaboration protects against loneliness. Team-based care therefore becomes a platform for supporting other team members as well as patients by modeling connection, hope, and healing to patients who suffer from illnesses perceived to be hopeless. Leaders should foster an environment that supports team members and gives them space to express fears or uncertainty in complex cases. Uncertainty should be an accepted cultural value on an interprofessional team that is met with curiosity and teamwork [8].

One of the advanced practice nurses working with ACT who facilitates a weekly holistic yoga group for patients, shares the following observations: "Due to the many medical, emotional, and practical challenges a person with active addiction faces, the work can feel overwhelming. In our regular collaborations, we can pool our knowledge and ideas and come up with creative approaches to the most complex situations. We assess, treat, and connect to care with efficiency generated by close collaborations, and as a result, I feel entirely supported in my work. I know that if I encounter a patient concern that I don't have an immediate resolution for that, I can bring my questions and worries to the team. Often, I come away with a new strategy, if not an outright solution. Belonging to a multidisciplinary team, however, allows me and every other member of the team to share the burden of responsibility rather than try and shoulder it alone. We share the outcomes, as well, experiencing together the emotional highs and the lows that are an inevitable part of caring for patients with OUD."

The work of the team includes supporting patients, teaching and promoting health and wellness, and ensuring patient education is complete. Team members may each address a patient's needs and problems differently, offering a range of perspectives on each patient. These ongoing communications and discussions take time and commitment and can be done formally, informally, or both. Team rounds are an important venue where the group can consider a patient's risks, identify barriers, and explore treatment options. These valuable team discussions review and identify medical and mental health needs and explore engagement techniques to motivate and teach patients.

Engagement and Treatment Planning

A critical component in caring for hospitalized patients with OUD is ensuring the interprofessional team is individualizing treatment plans based on patient preferences. Developing direct linkage to aftercare is essential and planning begins upon hospital admission to ensure the plan is patient-centered and guided and that the whole interprofessional team has time to collaboratively develop a realistic plan with the patient. To facilitate these direct linkages, ACT connects patients with addiction medicine providers in the community, individual and group therapy, intensive outpatient treatment, residential care, psychiatric care, recovery coaching, and peer support meetings.

ACT utilizes the inpatient general hospital admission as a unique opportunity to engage a patient and to develop a therapeutic alliance with them. The acute phase of the patient's illness can increase the possibility of connection and engagement to a person who is experiencing negative consequences related to opioid use in order to reduce harm, promote patient dignity and health, and engage in ongoing care. In 2017, over 70% of adults diagnosed OUD did not receive any treatment [10] so any positive engagement with patients is worthwhile. There are no hard and fast calls or demands for a person to recover. A goal for stabilization and comfort in the immediate moment is the most critical consideration while promoting positive connections with the healthcare system. ACT staff members fully appreciate the potential for change; however, the timing of this can never be certain.

Medication for OUD (MOUD) can be started and continued during a hospitalization, and linkages to aftercare are crucial to ensure ongoing engagement and retention. A robust healthcare team supporting a patient and encouraging them to consider medication and to ensure treatment access can help build a patient's confidence and help them to believe in themselves. One of the team's recovery coaches often cautions other members on the team that patients with OUD have experienced stigma in most medical settings, and "they come to us with low expectations of the treatment they will get." It may take time for patients to trust a healthcare system that has often shunned them. ACT recognizes the particular challenges that patients with OUD encounter and the ongoing health risks they face, including overdose and infectious disease complications in part due to our ongoing punitive approaches and policies toward people with OUD [11]. Engaging them in care, focusing on patient-identified health goals, and expanding their access to treatment is essential.

Even beyond the hospital encounter, there are opportunities for continued engagement. Each September, members from ACT participate with patients and community members in National Recovery Month activities, standing together to combat social stigma, promote awareness, and celebrate recovery as defined by each human being.

The Bidirectional Benefit of a Patient's Story

One of the most potent interventions ACT staff can provide to a patient is listening carefully and respectfully to their story. When care is organized around the patient story the essential goals and priorities quickly emerge [8]. It is not uncommon for patients with OUD to have significant trauma histories and multiple adverse childhood events [12–15]. Many individuals we serve on ACT who are struggling with OUD are also experiencing homelessness, may struggle with co-occurring mental health conditions/trauma, comorbid medical conditions, structural barriers, discrimination, and racism. Therefore, an effective treatment plan must account for all of these factors and take a multimodal approach, which is afforded by the interdisciplinary team.

ACT staff seeks to model for hospital staff a regular practice of trauma-informed care. It is imperative to employ trauma-informed principles in working with patients. Having the space to engage with and hear each patient's story is one of the most powerful tools ACT members utilize. Connecting with a patient through their story fosters a better understanding of the patient and can help a patient to establish trust in a team member. A patient who has experienced an overdose or is hospitalized for complications of injection drug use (IDU) is at massive risk for imminent death [16]. When evidence-based medication that keeps them from suffering the pain of withdrawal offered, a welcome hand is extended, and kindness is administered. It can increase a person's hope and their desire to live.

Cross-Collaboration with Other Care Teams and Specialties

ACT regularly collaborates with a range of other specialty groups, the primary medical team, and other services caring for a patient. For example, ACT works closely with infectious disease colleagues to ensure a patient's untreated Hepatitis C or HIV infection can be evaluated during the inpatient stay. ACT providers, social workers, and recovery coaches also attend monthly meetings with cardiac surgery and infectious disease colleagues to discuss patients with infectious endocarditis in need of valve repair, and to advocate on a patient's behalf. Having a better understanding of a patient's support systems, readiness, and motivation for change can change the calculus of other specialists in deciding about timing and offering of needed interventions. Being able to receive these medical and surgical interventions that patients may not have thought possible due to their OUD can be hugely motivating for them to stay in care. This model of holding regular, interprofessional case conferences to discuss high-risk, shared patients and to provide addiction expertise and education has been utilized effectively by ACT with a range of other teams including Burns and Trauma, Obstetrics, the Cystic Fibrosis team, the Transplant Center, Hepatology, Oncology, Palliative Care, Psychiatry, Primary Care, Emergency Medicine, and the Pain Center.

Research by Kerr et al. [18] has shown that people who inject drugs present for care to emergency departments later in the course of their illness and, in turn, incur higher admission rates to hospitals. They also have a higher incidence of leaving the hospital prematurely, or "against medical advice" (AMA) and, therefore, not completing the recommended treatment. Their indications for admission most often are related to painful soft tissue infections and other even more serious infections, raising the likelihood of readmission with worsening illness. These cycles of leaving, returning, and readmission are perpetuated by stigma and discrimination, by ineffective withdrawal management, and by staff expectations that patients remain abstinent from use in hospital settings. These habitual expectations are unrealistic and nearly impossible to achieve, and staff require substantial education in harm reduction concepts. Ongoing collaboration between ACT and other care teams can help provide education and training to other healthcare team members, in addition to providing direct clinical care to patients.

Stigma and Harm Reduction

Emergency departments and general hospitals are a unique access point for populations at high risk of overdose, however incorporation of harm reduction strategies in the emergency department and inpatient settings is a woefully neglected topic and one that requires reinforcing [17]. It is important to recognize the unfamiliarity with or frank bias toward harm reduction that healthcare providers may have, especially those who have received little to no training in harm reduction concepts. To combat this, ACT seeks to incorporate harm reduction in their day-to-day interactions with patients and modeling these approaches for frontline staff. A delay in care or in providing harm reduction teaching can result in missed opportunities to optimize health, which is critical in treating illness. If a patient with hypertension has chest pain or with chronic obstructive pulmonary disease (COPD) cannot breathe, delays in treatment could have deadly consequences. It is unlikely that a patient with these illnesses confronts a level of stigma that prevents them from seeking help. For patients with stigmatizing diseases such as OUD, fear of discrimination may delay individuals from reporting symptoms, which can result in lethal consequences [11]. Interprofessional presence and access for patients is essential as it widens the space for a patient to connect and land, reducing the likelihood of missed opportunities for intervention.

Interprofessional Learning

In addition to minimizing stigma, having an inpatient, interprofessional addiction consult team promotes a paradigm shift among hospital staff and other services. ACT members work with hospital-wide staff and identify the learning deficits and educational needs of staff. Carney et al. [19] defines interprofessional learning as "learning arising from interactions between members (or students) of two or more professions" that can happen spontaneously in the workplace or as a product of formal interprofessional education.

Ongoing learning is essential for all staff. Project MAINSTREAM (Multi-Agency Initiative on Substance Abuse Training and Education for America), a federally funded multisite project to study SUD training and education, identified successes and barriers for implementing interprofessional education and training [19]. Thirteen university healthcare settings incorporated interprofessional education of fellows from 14 different disciplines. The majority found the interprofessional approach provided a positive framework for instruction, and their institutions valued interdisciplinary education. However, there were significant barriers to implementing training. Institutional barriers such as scheduling conflicts and lack of rewards for faculty presented the most significant impediments to the implementation of interdisciplinary education [19]. Creating teams, such as ACT, which explicitly prioritize interprofessional care and collaboration naturally creates space for interprofessional education and training. This occurs informally through rounds and shared patient cases, but also formally through shared lecture series and case conferences.

The paucity of formal interdisciplinary OUD educational opportunities is a reality. The importance of relevant addiction education is critical for healthcare providers.

Interprofessional cross-education is ideal as members are prepared together and learn from each other. The Association for Medical Education and Research in Substance Abuse (AMERSA) identifies core competencies that are relevant for multidisciplinary teams with the caveat that specific skills may vary according to the role of distinct team members [19]. Haack et al. [20] emphasize that it is vital for all health professionals to be "equipped with the knowledge and skills to respond appropriately to the needs of patients and families affected by SUD" in order to accurately identify mental health challenges associated with SUD.

Due to the lack of formal education structures to promote interprofessional learning, less formalized teaching is also critical. The inpatient consult team provides excellent opportunities for this type of interprofessional training. Shadowing opportunities, journal clubs, and joint case conferences with other services are directly beneficial to staff and indirectly beneficial to patients with SUD. All of these opportunities can work toward increasing education and also reducing stigma among general medical providers.

Interprofessional Care Team's Role in Combating Stigma: Learning from HIV/AIDS

In the 1980s, healthcare workers faced the daunting challenges of confronting human immunodeficiency virus/autoimmune deficiency syndrome (HIV/AIDS), one of the most stigmatizing and lethal illnesses of all time [21]. Scientists, medical experts, and academic scholars led efforts to understand and attack the virus while patients diagnosed with the disease confronted stigma and ostracization. It was not uncommon for patients to find themselves banished from family, neighbors, and communities. In the United States and other parts of the world, patients faced beatings and even death at the hands of their community members. A patient's lifestyle was one of the most commonly used justifications for stigmatization; the biased notion that a person with HIV/AIDS had brought it on themselves. Even among healthcare workers, patients encountered stigma. Physicians and nurses, in particular, identified fear of contagion for their mistreatment or neglect of patients. However, other frontline health care staff did not waiver in their compassion and commitment and worked directly with patients, families, and communities affected by the illness [21].

In January 1983, the University of California San Francisco opened the first HIV-focused outpatient clinic in the country [21]. Its frontline staff included nurses, physicians, scientists, and activists. They collaborated regularly and utilized evidence-based research to inform their practice in the care and treatment of patients diagnosed with AIDS in the city of San Francisco. Their inpatient counterparts adopted similar models of interprofessional collaboration to treat patients with dignity [21]. Over time through the cooperation and extraordinary efforts and response of many healthcare disciplines, the stigma associated with HIV/AIDS decreased.

This team-based approach utilized in HIV-AIDS treatment provides an excellent example for treating OUD. Like HIV/AIDS, the OUD and overdose epidemic is a public health crisis and the associated illness is still stigmatized. Similar to the AIDS pandemic, the opioid overdose epidemic has resulted in hundreds of thousands of deaths [21–23]. Bureaucratic delays in both cases have caused needless death. Unlike the early years of HIV/AIDS, effective treatments for OUD are readily accessible. Yet barriers to utilizing science, funding research, and developing adequate clinical expertise to address OUD has led to more significant morbidity and mortality than even that of HIV/AIDS [23].

Evidence shows that positive outcomes increase when many people join together in support and care of patients [16]. Families and patients can also help galvanize communities to act. With the development of evidence-based antiretrovirals for the treatment of HIV, the Federal Drug Administration (FDA) fast tracked these medications for approval, saving many lives. With OUD, evidence-based medicine is available; however, a shortage of prescribers and outdated regulations causes delays in treatment access. Over 30 million people live in the US counties without any prescribers of buprenorphine [24]. Even where medication is available, there is stigma and misinformation regarding medication, which can prevent patients from opting to take them. Patients receiving MOUD often face discrimination in the medical system, with many post-acute care facilities refusing to accept patients on these medications [24]. Healthcare leaders must ensure that science and not stigma drives patients' decisions on whether or not to take medication [25].

Interprofessional OUD Care in Primary Care Settings

An interprofessional outpatient model of care that has been implemented to expand OUD treatment access is Office-Based Opioid Treatment (OBOT), which utilizes nurse care managers (NCM) playing the central role [26]. The OBOT Model relies on the interprofessional collaboration between (NCMs) and physicians in community primary care practices caring for patient with OUD, predominantly utilizing buprenorphine treatment. Many outpatient models for provision of MOUD care exist, nearly all agree on some degree of the following four essential key components: pharmacological therapy, access to psychosocial services, integration of care, and education and outreach [27].

Conclusion

Interprofessional care teams for OUD treatment offer vulnerable patients who have historically been marginalized in healthcare settings radical acceptance and advocacy, while promoting and expanding treatment access. This care model is rooted in appreciation for the diverse training, expertise, skills, and perspectives that all team members bring to the shared goal of partnering with patients to achieve their best quality of life, health, and self-defined recovery. In contrast to older models of care which required patients to demonstrate "readiness" or to meet stringent prerequisites, there should be no requirements for engagement with an interprofessional OUD care team. An example of this approach is the MGH ACT, which intentionally uses the range of disciplines represented in its team to incorporate multiple approaches to care and offer patients a holistic treatment approach that addresses the biological, psychological, and social components of addiction.

References

1. World Health Organization (WHO). Framework for action on interprofessional education & collaborative practice. [Internet]. Geneva: WHO; 2010 [cited 2020 Mar 21]. Available from: https://apps.who.int/iris/bitstream/handle/10665/70185/WHO_HRH_HPN_10.3_eng.pdf;jsessionid=1F4D8FACC7D79EA7AB880B9C8B2A20D7?sequence=1.
2. Eaton EF, Westfall AO, McClesky B, Paddock CS, Lane PS, Cropsey KL, Lee RA. In-hospital illicit drug use and patient directed discharge: barriers to care for patients with injection related infections: open forum infectious disease: IDSA. http://creativecommons.org/licenses/by-nc-nd/4.0/.
3. Hawk KF, Vaca FE, D'Onofrio G. Reducing fatal opioid overdose: prevention, treatment and harm reduction strategies. The Yale J Biol Med [Internet]. 2015 [cited 2020 Mar 21];88(3):235–45.
4. National Association of Social Workers (NASW). About social workers [Internet]. www.socialworkers.org. Washington, DC: NASW; 2020 [cited 2020 Apr 1]. Available from: https://www.socialworkers.org/news/facts.
5. American Society of Addiction Medicine (ASAM). Public Policy statement: definition of addiction [Internet]. Rockville: ASAM; 2011 [cited 2020 Mar 16]. Available from: https://www.asam.org/docs/default-source/public-policy-statements/1definition_of_addiction_long_4-11.pdf?sfvrsn=a8f64512_4.
6. Rollnick S, Miller WR, Butler C. Motivational interviewing in health care: helping patients change behavior. New York: Guilford Press; 2008.
7. Schuckit MA. Treatment of opioid-use disorders. New Engl J Med [Internet]. 2016 [cited 2020 Mar 21];375(16):1596–7. https://doi.org/10.1056/NEJMc1610830.
8. Robert Wood Johnson Foundation (RWJF). Lessons from the field: promising interprofessional collaboration practices. [Internet]. RWJF; 2015 [cited 2020 Mar 21]. Available from: https://www.rwjf.org/en/library/research/2015/03/lessons-from-the-field.html.
9. Hardin L, Kilian A, Spykerman K. Competing health care systems and complex patients: an inter-professional collaboration to improve outcomes and reduce health care costs. J Interprof Educ Pract [Internet]. 2017 [cited 2020 Mar 16];7:5–10. https://doi.org/10.1016/j.xjep.2017.01.002.

10. U.S. Department of Health and Human Services (HHS), Office of the Surgeon General. Facing addiction in America: the surgeon general's report on alcohol, drugs and health. HHS publication: no. (SMA) 16-4991. [internet]. Washington, DC: HHS; 2016 [cited 2020 Mar 21]. Available from: https://addiction.surgeongeneral.gov/sites/default/files/surgeon-generals-report.pdf.

11. Madras BK, Ahmad N, Wen J, Sharfstein J. Improving access to evidence-based medical treatment for opioid use disorder: strategies to address key barriers within the treatment system. NAM perspectives. Discussion paper, Washington, DC. https://doi.org/10.31478/202004b.

12. Ayello EA, Sibbald RG. Treating persons who inject drugs: the need for holistic and respectful care. Adv Skin Wound Care [Internet]. 2019 Jul [cited 2020 Mar 16];32(7):293. https://doi.org/10.1097/01.ASW.0000558412.90463.af.

13. SAMHSA. SAMHSA's concept of trauma and guidance for a trauma-informed approach. [internet]. HHS Publication No. (SMA) 14-4884. Rockville: Substance Abuse and Mental Health Services Administration; 2014 [cited 2020 Mar 21]. Available from: https://store.samhsa.gov/product/SAMHSA-s-Concept-of-Trauma-and-Guidance-for-a-Trauma-Informed-Approach/SMA14-4884.html.

14. Allem J-P, Soto DW, Baezconde-Garbanati L, Unger JB. Adverse childhood experiences and substance use among Hispanic emerging adults in Southern California. Add Behav [Internet]. 2015 [cited 2020 Mar 21];50:199–204. https://doi.org/10.1016/j.addbeh.2015.06.038.

15. Gielen N, Havermans RC, Tekelenburg M, Jansen A. Prevalence of post-traumatic stress disorder among patients with substance use disorder: it is higher than clinicians think it is. Eur J Psychotraumatol [Internet]. 2012 [cited 2020 Mar 16];(0):1. https://doi.org/10.3402/ejpt.v3i0.17734.

16. Hassan AN, Foll BL, Imtiaz S, Rehm J, Le Foll B. The effect of post-traumatic stress disorder on the risk of developing prescription opioid use disorder: results from the National Epidemiologic Survey on Alcohol and Related Conditions III. Drug Alcohol Depend [Internet]. 2017 [cited 2020 Mar 21];179:260–6. https://doi.org/10.1016/j.drugalcdep.2017.07.012.

17. Bassuk EL, Hanson J, Greene RN, Richard M, Laudet A. Peer-delivered recovery support services for addictions in the United States: a systematic review. J Subst Abuse Treat [Internet]. 2016 [cited 2020 Mar 21];63:1–9. https://doi.org/10.1016/j.jsat.2016.01.003.

18. Kerr T, Rachlis BS, Montaner Julio SG, Wood E. Harm reduction in hospitals: is it time? Harm Reduct J [Internet]. 2009 [cited 2020 Mar 21];(1):19. https://doi.org/10.1186/1477-7517-6-19.

19. Carney PA, Thayer EK, Palmer R, Galper AB, Zierler B, Eiff PM. The benefits of interprofessional learning and teamwork in primary care ambulatory training setting. J Interprof Educ Pract [Internet]. 2019 [cited 2020 mar 16];15:119–126. https://doi.org/10.1016/j.xjep.2019.03.011.

20. Haack MR, Adger H Jr, editors. Strategic plan for interdisciplinary faculty development: arming the nation's health professional workforce for a new approach to substance use disorders. Subst Abuse [Internet]. 2002 [cited 2020 Mar 16];23(sup1):1–21. https://doi.org/10.1080/08897070209511505.

21. Austin D. The unbroken chain: three decades of HIV/AIDS nursing [Internet]. The unbroken chain: three decades of HIV/AIDS nursing | UCSF Science of Caring. University of California San Francisco; 2014 [cited 2020Apr3]. Available from: https://scienceofcaring.ucsf.edu/patient-care/unbroken-chain-three-decades-hivaids-nursing.

22. Center for Behavioral Health Statistics and Quality. Key substance use and mental health indicators in the United States: results from the 2015 National Survey on Drug Use and Health. HHS Publication No. SMA 16-4984, NSDUH Series H-51. [Internet]. Rockville: SAMHSA; 2016 [cited 2020 Mar 16]. Available from: https://www.samhsa.gov/data/sites/default/files/NSDUH-FFR1-2015/NSDUH-FFR1-2015/NSDUH-FFR1-2015.pdf.

23. American Society of Addiction Medicine (ASAM). Opioid addiction 2016 facts & figures [Internet]. Rockville: ASAM; 2017 [cited 2020 Mar 16]. Available from: https://www.asam.org/docs/default-source/advocacy/opioid-addiction-disease-facts-figures.pdf.

24. CDC. National Center for Health Statistics: FastStats – Injuries. [Internet]. Centers for Disease Control and Prevention; 2017 [cited 2020 Mar 21]. Available from: https://www.cdc.gov/nchs/fastats/injury.htm.

25. Wakeman SE, Rich JD. Barriers to medications for addiction treatment: how stigma kills. Subst Use Misuse [Internet]. 2018 [cited 2020 Apr 2];53(2):330–3. https://doi.org/10.108 0/10826084.2017.1363238.
26. Wakeman SE. Using science to battle stigma in addressing the opioid epidemic: opioid agonist therapy saves lives. Am J Med [Internet]. 2016 [cited 2020 Mar 21];129(5):455–6. https://doi.org/10.1016/j.amjmed.2015.12.028.
27. Korthuis TP, McCarty D, Weimer M, Bougatsos C, Blazina I, Zakher B, Grusing S, Devine B, Chou R. Primary care–based models for the treatment of opioid use disorder a scoping review. Ann Intern Med. 2017. https://doi.org/10.7326/M16-2149; Wyllie AH, Kerr JFR, Currie AR. Cell death: the significance of apoptosis. In: Bourne GH, Danielli JF, Jeon KW, editors. International review of cytology. London: Academic; 1980. p. 251–306.

Further Reading

Alcoholics Anonymous. The story of how many thousands of men and women have recovered from alcoholism. 4th ed. New York: Alcoholics Anonymous World Services, Inc.; 2001.
American Psychiatric Association (APA). Diagnostic and statistical manual of mental disorders: DSM-5. 5th ed. Arlington: American Psychiatric Association; 2013.
Babor TF, Del Boca F, Bray JW. Screening, brief intervention and referral to treatment: implications of SAMHSA's SBIRT initiative for substance abuse policy and practice. Addiction [Internet]. 2017 [cited 2020 Mar 21];112:110–7. https://doi.org/10.1111/add.13675.
Barrett K, Chang Y. Behavioral interventions targeting chronic pain, depression, and substance use disorder in primary care. J Nurs Scholarsh [Internet]. 2016 [cited 2020 Mar 21];48(4):345–53. https://doi.org/10.1111/jnu.12213.
Galanter M. Combining medically assisted treatment and Twelve-Step programming: a perspective and review. Am J Drug Alcohol Abuse [Internet]. 2018 [cited 2020 Mar 16];44(2):151–9. https://doi.org/10.1080/00952990.2017.1306747.
Herron A, Brennan TK. The ASAM essentials of addiction medicine. 2nd ed. Philadelphia: Wolters Kluwer Health; 2015.
Hunt GE, Siegfried N, Morley K, Sitharthan T, Cleary M. Psychosocial interventions for people with both severe mental illness and substance misuse. Schizophr Bull [Internet]. 2014 [cited 2020 Mar 21];40(1):18–20. https://doi.org/10.1093/schbul/sbt160.
Jordan CJ, Andersen SL. Sensitive periods of substance abuse: early risk for the transition to dependence. Dev Cogn Neurosci [Internet]. 2017 [cited 2020 Mar 21];(29–44):29. https://doi.org/10.1016/j.dcn.2016.10.004.
Kelly JF, Saitz R, Wakeman S. Language, substance use disorders, and policy: the need to reach consensus on an "addiction-ary." Alcohol Treat Q [Internet]. 2016 [cited 2020 Mar 16];34(1):116–23. https://doi.org/10.1080/07347324.2016.1113103.
Kourrich S, Calu DJ, Bonci A. Intrinsic plasticity: an emerging player in addiction. Nat Rev Neurosci [Internet]. 2015 [cited 2020 Mar 21];16(3):173–84. https://doi.org/10.1038/nrn3877.
Kowalchuk A, Reed B. Substance use disorders. In: Rakel RE, Rakel D, editors. Textbook of family medicine. 9th ed. Philadelphia: Elsevier; 2016. p. 1152–63.
LaBelle CT, Han SC, Bergeron A, Samet JH. Office-based opioid treatment with buprenorphine (OBOT-B): statewide implementation of the Massachusetts Collaborative Care Model in Community Health Centers. J Subst Abuse Treat [Internet]. 2016 [cited 2020 Mar 21];60:6–13. https://doi.org/10.1016/j.jsat.2015.06.010.
Mennis J, Stahler GJ. Racial and ethnic disparities in outpatient substance use disorder treatment episode completion for different substances. J Subst Abuse Treat [Internet]. 2016 [cited 2020 Mar 16];63:25–33. https://doi.org/10.1016/j.jsat.2015.12.007.
Park-Lee E, Lipari RN, Hedden SL, Copello EA, Kroutil LA. Receipt of services for substance use and mental health issues among adults: results from the 2015 National Survey on Drug Use and Health. [Internet]. [place unknown]: SAMHSA; 2016 [cited 2020 Mar 16]. Available from:

https://www.samhsa.gov/data/sites/default/files/NSDUH-ServiceUseAdult-2015/NSDUH-ServiceUseAdult-2015/NSDUH-ServiceUseAdult-2015.pdf.

SAMHSA. Advisory: complementary health approaches: advising clients about evidence and risks. [internet]. HHS Publication No. (SMA) 15-4921. Rockville: Substance Abuse and Mental Health Services Administration; 2015 [cited 2020 Mar 21]. Available from: https://store.samhsa.gov/shin/content//SMA15-4921/SMA15-4921.pdf.

Volkow ND, Koob GF, McLellan AT. Neurobiologic advances from the brain disease model of addiction. N Engl J Med [Internet]. 2016 [cited 2020 Mar 21];374(4):363–71. https://doi.org/10.1056/NEJMra1511480.

Integrating Recovery Coaches into Primary Care Teams

Martha T. Kane and Windia Rodriguez

In the face of the rising opioid overdose epidemic, it has become increasingly clear that despite recognition that opioid use disorder, like all substance use disorders (SUD), is a chronic condition, many treatment models do not incorporate a Chronic Disease Management approach in design or execution. Chronic care models incorporate a number of elements not typically part of traditional SUD care, including routine screening, early intervention, education, integrated and coordinated care delivery between medical and specialty care, long-term care delivery with variation in treatment intensity depending on patient need, and thoughtful delivery of evidence-based care with changes in treatment plan as needed based on variations in disease severity [1, 2]. The key frame shift in this approach is transitioning from an acute, episodic care model to a chronic care management approach. Managing SUD requires long-term engagement in treatment, but perhaps even more importantly an investment and the tools to rebuild one's life, supported by active engagement with recovery supports over the lifetime. Others who have experienced this process and actively engaged in the process are often extremely helpful in successfully entering and sustaining this lifelong process.

The essence of this shift is captured in the concept of Recovery-Oriented Systems of Care (ROSC) [2]. ROSC refers to a system of care adapted to incorporate a recovery-based approach focused on early identification and engagement in treatment that is easily accessed and adapted to match the needs of someone early in the disease process. This model also utilizes active outreach to identify and reduce any obstacles to engaging in care. Services are delivered in an environment as devoid of stigmatizing elements as possible, allowing patients to seek care for a chronic medical condition rather than a moral fault or behavioral problem. Certainly, the primary care setting could offer the ideal opportunity to provide the early engagement, support through acute episodes, and close monitoring in follow-up necessary to manage

M. T. Kane (✉) · W. Rodriguez
Department of Psychiatry, Massachusetts General Hospital, Boston, MA, USA
e-mail: kane.martha@mgh.harvard.edu; wrodriguez1@partners.org

© Springer Nature Switzerland AG 2021
S. E. Wakeman, J. D. Rich (eds.), *Treating Opioid Use Disorder in General Medical Settings*, https://doi.org/10.1007/978-3-030-80818-1_9

a chronic relapsing condition. The addition of peer support services for patients receiving SUD treatment in the primary care setting has been identified as a key support to both medical providers and patients working through the recovery process [3, 4].

State and local governments have recently provided financial support and training resources to develop a peer-based workforce able to deliver recovery-focused approaches to SUD care. The move toward peer involvement draws on a history of effective involvement of peers in caring for those in recovery utilizing multiple recovery pathways. Peer support services (PSS) in the form of mutual aid groups such as Alcoholics Anonymous (AA) and Narcotics Anonymous (NA) have long been an essential part of the care spectrum for persons with SUD, but have not typically been integrated into either medical or behavioral health treatment. However, peer-based support for other chronic diseases, such as diabetes, HIV, and depression, is utilized in both medical and behavioral settings to great effect. Over the last 10 years, peer support services have increasingly been incorporated into substance use treatment programs and have been rapidly expanding to medical settings with the shift to chronic disease management models. Although the data is limited to date, there is a consensus that peer support services are generally effective, though it remains unclear which peer support models are most effective and for whom [5, 6].

Peer Support in Medical and Behavioral Health Settings

The notion of peers providing positive support to others with shared experience draws on well-established principles from social psychology, and almost seems like common sense. The Center for Medicare and Medicaid Services declared peer support services to be an evidence-based practice in 2007 [7], based on findings in several studies that suggested peer support improved a variety of outcomes in a range of settings, both medical and behavioral health [8].

The effectiveness of peer involvement in primary care is well established as part of the treatment approach for many medical conditions with significant behavioral health components, such as diabetes, HIV, and HCV. Peer support to patients with diabetes has been found to be helpful in many ways. Peer-led groups are often well attended, and patients report that they prefer to turn first to a peer for information. Patients also report that they appreciate the structured network of support [9]. When added to treatment as usual, peer-led, group-based focused discussions have been shown to contribute to reduced A1C levels, increased self-management and self-care activities, and improved quality of life scores for patient with Type 2 Diabetes Mellitus (DM) [10]. Peer support group meetings combined with peer-led activities were additionally associated with reduced inpatient hospital utilization and lower overall hospital costs for patients with Type 2 DM [11]. The Substance Abuse and Mental Health Services Administration and Health Resources Services Administration (SAMHSA–HRSA) both recommend the use of peers to support diabetes care [4], describing a program that links patients with chronic diseases to others who share the condition, learning from others' lived experience of diabetes.

These services can be provided in several settings, including group meetings or home visits, and phone contacts can be utilized to either provide support or to augment supports offered via other service types. These services are generally delivered as a complement to ongoing traditional services, and are structured as nonhierarchical, providing an opportunity for more frequent contact and support with more flexibility and accessibility. It also seems that peers who provide support to others benefit from this work to assist them in increased effectiveness at managing their own disease, with increased likelihood of improving their own long-term self-care and glycemic control [12].

Similarly, there is a growing indication in the literature for the effectiveness of peer support services for patients living with HIV and those living with HCV. Peers are often called on to provide services to support patients' behavioral change efforts resulting in improved health outcomes. Harm reduction–focused individual and group support was found to be more effective than traditional support services in reducing unsafe injection use in people living with HCV [13]. Velasquez et al. [14] trained peer counselors and therapists to deliver an intervention designed to reduce drinking and risky sex behaviors for men living with HIV. Men in the intervention condition reduced both the number of drinks overall, the number of heavy drinking days, and the number of days of risky sexual behavior. Peers were trained to deliver the protocol and performed the intervention as effectively as trained therapists. In some more recent work, peer support groups delivered patient education and navigation services to supplement routine primary care for persons from historically marginalized ethnic/racial groups living with HIV. For those who were stably housed, the intervention enhanced the likelihood of treatment retention as measured by fewer 4-month gaps in care and for those participants who completed all peer-led sessions, there was an even stronger effect on retention in care [15]. Based on several studies of peer involvement in programs for youth living with HIV in sub-Saharan Africa [16], several recommendations for likely best practices emerged. Successful peer-based interventions with youth recruited peers from the community to provide services that enhanced existing medical services. Recommended services varied in intensity and duration, and included health education, individual and group counseling for adherence and social supports, and linkage to other referral services as needed.

Peer support roles have also been integrated into mental health care settings with positive effect and have been recognized as an important component of mental healthcare for more than a decade [17]. Peers provide a variety of services in differing roles depending on the mental health needs of the patient population and type of service delivered. In general, peer support services are used to provide empathic, emotional support to reduce isolation and increase sense of connection to others. Providing informational support and linking patients to concrete community resources to address a wide range of needs are also common and essential roles for peers. Skills-based support services are often offered to help people develop improved coping and disease self-management skills. Over a broad range of studies with variable rigor, there is a strong suggestion that peer support activities are associated with reduced medical and psychiatric hospitalizations, improved engagement with ongoing care, better relationships with providers, and increased patient activation and hopefulness [18]. In a randomized controlled trial of peer support services delivered to depressed patients as compared to usual care, Pfeiffer and Heisler [19] demonstrated that peer support services were associated with greater reductions in depressive symptoms than the treatment as usual condition. In addition, there were not significant differences in outcomes between peer-based services and formal Cognitive Behavioral Therapy for depression. The authors hypothesized that by reducing isolation, increasing access to information, reducing the impact of stressors, providing a positive role model, and empowering patients to be a more active participants in recovery, peer support interventions had a significant impact on symptoms of depression. In an age where there are only limited behavioral health services and access to treatment services is one of the most difficult challenges, the effectiveness and comparability of peer-provided interventions is noteworthy and opens new care design possibilities.

Peer Support in Context of Substance Use Disorder

The importance and effectiveness of peers supporting peers in the work of recovery has long been recognized [20, 21]. Peer-based supports were first described in the 19th century, largely originating in missionary work and other spiritual contexts. Beginning in 1935, Alcoholics Anonymous has become a peer-based cornerstone with long history of effective support for those in recovery [22]. For people with substance use disorder who attend AA, attendance is associated with higher rates of reported abstinence even for those with other co-occurring mental health issues [23].

With the recognition of substance use disorder as chronic condition with a waxing and waning course of symptoms, the focus must shift from treating SUD as an acute illness to treating recovery as a process of symptom management over time. With the shift to a long-term focus on recovery, treatment targets must also shift to focus on long-term engagement in the treatment process, supported by a community of care providers. In this model, there is an expanded opportunity for others who are in recovery from the disorder to support those who are currently suffering. Over the last several years, the role of peer support expanded beyond mutual aid groups to include a wide scope of recovery supports with peers serving in a number of roles essentially based in peer mentorship [21]. These newer models are drawn in part from models of the patient navigator and community health worker roles that have been developed to support models of integrated care in medical settings and the mental health world [6].

Expanded peer recovery support services began to develop in the early part of this century as a number of factors came together, according to William White [21], a leading advocate of the peer-based movement. He attributes the expansion to a fundamental shift in understanding of substance use disorder, shifting away from episodic treatment of acute symptoms to a notion of longer-term treatment of variable intensity to manage a chronic, recurring disorder. There was a concurrent expansion of community-based recovery resources such as recovery homes and school-based supports as it began to be increasingly clear that there are many components to recovery support and no single set of treatment experiences was adequate to address the needs of the entire population with SUD. In addition, there was a surge in interest in mutual aid support groups and a broad-based, fundamental movement toward recovery advocacy. Numerous state and federal initiatives were undertaken as well to provide financial support to expanding service access. The Center for Substance Abuse Treatment (CSAT) developed the Recovery Community Services Program and Access to Recovery (ATR), both which provided resources to assist persons with SUD in accessing needed recovery support services. Treatment for SUD began to expand to a more recovery services-oriented framework rather than an exclusively clinically oriented framework [24].

In many ways earlier perceptions of substance use disorder as an acute condition led to a treatment system designed as a series of discrete treatment episodes, each one designed to lead to stable recovery, despite limited evidence of clinical effectiveness of this approach. This led to a treatment system in which each treatment episode (e.g., detox and rehabilitation) was expected to be effective in establishing abstinence and recurrence of use was understood essentially as a failure on the patient's part. The treatment system was not designed to provide an easily accessed continuum of care with the capacity for increased intensity when needed and gradual changes as person established recovery. Many roadblocks between levels of care resulted in a lack of continuity in care, inadequate length of treatment dose, lack of linkages to necessary supports in a gradually stepped-down approach, and treatment models that were not designed to address the complexities of a chronic condition. The result was often high levels of recurrence and readmission [21]. The concept of peer support services grew in response to the need for an adjunct to the treatment system supporting the shift from an acute care model to a culture of recovery. Peers with lived experience were particularly helpful in supporting people to develop resources and tools of recovery that allow them to move beyond a sense of failure, to engage in long-term recovery work that can adjust with the ebb and flow of the disorder, to link into supports and resources that enhance long-term outcomes, and gradually shift to successfully maintain a life of self-defined recovery. Essentially the goal is to utilize peers with lived experience to create essential supports that allow a shift to recovery-oriented system of care [2].

What Are Peer Support Services?

Peer support services are designed to support the process of recovery over time during which persons with SUD work to improve the quality of their lives, including health, purpose, and meaning. Like other chronic disease care models, peer support services are generally patient-centered and highly collaborative, acknowledging the patients as the experts on their own health and the experience of their disease. Recovery is approached from the strengths-based perspective, acknowledging that each person creates his or her own pathway into recovery. Persons entering recovery must build their own recovery resources and tools, called recovery capital, with the support of community and care providers [25].

Peers with lived experience are uniquely able to build strong collaborations with consumers working on recovery while supporting the process of building this "recovery capital" [2], a set of resources and supports that improve the overall quality of life, help create meaning and purpose, and support autonomy and self-determination [26, 27]. Shifting from a more traditional treatment approach, the model of peer support specialist is not equivalent to the more familiar 12-step or mutual aid approach. A peer support specialist differs significantly from a sponsor in that a sponsor represents an approach espoused by AA and NA. The peer support specialist role is also distinct from traditional medical or behavioral health clinical roles. It is also not a spiritual or pastoral role [21]. While each of these roles may have value for the recovery process, the peer support role is a distinct and valuable support that operates outside of the strictures of traditional care. Peer specialists can support persons considering recovery to explore the variety of diverse pathways that are available, including harm reduction. They can help persons with SUD locate and connect to essential resources, including family and community options, and help to establish needed recovery capital to support overall quality of life [6].

The peer support specialist (PSS) builds a collaborative relationship with the person they are working with, and there is no power differential in this relationship [24]. Traditional clinical relationships are based on a hierarchy of power, preventing true collaboration. PSS have different core functions and different accountabilities [28]. The role is designed to help the person with SUD discover their own pathway to recovery. Each consumer defines what recovery means to them and sets their own recovery goals; the PSS does not dictate any pathway, nor do they assume they know what is best for the participant. It is understood that each person with SUD is the expert on their own recovery process, and the work focuses on helping the consumer to sort through the options, consider next steps, and likely costs versus benefits. Recovery efforts are validated, and further courses of action are considered, evaluated, and implemented with peer support. Peers essentially act as consultants to the work of recovery and provide essential links to the culture of recovery [2, 21, 29]. Recovery supports are individualized to fit the needs of the person and will necessarily change over time as the person tests pathways to improving their lives and more clearly understands what works for them. PSS walk through this process offering support and counsel along the way.

Peers may have more credibility based on the expertise they have gained through their own lived experience and what they have observed in others [30]. Peers can create unique trust-based relationships rooted in compassion and commitment. They are well suited to help someone move from hopelessness to hope, and to learn essential tools for self-management and increased self-awareness. In addition, those with their own lived experience most clearly comprehend the experience of stigma, from both society and from internalized guilt and shame. They are uniquely able to help others with SUD cope with these complicated realities [8].

The presence of peers on the clinical care team offers an obvious opportunity to provide important support to the person over the long-term course to stable recovery. However, this perspective necessitates an approach to peer support that isn't specifically abstinence based; much of the work is done while persons continue to be actively engaged with substances. As the person with SUD works through the process of gradual problem recognition leading to change initiation, followed by stabilization and maintenance of a recovered lifestyle, peers have the opportunity to provide support in every aspect of the work, including the process of recurrence of use and return to self-defined recovery [28]. Peers have the insight and credibility to enter collaborative relationships with persons as they consider how to meet their goals and succeed at recover as they define it.

Peer Support Specialist Model

Gradually over the last two decades awareness of the value of incorporating peers as specialists augmenting traditional models of treatment has grown. This approach to care developed in response to escalating needs of patients, particularly most recently in the context of the opioid use disorder crisis. Despite the variety of settings and locations where peer support services have been developed in recent years, there seems to be a broad consensus on the role, function, and specific competencies for peer support specialists. According to recommendations from SAMHSA's technical website for peer service support, BRSS TACS [8], peer support specialists focus on four major dimensions of recovery capital that assist to improve the quality of life and create stable recovery as the person defines it. Peer support targets general health-related issues, including treating current issues and supporting making healthy choices that facilitate improved mental and physical health. They work on assisting with stable, safe housing, and linkage to communities that promote social networks and relationships to help persons develop friendships and create hope. Finally, PSS support persons to develop a meaningful life, driven by purpose, featuring relevant activities [31]. William White [28] described the role similarly, including providing emotional support via empathy and mentoring, and companionship to help support connection to others. He also highlighted informational support provided via knowledge sharing and skills acquisition enhanced by instrumental support defined as concrete assistance in tasks such as arranging transportation and removing other barriers. In addition, peer service delivery models often utilize non-traditional settings, where people coping with SUD can access services without encountering barriers. Depending on the resources and location of the provider, services may be delivered in more convenient non-traditional and nonclinical locations. The ability to meet in the community strengthens the trust and nonhierarchal nature of the relationship.

The role of the PSS is flexible and able to adapt to the needs of the person. The PSS may be a mentor or role model who provides key emotional and/or social support. They may help the person to set goals or design recovery plans. They may provide coaching on how to build and sustain recovery capital by connecting to important resources or identifying key barriers to success. Discussions of coping skills or social experiences may increase success in implementing a recovery plan. The PSS can provide essential linkages to medical or mental health treatment or other recovery resources. Connections to other critical resources such as supports to manage criminal legal issues are also often part of the role of the PSS. In the end, the responsibility for the implementation and outcome of the recovery plan belongs to the consumer, but the PSS is an active consultant or guide [28].

According to the technical assistance website for conceptualizing peer support programs [32], there are several general competencies for peer workers caring for patients with behavioral health issues. Persons providing peer-based services need to operate from a recovery orientation that recognizes the many paths of recovery and that the chief architect is the person who is recovering. The peer must support the person to work with their own strengths and resources since these are the building blocks of a life of meaning and purpose. The work is voluntary; person centered; and directed by the individual's desires, hopes, and needs. Or course, to be successful the PSS must form an empathic, collaborative relationship of mutual respect and trust with a person working on recovery. The PSS approach needs to be trauma-informed, emphasizing physical and emotional safety.

These general competencies require a set of specific core competencies that include a primary focus on creating collaborative relationships that help the person recognize themselves as an expert in their own lives and encourage them to explore and develop concrete recovery plans. Relationships are often built through outreach and gradual engagement with the person in need. Peers must be able to provide individualized and personalized support including concrete support and links to resources and services and may at times be responsible for seeking these resources in the community. PSS must be able to appropriately draw on their own recovery experiences and incorporate these experiences in a set boundary and useful way for persons working on the recovery process. Direct and honest communication skills are key to success for the PSS, and they must be able to function effectively in teams of colleagues from a variety of roles and settings. Peers in recovery need to share wellness and recovery skills with the person, and they need to be comfortable exploring values and emotions as well. Of course, PSS need to be familiar with trauma-informed care concepts and apply these to the recovery work, as well as comfortable helping a person to manage a crisis. Peers in this work must also be able to manage their own recovery effectively, seek support as needed, and utilize system-based supports such as supervision and additional training as available. They need to have a clear understanding of how to set and maintain appropriate boundaries with others. They need to have a keen awareness of their own strengths and weaknesses, and a clear sense of their own motivations for being involved in this work [2, 30]. Increasingly PSS also are required to obtain certification via completion of a training course and supervised work hours, and these certifications are maintained through ongoing workshops and courses [6].

This peer support model offers several unique benefits to augment traditional care and may at times be a unique supplement when traditional approaches have not been effective. Since the peer support model recognizes the chronic nature of substance use disorder, persons coping with SUD may engage peer support specialists at any time in the process of recovering. Early in the process, peers may help with initial engagement, may be able to help instill hope, or may provide important linkages to community-based supports that help the individual address critical barriers to recovery. As the person proceeds through the journey of recovery, PSS can continue to provide support and perspective through the difficult process of determining goals and finding an effective pathway. Once a stable, productive recovery is established, their continued support may help with maintaining gains and coping with new barriers or issues as they arise. Different from the more familiar community health worker (CHW) who connects via shared experiences of community, peer support workers connect via shared lived experience of substance use disorder and have formal training in how to support others with the same issue [33]. The role of the CHW includes providing culturally appropriate outreach, information, and education, as well as advocacy with community and health services agencies. PSS incorporate these role dimensions while also focusing on recovery-oriented skill building and mentoring, linkage, and coordination based in relationships that are sustained over time. The context of PSS work is recovery driven from a person-centered recovery orientation with a relational focus.

The peer support model is distinct form traditional clinical models in important aspects. Unlike traditional clinical models, peer support work is not based on the hierarchy of the counseling relationship, and different boundaries must be observed, particularly in terms of self-disclosure. As suggested by White [34] professional models and peer-based recovery models can work in complementary ways to enhance possibilities of recovery. Each has a role and may be important at different points in the process of recovery. A clinical provider and a peer support provider have different core functions and different accountabilities, but recovery support specialist can likely be seamlessly integrated into the treatment continuum in a complementary role [21]. Each role may impact the other, for example, in a clinical setting, PSS may take on clinical tasks such as formal motivational interviewing protocols [35]. Clinicians may also appreciate peers' perspective from outside the norm in clinical setting and peers may be valued as role models and guides in helping to establish a more comfortable and engaging environment in the clinic setting [3]. The most effective balance of peer support and clinical services will likely vary depending on the patient population and the treatment setting, but in all settings, clear delineation of roles and efficient collaborations are essential to effective care. Further research is needed to explore the most effective models for peer support services, particularly in general medical settings [5, 6, 36].

This work is often very meaningful for the peer themselves and helps to sustain their own identity as a person in recovery [37]. They may be able to reframe past experiences with more self-forgiveness and achieve greater understanding of their own journey. New opportunities to pay forward the support they received are presented every day as they are more fully integrated into a community of others in need. Reduced isolation and increased acceptance by others may be fostered by a sense of a safety in their work environment. They are likely to be more motivated about their own self-care and to increase attention to sustaining their own recovery supports [29]. Overall, the role of peer support specialist offers many benefits for the peer as well as patients and the system overall.

Peer-Based Care Delivery Settings

The settings for peer-delivered services vary depending on the type and general purpose of the service being offered. Peer support services have historically been designed to be easy to access, delivered in a nonprofessional, nonclinical location [28]. Increasingly peer support services are being integrated within a medical or behavioral health settings. However, even when a PSS is a member of a medical or behavioral healthcare team, whenever possible meeting patients in community-based locations may be preferable as peer-based care is easily transferred to less formal settings. The agent of change is the connection to the recovery community in general, rather than a specific individual or setting [21]. An example of a community-based peer outreach model was designed to assist persons with Opioid Use Disorder (OUD) to access medication treatment. Peers initiated contact and then followed the person through the process of initial engagement in treatment. Outreach was informal with printed information and was followed up by phone calls using recovery management check-up (RMC) models [38]. Linkage using RMC model included peer-delivered motivational support, problem-solving, and assertive linkage to supports. Peers also worked to reduce barriers to access and ensure ongoing contact [39]. This type of approach might work well in primary care medical settings to increase engagement and retention in care.

PSS are frequently delivered via individual or group-based approaches as an element of team-based care in integrated healthcare settings. As Tracy and Wallace [40] summarize from their review of the literature on group-based approaches, it can be difficult to evaluate whether individual or group approaches are more effective since recovery support services are often delivered as part of a suite of integrated interventions. Associated benefits of peer-led groups include reductions in substance use and craving, along with increased treatment engagement in outpatient SUD and mental health treatment appointments. Participants also report an increased sense of self-efficacy in addressing the process of recovery, and reductions in HIV/HCV risk behaviors. In a study of a group-based intervention, persons with SUD were approached during an inpatient stay and randomly assigned to either peer led group only (Mentorship for Addiction Problems – MAP) or MAP plus more traditional treatment [41]. The MAP group approach involved mentors engaged in open-ended contact, beginning while inpatient and following through to outpatient services. Services provided by the mentors included a peer mentor–led support group plus linkage to community-based supports. The MAP-only intervention was as effective as MAP plus more traditional treatment in terms of numbers of patients who attended outpatient SUD treatment appointments, as well as medical and mental health appointments. MAP-only participants attended more than three times as many treatment appointments as the MAP plus usual treatment participants and sustained those gains for at least 9 months. Peers working as mentors in this study reported that mentorship supported their own recovery as well. Peer-based support groups have also been helpful for patients who felt judged for treatment with medications for OUD (MOUD) in other more traditional mutual aid groups. Groups were run by peers and allowed participants to freely discuss the fact that their path to recovery included medication treatment. Participants reported this approach was helpful in three ways: (1) shame and self-loathing were reduced by the respectful nonjudgmental environment; (2) overall holistic approach helped participants in recognizing the importance of physical and mental health in stable recovery; and (3) core values of more traditional mutual aid approaches were retained, including spirituality, sharing, and celebration [42].

Peers have also recently been deployed in Emergency Departments (ED) to provide rapid intervention with patients admitted due to opioid overdose. Limited research exists on the effectiveness of peer intervention in the emergency setting but peer services are being implemented anyway due to the severity of the overdose crisis. The primary services peers provide include linkage to MOUD and other treatment and peer-based supports [43]. Waye and Goyer [44] reported on the ED-based model in use in Rhode Island. The intervention is initiated via 20–30-min contact with person while in the ED, focused on overdose education, and naloxone training plus treatment referrals. After 10 days, patients are referred to a Recovery Center, with 87% agreeing to post-ED engagement, 51% receiving service referrals, and 45% sustaining involvement over following months.

Finally, in an era of expanding use of apps and other web-based approaches, there is growing interest in delivering peer-based services virtually. Online, web-based recovery support groups have grown in recent years, including both AA and NA groups offered entirely in a virtual format. This has become particularly relevant in the context of the global COVID-19 pandemic. Other types of SUD-focused groups offer targeted supportive content, information sharing, and guidance, offered altruistically [45]. Possemato et al. [46] trained peers to support digitally delivered Cognitive Behavioral Treatment (CBT) to veterans with both post-traumatic stress disorder (PTSD) and hazardous drinking. Peers were trained to support a web-based CBT protocol. Both groups improved equally on PTSD symptoms, quality of life, and overall coping. Peer sessions were delivered in person or on phone weekly for 20 min (adapted to patient's needs). Peers demonstrated fidelity to the protocol, and satisfaction was rated good for both peers and participants. Participants reported liking content related to real-life application of skills and goal setting, liked feeling cared for, and appreciated feeling accountable to their peer. Engagement in peer support sessions was comparable to the typical number of sessions delivered by mental health providers in the primary care setting. The authors concluded that peers can be trained to deliver semi-structured interventions utilizing telemedicine or mobile applications with fidelity. The role of peers in supporting consumers to benefit from an app-based intervention for hazardous drinking in veterans in a primary care setting was considered by Blonigan et al. [47] They recommended that peers might be helpful in increasing patients' motivation for use of the app, help patients to use the app-based work to increase progress toward recovery goals, and assist in helping patients to persist in completing the work.

Effectiveness of the Peer Support Specialist Model

Since the use of peer support models is a relatively new SUD treatment approach, the field is just beginning to consider how to most effectively deploy peers in medical or mental health settings. Overall, peer involvement seems to have a positive effect on several key recovery-related outcomes. Peers are uniquely able to help patients engage in recovery work [3] and their involvement is associated with reduced substance use [48–50]. A study evaluating the impact of integrated SUD treatment in primary care which included the use of PSS demonstrated improved outpatient treatment utilization and retention, both primary care and mental health, and reduced length of inpatient hospitalizations and emergency room visits [51]. Patients who work with peers in clinical settings have also been shown to report increased treatment satisfaction [52]. Factors deemed to be the social determinants of health and general measures of social stability, such as housing and legal issues, have also been shown to generally improve in association with PSS involvement [50]. Other studies have shown that quality of life ratings increase alongside increased sense of empowerment and hope [18]. Taken together the accumulating data suggests that peer support specialists increase the likelihood of improved outcomes for people with SUD. Data also suggest that peers who work as support specialists experience benefits, including opportunities to reframe their own suffering and give back to the community who supported them [29].

Systematic reviews of peer support services suggest a more cautious outlook. In independent reviews, Reif et al. [36] and Bassuk and colleagues [5] suggested that taken together, data across the many studies provide a moderate level of support that peer involvement was generally effective and specific positive effects were seen in several key recovery factors. More recently, Eddie et al. [6] concurred that results continue to imply the apparent efficacy of peer support in the recovery process. However, all three systematic reviews emphasize the need for more rigorous research since many of the studies have important methodological limitations. It is very difficult to distinguish the distinct impact of peer support specialists from other types of recovery support or treatment. It remains difficult to identify which interventions are most useful in which settings, whether patient-specific or PSS-specific characteristics predict success with the model, and the key mechanisms of change are as yet unidentified.

Peer Support Services in Primary Care Settings

As the opioid overdose crisis has developed over the last several years, it has become increasingly clear that medical providers have a unique and critical role in the spectrum of treatment services available for substance use disorders. Primary care holds a central management role in the care of most chronic diseases, particularly between episodes of acute symptom exacerbation. Treatment for substance use disorder also benefits from engaging primary care doctors in the process. The outpatient medical setting is ideally suited for patients who come for SUD-related medical problems, particularly early in the course of the disorder. Medical sequelae will likely cause patients to recognize the impact of substances in their lives before other symptoms appear. Patients may be more open to engagement and eventually treatment referral [5]. In addition, primary care treatment models are well suited to address the chronic recurring nature of substance use disorders and primary care doctors are likely to be willing to continue to work with patients even when symptoms such as return to substance use persist. Patients may be more likely to seek care from their primary care doctors, or at the very least, it may be that the PCP is the first treatment professional with whom the patient shares this information. However prior studies have found that PCPs identify a need for greater supports for patients as a barrier to offering SUD treatment, particularly MOUD. Access to traditional mental health and substance use services is often quite limited with many barriers to treatment. Options for treatment other than medication may be difficult for a primary care provider to access. A peer support specialist thus may offer a reasonable solution to provide the additional support needed for both doctor and patient. Peer support workers represent a previously unused resource to support the patient, the healthcare staff and the providers, particularly for patients whose care needs do not fall within usual primary care treatment protocols [53].

As primary care providers expand usual care to incorporate targeted care for substance use disorder, some have opted to include peer support specialists into care models. Utilizing social network analyses of qualitative data, Siantz and Rice [1] explored the roles peer support specialists can play in integrated primary care/ behavioral health teams. The primary activities included wellness coaching, using education and support to facilitate chronic disease management, and helping patients to navigate the health system. In the community-based primary care health centers affiliated with Massachusetts General Hospital, peer support specialists, called Recovery Coaches, were assigned four core responsibilities identified via semi-structured interviews [30]. Each of the major primary care practices was assigned a peer support specialist to work with the patients in that practice. These relationships were initiated via referrals from PCPs or other staff in the practice. Peers' primary goal was to build and maintain collaborative, trust-based relationships with the patients. Once a connection was established, the recovery coaches worked to support behavior change toward goals identified by the patient, assisted patients to employ harm reduction interventions and self-care, and assisted patients to navigate the system, promoting patients' access to medical and other appointments. Wakeman et al. [51] reported outcomes of this model based on a nonrandomized retrospective assessment and demonstrated that patients in a primary care practice with a recovery coach had fewer emergency department visits, and fewer days spent admitted to the hospital, though there were no differences in the number of hospitalizations. Patients in these practices were more likely to be prescribed medications for addiction treatment, and providers in the practices were more likely to prescribe addiction pharmacotherapy given this increased level of support.

Another peer-delivered approach is the Wellness Recovery Action Plan (WRAP) model. In this model, peers are trained to deliver 8–10 weekly sessions of group-based education and support to increase disease self-management. The goal is to help participants take ownership of their own well-being by developing skills to manage symptoms and creating strong support networks to help create and sustain an improved quality of life. The goal is to encourage increased resiliency and well-ness in context of self-directed goal setting and monitoring, with peer support and relaxation response training. Cook and colleagues published studies of RCT using the peer-supported model versus an alternative intervention [54, 55]. In both stud-ies, patients receiving the peer-delivered group intervention model reported an increased ability to cope with challenges and more confidence in their ability to define and reach goals. Objectively, patients in the peer-delivered intervention reported lower need for services and utilized fewer services, including both group and individual treatment. A review of several trials of the WRAP model suggest a reliable positive effect on the participants, particularly in terms of their perceived recovery outcomes. Participants reported increased hope, sense of self-efficacy and overall sense of well-being [56]. However, there was no evidence of sustained improvements in clinical symptoms, which emphasizes the need for ongoing sup-port as patients are learning to manage and cope with these chronic diseases.

In a qualitative study of patient experience in a primary care–based MOUD pro-gram providing buprenorphine, patients report that having someone to deliver psy-chosocial support as part of the program improved the overall experience of care [57]. Patients are more comfortable when the treatment model is patient centered and the patient collaborates closely with the doctor in developing the treatment plan. Peers in recovery have a valuable role in helping the team to develop an effective plan for person-centered care. In a patient-centered approach, the office becomes a non-judgmental space for confidential self-disclosure, especially important when active symptoms of disease such as recurrence of use need to be discussed. Having peers in recovery as part of the team is particularly helpful in these situations, essential in helping to validate the participants' experience of shame and frustration. There may even be a role for peers in helping medical professionals to better understand the lived experience of SUD and to model more effective ways for medical staff to engage with patients. In fact, a study of MOUD implementation in a rural setting highlighted the importance of care management specialists in helping primary care practices develop and manage a successful program [58]. Specialists facilitated access to community-based supports including housing, food access, and transporta-tion. They provided support to navigate through the complex treatment system and their support was associated with greater treatment retention and more effective self-management. While in this study the care management specialists were not identified as peers in recovery, the identified functions of the care management specialists have often been conducted with much success by peer support specialists. The support of peers helps to facilitate the implementation of MOUD in primary care, providing essential support services for both participants and primary care staff.

Considerations and Issues in Implementing Peer Support Services

While peer support specialists add a valuable resource to the primary care team, there are several considerations in designing and integrating PSS services into a primary care practice. Perhaps most importantly, the program must be designed with clear role definitions and expectations of the peer providing the service. Duties and expectations need to be explicit, and there must be clarity about how the peer support work will be integrated into ongoing medical care. Peers need to be an integrated, nonclinical part of the team and viewed by other team members as having a legitimate role and function on the team. Peers' roles and functions need to fit with the team's understanding and beliefs about SUD and treatment [59]. Issues frequently arise when the specifics of the role are not clear to both the medical professionals and the peer, and may also then be unclear to the patient. Will the peer provide linkage to community resources and navigation of the external treatment system or will they primarily be involved in running peer groups in the practice and encouraging treatment adherence? Is the primary responsibility to engage with the patient and provide patient-centered support? Do the medical professionals understand the importance of peer-to-peer confidentiality and trust (outside of mandated reporting for safety)? Are the peer-based resources enough to meet patient need in terms of intensity and duration of contact? [6] When the role of the peer is not clearly defined at the outset, peers can feel disconnected and underutilized [29], which may translate to feeling undervalued. Or peers may feel overwhelmed by an expectation to manage patient needs that exceed their training and experience, in particular mental health needs [30]. It is essential that the role of the PSS on the team, including both expectations and boundaries, is clear to all team members. If not, it will be difficult for peers to understand the boundaries and purpose of engaging with a patient and they may be unable to create an identity as either staff person or peer worker. It will be equally difficult for the care team to integrate the peer effectively.

There may be significant differences between the peer support model and traditional primary care medical models. Conflicts in models operating concurrently on the same team will disrupt care and create tensions. In general, the traditional medical model is inconsistent with recovery principles [25]. Peers introduce and lead change from a strengths-based perspective, supporting the participant to rely on these strengths as they seek to achieve participant-defined goals [59]. In contrast, traditional clinical models are founded on framework of diagnosis and treatment of acute symptoms, and the goal is often framed by a concept of cure. The participant is expected to take a more dependent role rather than to pursue their own goals toward self-management with the support and collaboration of the medical team. The traditional power differential that underpins the medical model interferes with building collaborative work between participant and medical team. The word "patient" itself implies a difference of power and autonomy and is in direct conflict with the principles of the recovery movement. Coercion is not consistent with a recovery environment since forcing compliance implies the patient is not in agreement with the goal or process. Emphasis on traditional boundaries in the clinical setting may also limit peer effectiveness by reducing the peers' ability to use their personal story, thereby reducing participation in the team and limiting their own unique value to the team [3]. This conflict in models can even extend into the documentation process, as peers may to be uncomfortable documenting in an electronic medical record due to trusting relationships with the participants. Peers working in the medical setting may feel as though they are trapped between two worlds that are in conflict as they try to implement recovery support work in a medical setting [25]. To increase the likelihood of a successful recovery process, medical providers must shift from a more traditional "doctor–patient" relationship to a provider–patient collaboration based on shared expertise about the participant's health [25]. The beauty of integrating care for addiction into primary care is that PCPs are more than familiar with providing chronic disease treatment where comanaging symptoms with patients to enhance recurrence prevention is consistent with routine care models.

Success in the PSS role requires adequate preparation and ongoing supportive supervision. Training is now offered in certificate programs, with requirements for many hours of supervised practice post training in order to obtain the certificate. Ongoing professional training is required to maintain the certificate. Training content typically includes developing clear understanding of the culture of recovery and the role of the peer as a support person, an evidence-based understanding of addiction, a general understanding of effective treatment modalities, strong communication skills with different role groups as well as patients, group management skills, and a clear recognition of the importance of understanding and maintaining boundaries [9]. Peers need ongoing supportive supervision from practice staff as well as networks of others in peer-based service roles. Issues like time management, clarifying role expectations, and managing boundaries require ongoing supervisory support [1]. It is essential that peers feel safe and supported in order to function effectively in the medical environment [29]. It has been noted that at times physicians and others remain uncertain about the role of peers in a medical setting, causing them to feel undervalued and dismissed. Peers feel stigmatized and shamed when medical staff lack adequate information and perspective on substance use disorder as a chronic disease [30]. In these situations, team cohesion and collaboration are negatively impacted, possibly compromising team effectiveness and efficiency [60]. Taken together these factors become barriers to effectively integrating peer support staff into medical care teams. In addition, for peers, there is a need to ensure they are continuing to feel supported in their own recovery, highlighting the need for clear role definition, training, guidelines, and oversight.

Administrative support is key to the success of a peer support program in any setting, essential to both program start-up and long-term maintenance [60]. Key stakeholders, including administrative service providers, nursing, security, facility support providers, and clinic leadership must all be willing to support patient-centered, patient-driven care for a peer support program to be successfully integrated. The PSS work will touch employees from across the health system or primary care practice and all must be on board to support the care of the patent with substance use disorder [59]. It is essential to carefully consider the role the PSS will play in the practice model in order to ensure comfort for all team members. Guidelines and policies related to the work of the peer support staff must be carefully considered and modified if needed. Beginning with the initial hiring process continuing throughout the period of employment key aspects of work conditions must be reconsidered in light of the role of a peer, including day-to-day work conditions and expectations, the ongoing supervision and evaluation activities, development of a career path, and support for the wellness of employees in the new role. All policies and procedures must be accessible to both staff and PSS providers.

A number of key factors need to be considered to ensure fairness and equity for the PSS staff. The hiring process needs to be free of subtle forms of racism and inequity, creating a diverse and representative PSS workforce with cultural and linguistic capacity to match the needs of the client/participants. Issues related to previous criminal charges or imprisonment must be addressed as these factors are often a part of the rich history and experience the PSS employee brings to the work. PSS staff may not have extensive typical work histories and may not have experience with the common customs or culture in a clinical or medical workplace. Some may even have had traumatic experiences in these settings. Supportive nonjudgmental conversations to help identify areas of growth or concern need to be part of the planned supervision and oversight for PSS staff, as well as a longer orientation period if needed to help them adjust to the environment. Accommodations might need to be made at times to support the PSS role. On a day-to-day basis, the PSS providers will need basic office resources such as private space to meet a patient, access to private phones, and access to basic equipment such as computer and fax resources. To maximize the impact of the PSS role, all employees in the health center or physicians' office should be familiar with the peer service providers and should know how to access their services since anyone may become aware that a patient is in need. All communication avenues, including text and email communications should be used to help create more opportunities for medical and support staff to link patients to PSS.

PSS health and wellness are key to creating effective peer-based support in the practice. Like all other employees, PSS need to have private, self-initiated access to Employee Assistance Programs (EAP) so they can access supports and services as needed. It can be difficult to seek support when you are identified as a caregiver, so it may be important to introduce PSS staff to EAP services or identify specific EAP providers who facilitate the outreach. In addition, it is necessary to plan how to support PSS staff when they need time out of the office to seek care. Generally available resources, such as time provided by the Family and Medical Leave Act (FMLA), should be explicitly reviewed with PSS providers and easily accessed when needed, either in blocks of time or in a more distributed model, for example, 2 h/week over a longer period to facilitate obtaining care. Human resources and occupational health policies and procedures need to be reviewed carefully to be correctly interpreted and applied to this novel group of employees.

Over time, it is important to explicitly consider the effectiveness of the role, and to redefine and modify the role as opportunities to improve the service become clear. Communication between team members including peer team members is essential for developing and refining effective, coordinated care [60]. Ongoing oversight is also essential to guide the program through challenges. Sustaining adequate funding becomes an important challenge to insure the program continues. Once the program is underway, commitment must be sustained in order to maintain the program.

A Word About Financing Peer Support Services

Financial sustainability is a concern in establishing any program. Peer-based services were initially largely volunteer services, but beginning in 2002, federal and state grants and other funding programs have been available to support peer-based services. Beginning in 2007, peer support services were recognized as billable services by the Center for Medicaid and Medicare. In 2014, reimbursable peer delivered services were expanded to include preventive services [61]. Programs have largely been funded and administered by SAMHSA, including Recovery Community Services Program, Access to Recovery (ATR), and Community Peer Support Centers. These programs have led the way in supporting innovative efforts to incorporate peer-based roles into appropriate settings. Many of these initiatives have been extended and expanded through a variety of innovative funding mechanisms including state and municipal resources like block grants and general funds, private and managed healthcare entities, and medical/behavioral health providers [7, 62]. To date, despite wide acceptance and expansion of peer-based services the balance on the cost–benefit ratio remains uncertain and additional research is needed for clarification [6]. With the rising opioid overdose crisis, there has been increasing concern about the fragmented care delivery system in place for substance use disorders. As discussed previously, this fragmentation in part sparked the expansion of peer support services [21]. As White and Smith [63] note, the system incentivizes care for the most acutely ill but inadequately supports the long-term care needed to manage a chronic condition like substance use disorder. Perhaps a more effective approach would be to create incentives for outcomes-based care across the care continuum, supporting participants to manage the course of recovery most effectively. They suggest the creation of care recovery teams, including medical and mental health providers, and featuring a central role for peer support specialists. These teams would be integrated and would coordinate care between medical and community-based resources. The person seeking recovery would have a comprehensive treatment plan created collaboratively with the care team. This would require a multiyear economic model, recognizing the value of a variety of supports. Primary care providers would be central to this sort of approach, and peer support specialists would drive much of the implementation for the medical and/or behavioral health providers. This plan draws on the unique role of peers in the recovery process, and the cost of the PSS would be essentially underwritten by the offset of reduced acute medical care costs. Perhaps the time is right to explore the utility of this sort of approach.

Conclusion

Peer support for the process of recovery, as defined by the participant, is an old idea reimagined and made new again. In a variety of settings providing both medical and behavioral healthcare, connection to others with lived experience provides essential support and guidance through a complicated process of recovery to wellness.

Employing a strengths-based perspective, peer support professionals help participants develop recovery resources and skills to achieve and maintain their recovery goals. Those who have lived with substance use disorder bring a level of understanding and credibility to the work that allows for greater hope and trust to develop with participants. Peers can also be a highly valuable resource for the care team, offering insight and guidance as key members of the team.

Although much more research is needed to clarify the best models for peer support in different settings, there is a growing consensus on the role, function, and general competencies for an effective peer support service. Peers provide collaborative support to help participants achieve improved general health, stable housing and environmental supports, linkage to community and social supports, and clarify their personal meaning and purpose in life. Peers are a key part of the care team, utilizing their own recovery experiences to provide understanding support and guidance while being role models as they manage and sustain their own recoveries. Employers must provide adequate tools and space for peers to conduct their work, in addition to essential supervision and unflagging support as peers collaborate with care teams to build these new approaches and treatment models.

Primary care settings offer a particularly rich opportunity to employ PSS in the work of helping patients achieve stable recovery. With an orientation to helping people achieve and sustain health and wellness over time, primary care settings are an ideal setting to incorporate peer-based services in collaboration with ongoing medical care. Although there are implementation challenges with integrating this novel role in a medical setting, management of chronic disease is a core element to any primary care practice, and substance use disorder care is well suited to this approach. Peers offer a largely untapped opportunity to help support PCPs in providing the best, long-term care possible for substance use disorders. As the battle with opioid use disorder as well as other substance use disorders rages on, the opportunity to enlist peers who have lived experience in the care of patients currently coping with active substance use problems provides a hopeful addition to the existing care options.

References

1. Siantz E, Rice E, Henwood B, Palinkas L. Where do peer providers fit into newly integrated mental health and primary care teams? A mixed methods study. Admin Pol Ment Health. 2018;45(4):538–49.
2. Kelly JF, White W, editors. Addiction recovery management: theory, research and practice. Humana Press: New York; 2011. p. 67–84.
3. Gillard SG, Edwards C, Gibson SL, Owen K, Wright C. Introducing peer worker roles into United Kingdom mental health service teams: a qualitative analysis of the organizational benefits and challenges. BMC Health Serv Res. 2013;13:188.
4. Peer providers [Internet]. Washington DC: SAMSHA-hrsa center for integrated health solutions. Roles of peer providers in integrated health. 2018 (Cited 2019 December 18). Available from: https://www.integration.samhsa.gov/workforce/team-members/peer-providers
5. Bassuk EL, Hanson J, Greene RN, Richard M, Laudet A. Peer-delivered recovery support services for addictions in the United States: a systematic review. J Subst Abus Treat. 2016;63:1–9.

6. Eddie D, Hoffman L, Vilsaint C, Abry A, Bergman B, Hoeppner B, Weinstein C, Kelly JF. Lived experience in new models of care for substance use disorder: a systematic review of peer recovery support services and recovery coaching. Front Psychol. 2019;10:1052. https://doi.org/10.3389/fpsyg.2019.01052.

7. Myrick K, Del Vecchio O. Peer support services in the behavioral healthcare workforce: state of the field. Psych Rehab J. 2016;39(3):197–203.

8. Substance abuse and mental health services administration [Internet]. Washington, DC: bringing recovery supports to scale – technical assistance center; 2017. Peers supporting recovery from substance use disorders. [Cited 2020 February 5]. Available from: https://www.samhsa.gov/sites/default/files/programs_campaigns/brss_tacs/peers-supporting-recovery-substance-use-disorders-2017.pdf

9. Paul G, Smith SM, Whitford D, O'Kelly F, Dowd T. Development of a complex intervention to test the effectiveness of peer support in type 2 diabetes. BMC Health Serv Res. 2007;7:136.

10. Peimani M, Monjazebi F, Ghodssi-Ghassemabadi R. A peer support intervention in improving glycemic control in patients with type 2 diabetes. Patient Educ Couns. 2018;101:460–6.

11. Johansson T, Keller S, Sonnichsen AC, Weitgasser R. Cost analysis of a peer support programme for patients with type 2 diabetes: a secondary analysis of a controlled trial. Eur J Pub Health. 2017;27(2):256–61.

12. Yin J, Wong R, Shimen A, Chung H, Lau M, Lin L, Tsang C, Lau K, Ozaki R, So W, Ko G, Luk A, Yueng R, Chan JCN. Effects of providing peer support on diabetes management in people with type 2 diabetes. Ann Fam Med. 2015;13(Suppl 1):S42–9.

13. Latka MH, Hagan H, Kapadia F, Golub ET, Bonner S, Campbell JV, Coady MH, Garfein RS, Pu M, Thomas DL, Thiel TK, Strathdee SA. A randomized intervention trial to reduce the lending of used injection equipment among injection drug users infected with hepatitis C. Am J Public Health. 2008;98:853–61.

14. Velasquez MM, von Sternberg K, Johnson DH, Green C, Carbonari JP, Parsons JT. Reducing sexual risk behaviors and alcohol use among HIV-positive men who have sex with men: a randomized control trial. J Consult Clin Psych. 2009 Aug;77(4):657–67.

15. Cabral HJ, Davis-Plourde K, Sarango M, Fox J, Palmisano J, Rajabium S. Peer support and the HIV continuum of care: results from a multi-site randomized clinical trial in three urban clinics in the United States. AIDS Behav. 2018;22:2627–39.

16. Mark D, Hrapcak S, Ameyan W, Lovich R, Ronan A, Schmitz K, Hatane L. Peer support for adolescents and young people living with HIV in sub-Saharan Africa: emerging insights and a methodological agenda. Cur HIV/AIDS Rep. 2019;16:467–74.

17. Substance abuse and mental health services administration [Internet]. Washington, DC: bringing recovery supports to scale – technical assistance center; 2017. Peers supporting recovery from mental health disorders. [Cited 2020 February 5]. Available from: https://www.samhsa.gov/sites/default/files/programs_campaigns/brss_tacs/peers-supporting-recovery-mental-health-conditions-2017.pdf

18. Chinman M, George P, Dougherty RH, Daniels AS, Ghose SS, Swift A, Delphin-Rittmon ME. Peer support services for individuals with serious mental illnesses: assessing the evidence. Psychiatr Serv. 2014;65(4):429–41.

19. Pfeiffer PN, Heisler M, Piette JD, Rogers MAM, Valenstein M. Efficacy of peer support interventions for depression. Gen Hosp Psychiatry. 2010;33:29–36.

20. Kelly JF, Stout R, Magill M, Tonigan JS. The role of Alcoholics Anonymous in mobilizing adaptive social network changes: a prospective lagged mediational analysis. Drug Alcohol Depend. 2011;114:119–26.

21. White WL. Nonclinical addiction recovery support services: history, rationale, models, potentials, and pitfalls. Alcohol Treat Q. 2010;28(3):256–72.

22. Krentzman AR, Robinson EA, Moore BC, Kelly JF, Laudet AB, White WL, Zemore SE, Kurtz E, Strobbe S. How Alcoholics Anonymous (AA) and Narcotics Anonymous (NA) work: cross-disciplinary perspectives. Alcohol Treat Q. 2010;29(1):75–84.

23. Tonigan JS, Pearson MR, Magill M, Hagler KJ. AA attendance and abstinence for dually diagnosed patients: a meta-analytic review. Addiction. 2018;113:1970–81.

24. Caldwell BA, Sclafani M, Swarbrick M, Piren K. Psychiatric nursing practice and the recovery model of care. J Psychosoc Nurs Ment Health Serv. 2010;48(7):42–8.
25. Byrne L, Happell B, Reid-Searl K. Lived experience practitioners and the medical model: World's colliding? J Ment Health. 2016;25(3):217–23.
26. Burns J, Marks D. Can recovery capital predict addiction problem severity? Alcohol Treat Q. 2013;31(3):303–20.
27. Cano I, Best D, Edwards M, Lehman J. Recovery capital pathways: modelling the components of recovery wellbeing. Drug Alcohol Depend. 2017;181:11–9.
28. White WL, The PRO-ACT ethic workshop, with legal discussion, Popovits R, Donahue B. Ethical guidelines for the delivery of peer-based recovery support services. Philadelphia: Philadelphia Department of Behavioral Health and Mental Retardation Services; 2007.
29. MacLillan J, Surey J, Abubakar I, Stagg HR. Peer support workers in health: a qualitative metasynthesis of the experiences. PLoS One. 2015;10(10):e014112.
30. Jack H, Oller D, Kelly J, Magidson J, Wakeman S. Addressing substance use disorder in primary care: the role, integration, and impact of recovery coaches. Subst Abuse. 2018;39(3):307–14.
31. Substance abuse and mental health services administration [Internet]. Washington, DC: 2019. Recovery and recovery support. 2019. [Cited: 2020 January 3]. Available from: https://www.samhsa.gov/find-help/recovery
32. Substance abuse and mental health services administration [Internet]. Washington, DC: bringing recovery supports to scale – technical assistance center, 2017. Recovery support tools – core competencies for peer workers. 2018. [Cited 2020 January 21]. Available from: https://www.samhsa.gov/brss-tacs/recovery-support-tools/peers/core-competencies-peer-workers
33. Daniels AS, Bergeson S, Myrick KJ. Defining peer roles and status among community health workers and peer support specialists in integrated systems of care. Psychiatr Serv. 2017;68(12):1296–8.
34. White WL. Peer based addiction recovery support: history, theory, practice, and scientific evaluation. Great Lakes Addiction Technology Center: Philadelphia Department of Behavioral Health and Mental Retardation Services; 2009.
35. Miller WM, Rollnick SR. Motivational interviewing: helping people change. 3rd ed. New York: Guilford Press; 2013.
36. Reif S, Braude L, Lyman DR, Dougherty RH, Daniels AS, Ghose SS, Salim O, Delphin-Rittmon ME. Peer recovery support for individuals with substance use disorders: assessing the evidence. Psychiatr Serv. 2014;65(7):853–61.
37. Barker SL, Maguire N, Bishop FL, Stopa L. Peer support critical elements and experiences in supporting the homeless: a qualitative study. J Community Appl Soc Psychol. 2018;28(4):213–29.
38. Scott CK, Dennis ML, Foss MA. Utilizing recovery management checkups to shorten the cycle of relapse, treatment reentry, and recovery. Drug Alcohol Depend. 2005;78(3):325–38.
39. Scott CK, Dennis ML, Grella CE, Kurz R, Sumpter J, Nicholson L, Funk RR. A community outreach intervention to link individuals with Opioid Use Disorder to medication-assisted treatment. J Subst Abus Treat. 2020;108:75–81.
40. Tracy K, Wallace SP. Benefits of peer support groups in treatment of addiction. Subst Abus Rehabil. 2016;7:143–54.
41. Tracy K, Burton M, Nich C, Rousaville B. Utilizing peer mentorship to engage high recidivism substance abusing patients in treatment. Am J Drug Alcohol Abuse. 2011;37(6):525–31.
42. Krawczyk N, Negron T, Nieto M, Agus D, Fingerhood MI. Overcoming medication stigma in peer recovery: a new paradigm. Subst Abus. 2018;39(4):404–9.
43. McGuire AB, Powell KG, Treitler PC, Wagner KD, Smith KP, Cooperman N, Robinson L, Carter J, Ray B, Watson DP. Emergency department peer-based support for opioid use disorder: emergent functions and forms. J Subst Abuse Treat. 2020;108:82–7.
44. Waye KM, Goyer J, Dettor D, Mahoney L, Samuels EA, Yedinak JL, Marshall BDL. Implementing peer recovery services for overdose prevention in Rhode Island: an examination of two outreach -based approaches. Addic Behav. 2019;89:85–91.

45. D'Agostino AR, Optican AR, Sowles SJ, Krauss MJ, Lee KE, Cavazos-Rehg PA. Social networking online to recover from opioid use disorder: a study of community interactions. Drug Alcohol Depend. 2017;181:5–10.
46. Possemato K, Johnson EM, Bronte Emery J, Wade M, Acosta MC, Marsch LA, Rosenblum A, Maisto SA. A pilot study of comparing peer supported web-based CBT to self-managed web CBT for primary care veterans with PTSD and hazardous alcohol use. Psychiatr Rehabil J. 2019;42(3):305–13.
47. Blonigan DM, Harris-Olenak B, Haber JR, Kuhn E, Timko C, Humphries K, Dulin P. Customizing a clinical app to reduce hazardous drinking among veterans in primary care. Psychol Serv. 2018;16(2):250–4.
48. O'Connell MJ, Flanagan EH, Delphin-Rittmon ME, Davidson L. Enhancing outcomes for persons with co-occurring disorders through skills training and peer recovery support. J Ment Health. 2017;29(1):6–11.
49. Smelson DA, Kline A, Kuhn J, Rodrigues S, O'Connor K, Fisher W, Sawh L, Kane V. A wrap-around treatment engagement intervention for homeless veterans with co-occurring disorders. Psychol Serv. 2013;10(2):161–7.
50. Rowe M, Bellamy C, Baranoski M, Wieland M, O'Connell MJ, Benedict P, Davidson L, Buchanan J, Sells D. A peer-support group intervention to reduce substance use and criminality among persons with severe mental illness. Psychiatr Serv. 2007;58(7):955–61.
51. Wakeman SE, Rigotti NA, Change Y, Herman GE, Erwin A, Regan S, Metlay J. Effect of integrating substance use disorder treatment into primary care on inpatient and emergency departments utilization. J Gen Intern Med. 2019;34(6):871–7.
52. Kulik W, Shah A. Role of peer support workers in improving patient experience in Tower Hamlets Specialist Addiction Unit. BMJ Qual Improv Rep. 2016;5(1):u205967.w2458. https://doi.org/10.1136/bmjquality.u205967.w2458.
53. Perez J, Kidd J. Peer support workers : an untapped resource in primary mental health care. J Prim Health Care. 2015;7(1):84–7.
54. Cook JA, Copeland ME, Jonikas JA, Hamilton M, Razzano LA, Grey DD. Results of a randomized controlled trial of mental illness self-management using Wellness Recovery Action Planning. Schizophr Bull. 2012;38(4):881–91.
55. Cook JA, Jonikas JA, Hamilton MM, Goldrick V, Steigman PJ, Grey DD, Burke L, Carter TM, Razzano LA, Copeland ME. Impact of wellness recovery action planning on service utilization and need in a randomized controlled trial. Psychiatr Rehabil J. 2013;36(4):250–7.
56. Canacott L, Moghaddam N, Tickle A. Is the wellness recovery action plan (WRAP) efficacious for improving personal and clinical recovery outcomes? A systematic review and meta-analysis. Psychiatr Rehabil J. 2019;42(4):372–81.
57. Fox AD, Masyukova M, Cunningham CO. Optimizing psychosocial support during office-based buprenorphine treatment in primary care: patients' experiences and preferences. Subst Abus. 2016;37(1):70–5.
58. Cochran C, Cole EC, Warwick J, Donohue JM, Gordon AJ, Gellad WF, Bear T, Kelley D, DiDomenico E, Pringle J. Rural access to MAT in Pennsylvania (RAMP): a hybrid implementation study protocol for medication assisted treatment adoption among rural primary care providers. Addict Sci Clin Pract. 2019;14(1):25.
59. Ehrlich C, Slattery M, Vilic C, Chester P, Crompton D. What happens when peer support workers are introduced as members of community-based clinical mental health service delivery teams: a qualitative study. J Interprof Care. 2020;34(1):107–15.
60. Shepardson RL, Johnson EM, Possemato K, Arigo D, Funderburk JS. Perceived barriers and facilitators to implementation of peer support in veterans' health administration primary care-mental health integration settings. Psychol Serv. 2019;16(3):433–44.
61. Center for integrated health solutions [Internet]. Washington DC: substance use and mental health services administration-health resources services administration. Peer providers: billing for peer provided integrated health services. Cited 2020 Mar. Available from https://www.integration.samhsa.gov/workforce/team-members/peer-providers

62. Faces and voices of recovery [Internet]. Washington DC: faces and voices of recovery; 2010 sept. Addiction recovery peer service roles: recovery management in health reform. [Cited 2020 Jan 10]. Available from www.facesandvoicesofrecovery.org
63. Williams G, Smith DE. Treatment of addiction: incentivizing recovery, not relapse. Healthc Financ Manage. 2019;25:1–6.

Supporting Any Positive Change: Harm Reduction as an Integral Pillar of Opioid Use Disorder Treatment

Kimberly L. Sue

Philosophy and Principles of Harm Reduction

"Harm reduction" is both a philosophy and a set of concrete practices and interventions that can be applied to substance use as well as other behaviors that have health-related harms. Principles of harm reduction include health and dignity, participant-centered services, participant involvement, participant autonomy, addressing sociocultural factors, and pragmatism and realism. Many clinicians have rightly pointed out that the provision of excellent clinical care entails harm reduction principles generally and could otherwise be called safety optimization or risk reduction. As clinicians across all fields of medicine, we attempt to ascertain what exact behaviors patients are engaging in and we work with patients to educate them and develop plans to minimize possible harms. Stopping these behaviors entirely may be the safest but not feasible or viable for the patient; our mandate is to educate and support patients.

Harm reduction understands substance use occurs along a spectrum ranging from and inclusive of abstinence to managed use to chaotic use. Using patient's goals and direction for their own individual recovery, clinicians can help patients achieve safer use, higher levels of social functioning, and connection. Harm reduction is inclusive of abstinence and people who are in recovery and does not stand in opposition to treatment.

"Meeting people where they're at" is one way of understanding this philosophy with the caveat to "not leave them there." Dan Bigg of Chicago Recovery Alliance, a harm reduction pioneer, defined harm reduction as "any positive change." If a person is not interested or able to decrease injection heroin use but stops sharing syringes with other people or obtains new sterile syringes instead of reusing them, these are important steps toward healthier behaviors. Many people who use or have

K. L. Sue (✉)
Harm Reduction Coalition, New York, NY, USA
e-mail: sue@harmreduction.org

© Springer Nature Switzerland AG 2021
S. E. Wakeman, J. D. Rich (eds.), *Treating Opioid Use Disorder in General Medical Settings*, https://doi.org/10.1007/978-3-030-80818-1_10

used drugs have faced stigma, lack of empathy and compassion, neglect of pain, or even abuse at the hands of healthcare providers. In contrast, harm reduction programs do not proscribe specific behaviors but rather accept individuals with non-judgment, treat them with respect, dignity and compassion, and continue to offer stigma-free service provision.

The history of formal harm reduction programs for substance use began in Europe with a range of interventions from syringe exchange programs to supervised drug consumption rooms and heroin-assisted treatment. The first documented needle or syringe exchange programs began in Amsterdam in 1984 as a Hepatitis B and HIV prevention strategy; these programs soon made their way to the United States. The first pilot needle exchange program in New York City began in 1988 and others began at the same time in Tacoma, Washington, and New Haven, Connecticut, led by HIV activists, people who used drugs, and allied researchers [1].

It is important to frame harm reduction as an intersectional movement with racial justice, reproductive and gender justice, worker justice and disability justice frameworks as well as within broader campaigns for health access and equity [2]. The "War on Drugs" in the United States has been founded on racist and xenophobic beliefs that became writ into policy and law at local, state, and federal levels [3, 4]. Part of a harm reduction approach entails assessing and intervening on the structural violence and upstream social determinants of health, including adverse childhood experiences, poverty, racism, and trauma, that can contribute to risk of chaotic substance use and addiction.

Harm Reduction for Opioid Use Disorder

There are several possible routes of administration for opioids (insufflation; oral ingestion; intramuscular, subcutaneous, or intravenous injection; and rectal absorption). Each route of administration has specific onset, durations of action, and risks for users. Unfortunately, few studies have directly assessed different routes of administration for relative safety. Strategies for safer use are discussed below.

Insufflation

Intranasal use of opioids or insufflation (commonly known as sniffing or inhalation of drugs into the lower part of the nares, or snorting, where drugs are absorbed in the upper part of the nares through either use of a straw or a dollar bill) is a common route of administration. Snorting has relatively quick onset of effect, however, is slower onset than intravenous. Both snorting and sniffing can cause damage to nasal septum, including perforation, ulceration, and necrosis as well as damage to the palate and pharynx, with sinusitis, rhinitis, pain, and/or purulent sputum [5]. Insufflation of heroin has also been reported as a trigger for respiratory issues such as asthma exacerbation [6].

Insufflation of opioids is considered one of the safer routes of administration of opioids; however, overdose can still occur and transmission of Hepatitis C Virus (HCV) is possible if sharing equipment such as straws [7, 8]. Harm reduction strategies for people sniffing or snorting include going slowly, doing one-fourth to one-half of a bag to test the strength, and using with others that have naloxone. Recommendations for safer insufflation include alternating nostrils and keeping nares hydrated and nasal passages in good condition with ointment, as well as avoiding this route if there is bleeding or evidence of mucosal damage. Some harm reduction programs provide safer snorting kits that include unused plastic straws or spoons of a variety of colors to avoid sharing as well as small plastic cards to prepare drugs.

Enteral/Rectal Administration

Oral/enteral and rectal administration of opioids are other routes of administration. Some people who developed opioid use disorder began with swallowing or "eating" prescription opioid tablets. Rectal administration ("boofing, booty bumping, plugging") is a less utilized route of administration of opioids although some people use this route of administration for stimulants and alcohol [9]. The substance is made water soluble and injected or inserted into the rectum or anal canal via a needle-less syringe, where it is absorbed through rectal mucosal vasculature. Rectal administration of opioids has been used as a means of pain control for palliative care. Bioavailability of rectal administration is variable between individuals and depends on location of drug administration, since the lower part of the rectum avoids first-pass metabolism draining directly to the inferior vena cava (quicker onset of drug effect), while the upper rectal veins drain into the portal vein circulation [10, 11].

Harm reduction for rectal administration requires discussing that patients avoid this route of administration if there are obvious rectal tears or fissures, hemorrhoids, or tissue damage. Insertion of any foreign body into the gastrointestinal tract can damage tissues and surrounding structures as well as increase the risk of transmission of HIV or other STI. Hand hygiene, counseling on regular condom use, as well as Hepatitis A and B vaccinations are recommended for patients using this route of administration. Finally, it is important to counsel patients to use a one-fourth to one-half of what they would otherwise take in via insufflation especially as there can be unpredictable potency and effect.

Smoking

Smoking opioids is one route of administration that people utilize. Historically, in the 1800s, it was not uncommon for people to smoke opium with pipes; this entailed heating pieces of opium with coals, with subsequent vapor traveling down the pipe to be inhaled by the user. In many of the contemporary heroin-assisted treatment (HAT) programs, in the Netherlands, Switzerland, and Germany, some heroin users choose to smoke heroin. It is important to recognize the differences between forms of opioids regarding smoking and/or vaporization. Heroin available in the United States is usually either Colombian-sourced heroin hydrochloride salt or black tar heroin. Powder heroin hydrochloride salt tends to burn with heating, which destroys most of the active agent, while black tar will vaporize on gentle heating and can be consumed via inhalation [12].

The smoking/vaporization method is fairly quick in onset, bypassing first-pass metabolism of the gastrointestinal tract and getting extensive absorption within the lung capillary system. However, it is not an economical way to consume opioids as much of the substance can be lost in combustion. Some users prefer smoking in order to titrate or gauge the potency of a supply of a substance; Brugal et al. compared rates of overdose of daily heroin sniffers versus smokers in Spain and found no difference in rates; however, they did note an increased risk of sniffing and overdose than smoking and overdose among sporadic users, perhaps supporting this hypothesis of titratability [13].

Smoking any substance has possible pulmonary effects. Smoking heroin has been linked to cases of leukoencephalopathy, a condition that affects cerebral white matter, with symptoms of ataxia, dysarthria, cognitive changes, and possible coma/death, first reported in 1982 in the Netherlands [14].

Despite the potential harms, smoking has been proposed as a safer alternative to injection. One public health campaign in German drug consumption rooms called SMOKE-IT! found that of 165 participants using these rooms in five cities, two-thirds of the individuals sampled tried smoking/inhalation instead of injecting and many felt that smoking was healthier because of the decreased risk of hepatitis or HIV transmission and reduced risk of overdose associated with smoking compared to injecting [15]. People in this study also stated they preferred pre-cut foil squares that were uncoated and heavy duty.

Harm reduction techniques for users smoking/inhaling opioids include aggressive mouthcare with lip balms and hydration, good oral hygiene to prevent cracks or blisters to the mouth and using one's own tinfoil or smoking gear (some people use meth pipes to smoke fentanyl). It is important for users of opioids in any route of administration to go slow, avoid mixing, take turns using and to try to use with others who have naloxone and can administer it.

Injection

People who inject drugs use three main routes of administration: subcutaneous (SC), intramuscular (IM), or intravenous (IV). Medical harms related to injection can be both local and systemic. Local damage can include trauma to venous, arterial, or nerve structures as well as skin and soft tissue infections, such as abscess and cellulitis, pyomyositis, or even necrotizing fasciitis. Systemic complications can include viral infections, such as HIV, Hepatitis A, B, C, and endovascular infections, including bacteremia, infective endocarditis, osteomyelitis, and septic arthritis. In addition to direct infectious risks from skin or bloodstream infections, people who inject drugs are at increased risk for pulmonary disease (pneumonia, septic embolization, increased risk of tuberculosis), increased risks of accident/trauma, and nonfatal or fatal overdose. Common infectious complications (bacterial, viral, and fungal) related to injection drug use are reviewed in detail elsewhere [16]. All equipment used to prepare drugs including syringes (barrel and needles, fixed or detachable), cookers used to prepare or contain drug solutions and filters (cotton, sterifilt, wheel filters) can create an environment for HIV; Hepatitis B; Hepatitis C; and bacterial, viral, or fungal infections [17–19].

For clinicians taking care of people who are injecting drugs, it is critical to take a detailed nonjudgmental history of how, what substances are utilized, and where the person is injecting in order to counsel patients on risk reduction techniques. Risks of injection should take into account the "drug, set, and setting model" proposed by Norman Zinberg [20]. Some of the risks of both local and systemic harms of injection drug use can be mitigated if people have access to supplies, time, space, and education to practice sterile technique with every injection. Social, legal and environmental factors can all affect the ability of someone to practice optimal sterile technique.

Factors to consider and offer counseling and education around safer injection techniques regarding drug, set, and setting include does the person have time, light, space, knowledge to practice sterile technique (a supervised drug consumption room versus a public bathroom), is the person in withdrawal (discomfort could lead to rushed injecting), does the person have access to a steady supply of sterile supplies (is syringe access restrictive or illegal in the state the person lives, or has the person been able to access supplies at a local pharmacy), is the person using a quantity of drugs alone or with someone else (might influence sharing of syringes or other equipment), does the person have warrants or legal trouble (which could increase risk of using alone or not accessing sterile equipment), or is the person engaging in sex work for drugs or money and is there pressure to engage in sexual activity without condoms.

Finally, there is some evidence that risks depend on what the person is injecting. For example, risks might be very different for people injecting simulants and opioids in the same preparation or if the person is crushing and injecting pharmaceutical tablets such as hydromorphone or oxycodone. Researchers have suggested different risks depending on the local heroin supply: black tar heroin is more frequently used via skin popping or intramuscular injection and is associated with more rapid venous sclerosis and damage and subsequently higher risks of abscess and cellulitis, as opposed to white/brown powder heroin. Powder heroin may be associated with increased risks of HIV because of continued intravenous use [21].

Subcutaneous/Intramuscular Use

Some people use opioids by injecting into the subcutaneous tissue or muscle ("skin popping" or "muscling" respectively). This is sometimes because patients cannot find a vein from sclerosis and scar tissue, but some people may also prefer this route of administration to try to hide or prevent track marks on the skin.

Skin popping has mostly local but also systemic harms [22]. Binswanger et al. found in a study of people with injection drug use that those who skin popped were more likely to have an abscess than those who injected intravenously; the authors hypothesized that the subcutaneous space is particularly conducive to pathogenic bacteria, especially anaerobes [23]. Injecting opioids concurrently with stimulants has been associated with increased risk of abscess, possibly due to local ischemia [24]. Tetanus and wound botulism have been reported with black tar heroin. Most recently, in San Diego County in 2019, there were nine reported cases of botulism, seven whom reported black tar heroin use, and six who engaged in skin popping) [25].

Reducing Risk of Skin and Soft Tissue Infections

Abscess is extremely common, and many people who use drugs do not seek medical attention for abscesses and manage them on their own [26]. One study indicated that of 252 people surveyed with a history of injection drug use, at least 64% reported a skin or soft tissue infection in the previous year, of which one-third reported self-treatment [27]. Reasons cited for not seeking formal medical care included stigma or embarrassment, previous harmful treatment, and dislike or fear of healthcare professionals.

Despite the prevalence of abscess and skin infections, simple and cheap interventions such as hand washing and cleaning skin prior to injection effectively reduce risk and are not uniformly applied. A study in Baltimore of 1057 injectors found that 53% reported cleaning their skin prior to injection and only 31% cleaned the skin area "all the time"; those that reported more frequently skin cleaning noted lower rates of abscess and endocarditis [28].

Harm reduction techniques for patients who are engaging in any injection use include washing hands with hot soap and water for 30–60 s or alternatively using alcohol-based hand rubs, cleaning the skin area vigorously with alcohol wipes, and counseling to always using a new sterile syringe for each injection [29]. Patients who inject intramuscularly should be educated to use big muscle groups such as thighs and upper arms and all patients who inject drugs should be encouraged to avoid areas where there is a high concentration of nerves and bony structures present (wrists, elbows, feet, ankles). Rotating sites is important to allow tissue to heal. Licking needles or holding caps or drugs in the oral cavity while preparing injection should be discouraged as this increases the risk for introduction of oral flora and anaerobes into the bloodstream. Counsel patients not to share syringes, but if they are sharing to split drugs using a third sterile syringe to dispense drugs into two separate sterile syringes or split drugs dry before creating a solution. It is recommended that people heat their drug solution in cookers for at least 10 s or until bubbling which can possibly decrease HIV virus and bacterial inoculum and to try to avoid sharing if possible. Ensure all patients have updated vaccinations including tetanus and Hepatitis A and B.

In the era of pervasive fentanyl in the illicit street supply, recommend "universal fentanyl precautions," where individuals using any drug assume that the supply could be 100% fentanyl. Harm reduction strategies that individuals are using to reduce the higher overdose risk associated with fentanyl include injecting more slowly, using only half the quantity to gauge potency, and to do a "test" dose, where a person injects just a small amount first to test the potency [12]. Using a consistent dealer, fentanyl test strips, and using with others who have naloxone are additional important strategies people have employed [30].

HIV and Hepatitis C

As soon as people who injected drugs (PWID) were identified at risk for transmission in the evolving HIV outbreak of the 1980s in the United States, community activists and researchers worked to establish interventions to prevent HIV transmission. Beginning in the 1980s and 1990s, syringe service programs (SSPs) for PWID were established in cities like New York City, Boston, New Haven, Tacoma, and San Francisco as a means to prevent transmission of infectious disease [1]. In 1993, PWID comprised 31% of people living with HIV. In 2017, according to the CDC, PWID made up 9% of new diagnoses of HIV [31]. The CDC has currently deemed 220 counties across 26 states as currently vulnerable to or experiencing an HIV and HCV outbreaks [32].

Worldwide, syringe service programs are regarded as an evidence-based, effective public health strategy for prevention of HIV [33, 34]. HIV can live in syringes and associated equipment (cookers, rinse cottons used to filter drugs) for days to weeks [18]. Canadian researchers examined the survival of HIV in cookers, since it is a common practice for people to reuse a cooker for drugs left inside ("wash" or "rinse" shot). They found that by heating the drug solution for preferably 10 s or until bubbling, HIV virus was destroyed [19]. These authors further hypothesized that heating the equipment for 10 s effectively decreased inoculum of methicillin-resistant *Staphylococcus aureus* (MRSA) and methicillin-susceptible *Staphylococcus aureus* (MSSA) bacteria in cookers, possibly decreasing endocarditis risk [35].

Given the epidemiology of HIV risk for PWID, there is strong evidence for using post-exposure prophylaxis (PEP) and/or pre-exposure prophylaxis (PrEP) for these patients: good candidates include patients reporting any active injection use, sharing equipment or needles even infrequently, recent recovery, sex work, history of inconsistent or no condom use, or >1 episode of PEP for HIV in the last year, among other criteria outlined by the CDC.

Hepatitis C Virus (HCV) is also of epidemic proportions among people who use drugs. It is estimated that 2.7–5 million people are living with Hepatitis C Virus (HCV) and that 80% of new HCV infections worldwide are among PWID [36]. Untreated HCV has significant complications including progression to cirrhosis and development of hepatocellular carcinoma and subsequent mortality [37]. Unfortunately, diagnosing and linking people with HCV to treatment along the cascade of care in the United States with direct-acting antiviral (DAA) therapy remains low, with only 50% of people infected having a known diagnosis, 16% of patients prescribed treatment, and 9% achieving SVR [38].

HCV is a relatively robust virus that has been demonstrated to live in syringes, filters, cookers, and on injection surfaces for up to 2–9 weeks, depending on environmental conditions and size of equipment and amount of blood [39, 40]. Treating people who are actively injecting drugs and/or sharing injection equipment is not only feasible, it is critical to breaking the cycle of transmission. According to the American Association for the Study of Liver Diseases (AASLD) and Infectious Diseases Society of America (IDSA) guidelines, ongoing substance use or concern for reinfection is not a contraindication to treatment with DAAs [41, 42]. Combination opioid agonist therapy and DAA treatment has excellent, synergistic results for people with a history of injection opioid use and a high percentage of patients are able to achieve sustained virologic response at 12 weeks [43]. Hepatitis B virus also can also be transmitted via sharing syringes; vaccination for both Hepatitis A and B is strongly recommended [44].

Syringe Service Provision

Syringe service provision is not only necessary for prevention of HIV, Hepatitis C, and other infectious diseases, but also for generally improving the care of people who use drugs. However, the legality of syringe service programs varies by municipality and state and federal funds currently cannot be used for the purchase of syringes. Syringe service provision takes many different models: fixed-site programs, mobile, mail-based, pharmacies, and even vending machines. Distribution policies and community relationships will also vary (see Useful Resources – National Alliance of State and Territorial Aids Directors [NASTAD]). Many storefront locations also have drop-in spaces, groups, on-site wound care, safe syringe disposal mechanisms, and access to other sterile supplies for drug preparation. Referrals to or care and treatment for HIV and hepatitis C, addiction treatment, as well as primary care and mental health care also occur routinely.

Federally Qualified Health Centers can become registered as secondary SSPs and can serve as critical access points for sterile supplies for patients who inject drugs. However, it is important for clinicians to know their state laws regarding syringe distribution and possession (see "useful resources"). Developing relationships with local syringe service providers can create a referral system as well as engage patients who might otherwise not access healthcare in traditional settings.

Case Study: Box 1 – Scott County, Indiana – HIV Outbreak and SSPs

In 2014–2015, an HIV outbreak was reported in Austin, Indiana, in a small rural county, Scott County, with 181 new HIV cases reported among a community of 4200 residents. Epidemiologists found that this HIV-1 cluster was linked to sharing syringes within a small community as individuals were crushing, dissolving, and injecting prescription oxymorphone extended-release (ER) tablets [45, 46]. Of these, 80% of those diagnosed with HIV reported injecting drugs and sharing syringes (all of the 108 people reported dissolving and injecting the tablets). Also, 7.4% endorsed engaging in commercial sex work and 84.4% of the people diagnosed with HIV had concurrent HCV coinfection.

Syringe exchange and syringe service provision were not authorized in 2015 in the state of Indiana, and HIV testing had not been available in that community as the local Planned Parenthood had closed in 2013 due to lack of funding. A public health emergency was declared authorizing syringe-service programs and HIV, HCV, and substance use programs. State legislation was passed that allowed counties to request permission to start programs, although local health departments had to declare states of emergency, hold a public hearing, and approve the program.

Upon evaluation of the syringe service programs that were established in Indiana, participants that were HIV-positive as well as HIV-negative indicated they were much more likely to use sterile syringes, dispose of them in official medical waste bins, and less likely to share syringes or equipment [47]. Public health modeling also suggested that sustained early epidemiologic assessment and intervention on an earlier HCV cluster in Indiana in 2010 as well as earlier response to the HIV cluster with sterile syringes, condoms, and contact tracing could have curtailed the number of infections [48, 49].

Naloxone

Naloxone hydrochloride, an opioid antagonist, was first patented in 1961 by Moses Lewenstein and Jack Fishman and approved in 1971 by the FDA for the reversal of opioid overdoses. Naloxone acts as a competitive inhibitor at delta-, kappa-, and mu-opioid binding sites in the brain and throughout the body; the reversal of mu-opioid receptors in the brain can effectively reverse respiratory depression and can prevent subsequent anoxia, cardiac arrest and death caused by opioid overdose. Naloxone works within seconds of administration (with IV, IM, intranasal all providing rapid onset of drug effect). Naloxone has an excellent safety profile: It has very few to no adverse reactions or side effects, no potential for misuse, and causes no harm if opioids are not present.

Common formulations available to laypeople include intramuscular and intranasal, with standard doses of 0.4 mg to 2 mg for the initial dose. Most naloxone kits come with two doses. An autoinjector formulation was approved by the FDA in 2014 at a dose of 2 mg and can deliver additional doses, however, it is not widely available because of cost. Naloxone can be safely administered by members of the lay community who have been trained in opioid overdose prevention as well as by emergency medical services (EMS), police, first responders, nurses, and other healthcare professionals. Despite an ongoing effort by many in the community to make naloxone over the counter, naloxone is currently a prescription medication in the United States.

Widespread community naloxone distribution was pioneered in 1996 by the non-profit harm reduction organization Chicago Recovery Alliance after they lost one of their cofounders to opioid overdose. Vast distribution of naloxone by community advocates working with and led by people who use drugs has led to more than 1 million doses of naloxone distributed in 2019 [50]. It is both cost-effective and a feasible strategy to get naloxone into the hands of lay people in the community. Massachusetts published on its Overdose Education and Naloxone Distribution (OEND) program and demonstrated that among 19 different communities those that had an OEND program for naloxone distribution to bystanders had reduced opioid overdose death rates [51, 52].

In the outpatient setting, getting naloxone to patients with opioid use disorder as well as their friends and family is essential. According to CDC, naloxone prescription or direct dispensation during appointments should be considered for patients receiving >50 morphine milligram equivalents/day, have COPD or OSA, have a history of benzodiazepine use, or a history of substance use disorder [53]. Pharmacy dispensing of naloxone is another critical access point. As of 2016, 44 states allowed naloxone to be prescribed for administration to a person who is not directly that provider's patient; 42 states have some version of a standing order protocol, allowing dispensation that is not patient specific, and 5 states have programs where pharmacists have the authority to dispense naloxone [54]. Some have raised the concern of liability associated with prescribing naloxone. Public health legal review has indicated that legal risks of co-prescribing naloxone for patients receiving opioids are no higher than other medications and could even be lower [55].

For states with syringe service programs, naloxone should be distributed to people who are receiving supplies. Community-based programs can work with departments of health to get medication into the hands of those most likely to administer and utilize it. Innovative programs to get this medication into the hands of people at risk of experiencing or witnessing an overdose also include dispensing directly out of roman emergency department after overdose, EMS or fire leave-behind programs, mobile harm reduction services that deliver to houses, or mail-based distribution to people who cannot otherwise access or afford it. Even in the setting of illicitly manufactured fentanyl and fentanyl analogues in the street drug supply market, two doses of intramuscular or intranasal naloxone are most often sufficient to achieve overdose response [56].

It is important to counsel patients briefly about how to use naloxone and how to recognize signs of an opioid overdose and to engage with them in developing an overdose prevention plan. In the chaos of an overdose situation, individuals may forget to perform rescue breathing, a critical part of the resuscitation effort, or to call for additional support from EMS. It is useful for clinicians to know about whether their state has a Good Samaritan law and what the stipulations of that state law entails. Good Samaritan laws were passed in order to encourage people to get additional medical attention and offered some legal protection against arrest or prosecution (e.g., not arresting people for drug equipment on the scene or for simple drug possession) and have been shown to decrease opioid overdose deaths [57].

Drug Checking

"Drug checking" or drug monitoring programs allow individuals and communities to determine the specific forensic makeup of drugs obtained for personal use utilizing a variety of techniques, ranging from colorimetric reagents to gas chromatography, gas chromatography/mass spectrometry, thin layer chromatography or high-performance liquid chromatography (HPLC). These programs began in the Europe and Australia in the 1990s as part of an effort to determine the composition of drugs such as 3,4-Methylenedioxymethamphetamine (MDMA), lysergic acid diethylamide (LSD), cocaine, or other substances, wherein individuals could either send a sample of drugs to a fixed testing laboratory location or get them tested on-site at a mobile location [58].

Drug checking technology is now being applied to opioids or other psychoactive substances. While illicitly manufactured fentanyl (IMF) has been present for decades in the street drug supply, IMF and its numerous analogues, some of which fall into the category of novel psychoactive substances (NPS), appear to be resurging in street-based markets around the United States. According to the Centers for Disease Control, fentanyl was detected in half of opioid OD deaths in seven of ten states surveyed and potent fentanyl analogues such as carfentanil were detected in >10% of opioid OD deaths in four states [59]. IMF is also rarely but sometimes present in other nonopioids available on street drug markets, such as pills sold or labeled as benzodiazepines, cocaine, or methamphetamines [60].

The FORECAST study evaluated three different technologies to test samples of drugs provided by Baltimore and Provide Police Departments for the presence of fentanyl to determine both validity and feasibility of these tests [61]. The BTNX brand fentanyl test strips were found to have high sensitivity and specificity and are increasingly available in harm reduction programs around the country. They can be used as a qualitative point-of-care where individuals can test drug residue or urine for the presence of fentanyl.

Research from the FORECAST study and other sites has indicated that participants would modify their behavior based on results to include harm reduction practices (including discarding the substance, using with others who have naloxone, going slower, doing a test dose of the product, or changing dealers). Regardless of whether individuals change their behavior, providing education and empowerment for individuals using drugs to know the content of what they are using or consuming is important enough to justify the use of drug checking interventions. However, since this technology is still often not available for most people who are using street drugs, "fentanyl universal precautions" are recommended.

Safe Supply

The theory of the "Iron Law of Prohibition," coined by activist Richard Cowan in 1986, refers to a phenomenon where when a society makes consuming, regulating, or distributing a substance illegal in order to limit supply, paradoxically contributes to the production and transformation of more dangerous, compact, and potent substances in their place [62]. Examples of this theory include the transition from beer to potent spirits during alcohol prohibition, use of synthetic cannabinoids to evade detection of cannabis or marijuana, the emergence of crack cocaine instead of powder cocaine, and fentanyl instead of heroin [63].

The concept of safe supply takes into account this theory. Instead of trying to get patients to stop use of illicit opioids, proponents of safe supply believe that providing a pure and regulated form of the substance could decrease many of the harms related to uncertain potency, contamination, and additional social or legal harms associated with the illicit market. Heroin-assisted programs (HAT) demonstrate the effectiveness of this model by providing pharmaceutical diacetylmorphine for specific patients who were at risk of overdose, illicit use, and crime [64]. HAT has been pioneered in Western Europe for decades, with an early positive trial in Switzerland in 1994.

In North America, the North American Opiate Medication Initiative (NAOMI) and Study to Assess Longer-term Opioid Medication Effectiveness (SALOME) trials demonstrated feasibility of providing a safe supply with injectable full opioid agonists in this geopolitical context [65, 66]. SALOME was a double-blind, noninferiority trial of 200 patients comparing IV diacetylmorphine to IV hydromorphone in British Columbia, Canada, and demonstrated noninferiority of hydromorphone. Crossroads Clinic in Vancouver administers IV hydromorphone for a subset of patients who comes three times a day for self-administration of substances under monitored and observed conditions. Other physicians in Canada are piloting safe supply of opioid medications such as hydromorphone tablets either distributed as directly observed therapy in clinic spaces or even distribution via biometrically managed vending machines.

Supervised Consumption Spaces/Overdose Prevention Centers

Supervised consumption spaces, also known as safe injection facilities, drug consumption rooms, or overdose prevention centers, refer to locations where people bring previously purchased illicit substances to consume in a facility with formal peer or medical supervision. Staff can work quickly to prevent fatal opioid or polysubstance-related overdoses by the rapid administration of oxygen, naloxone, and emergency medical attention. In addition, many programs have low-barrier linkages to treatment programs for opioid agonist therapy, on-site HIV/HCV testing and treatment, access to wound care, and/or primary and mental healthcare or social service referrals.

The first supervised consumption space in the world was started in Berne, Switzerland, for people injecting heroin in 1986 [67]. Currently there are over 120 supervised consumption spaces across Europe, Australia, and Canada. Part of the momentum for such facilities came at the insistence of people actively using drugs who demanded safer spaces for use. An important study comparing overdose fatality rates before and after the opening of Insite, a Vancouver supervised injection facility, documented a significant decrease in fatal opioid mortality in the neighborhood where Insite opened (decreased by 35%), while other neighborhoods in the city saw smaller decreases in fatal overdose rates (9.3%) [68].

In the United States, such a site could technically be a breach of a statute of the federal Controlled Substances Act, wherein any individual who maintains a place for manufacture, distribution, or use of controlled substances could face up to 20 years in prison [69]. However, in 2019, a judge in Philadelphia ruled that a supervised injecting facility as a space that would provide medical care and treatment would not violate this statute. There also is a researched, unsanctioned facility that has been operating in the United States since fall 2014 with zero overdose fatalities at the site since its opening [70, 71].

Several different cost-effectiveness models in the United States have shown that municipalities can save money from this approach, mostly from preventing transmission of HIV/HCV, as well as potential hospitalizations and ambulance calls for overdose, overdose death, and other injection-related health harms [72, 73]. A systematic review found that the presence of a supervised injection site does not increase crime or drug use and that sites are helpful in engaging structurally marginalized people, increasing rates of primary care uptake and education of safer injection techniques [74].

Conclusion

There are many ways clinicians can engage with and improve the healthcare of people who use drugs. These include strategies within an office visit based on harm reduction principles as well as supporting and networking with local syringe service providers and community organizations serving people who use drugs. Recognizing that local and state policies vary, it is critical for clinicians to both become informed about regional laws (such as local syringe possession and Good Samaritan laws) and advocate for improved public health legislation.

Useful Resources

Law Atlas – Syringe Distribution Laws http://lawatlas.org/datasets/syringe-policies-laws-regulating-non-retail-distribution-of-drug-parapherna

NASTAD SSP Guidelines – https://www.nastad.org/sites/default/files/resources/docs/055419_NASTAD-SSP-Guidelines-August-2012.pdf

Getting Off Right – Harm Reduction Coalition https://harmreduction.org/drugs-and-drug-users/drug-tools/getting-off-right/

Quality Healthcare Is Your Right – Harm Reduction Coalition https://harmreduction.org/issue-area/issue-drugs-drug-users/quality-health-care-is-your-right/

Fentanyl test strips – Harm Reduction Coalition https://harmreduction.org/issues/fentanyl/

CDC PrEP for IVDU https://www.cdc.gov/hiv/pdf/risk/prep/cdc-hiv-prep-guidelines-2017.pdf

Bibliography

1. Des Jarlais DC. Harm reduction in the USA: the research perspective and an archive to David Purchase. Harm Reduct J. 2017;14(1):51.
2. Crenshaw K. Mapping the margins: intersectionality, identity politics, and violence against women of color. Stanford Law Rev. 1991;43(6):1241.
3. Courtwright DT. Dark paradise: a history of opiate addiction in America. Enlarged ed. Cambridge: Harvard University Press; 2001. p. 352.
4. Netherland J, Hansen HB. The war on drugs that wasn't: wasted whiteness, "dirty doctors," and race in media coverage of prescription opioid misuse. Cult Med Psychiatry. 2016;40(4):664–86.
5. Peyrière H, Léglise Y, Rousseau A, Cartier C, Gibaja V, Galland P. Necrosis of the intra-nasal structures and soft palate as a result of heroin snorting: a case series. Subst Abuse. 2013;34(4):409–14.
6. Krantz AJ, Hershow RC, Prachand N, Hayden DM, Franklin C, Hryhorczuk DO. Heroin insuf-flation as a trigger for patients with life-threatening asthma*. Chest. 2003;123(2):510–7.
7. Aaron S, McMahon JM, Milano D, Torres L, Clatts M, Tortu S, et al. Intranasal transmission of hepatitis C virus: virological and clinical evidence. Clin Infect Dis. 2008;47(7):931–4.
8. Fernandez N, Towers CV, Wolfe L, Hennessy MD, Weitz B, Porter S. Sharing of snorting straws and hepatitis C virus infection in pregnant women. Obstet Gynecol. 2016;128(2):234–7.
9. Rivers Allen J, Bridge W. Strange routes of administration for substances of abuse. Am J Psychiatry Resid J. 2017;12(12):7–11.
10. Stevens RA, Ghazi SM. Routes of opioid analgesic therapy in the management of cancer pain. Cancer Control. 2000;7(2):132–41.
11. Kestenbaum MG, Vilches AO, Messersmith S, Connor SR, Fine PG, Murphy B, et al. Alternative routes to oral opioid administration in palliative care: a review and clinical sum-mary. Pain Med. 2014;15(7):1129–53.
12. Mars SG, Ondocsin J, Ciccarone D. Toots, tastes and tester shots: user accounts of drug sam-pling methods for gauging heroin potency. Harm Reduct J. 2018;15:26.
13. Brugal MT, Barrio G, Fuente LDL, Regidor E, Royuela L, Suelves JM. Factors associated with non-fatal heroin overdose: assessing the effect of frequency and route of heroin administration. Addiction. 2002;97(3):319–27.
14. Buxton JA, Sebastian R, Clearsky L, Angus N, Shah L, Lem M, et al. Chasing the dragon – characterizing cases of leukoencephalopathy associated with heroin inhalation in British Columbia. Harm Reduct J. 2011;8(1):3.
15. Stöver HJ, Schäffer D. SMOKE IT! Promoting a change of opiate consumption pattern – from injecting to inhaling. Harm Reduct J. 2014;11(1):18.
16. Gordon RJ, Lowy FD. Bacterial infections in drug users. N Engl J Med. 2005;353(18):1945–54.
17. Keijzer L, Imbert E. The filter of choice: filtration method preference among injecting drug users. Harm Reduct J. 2011;8(1):20.
18. Abdala N, Reyes R, Carney JM, Heimer R. Survival of HIV-1 in syringes: effects of tempera-ture during storage. Subst Use Misuse. 2000;35(10):1369–83.
19. Ball LJ, Venner C, Tirona RG, Arts E, Gupta K, Wiener JC, et al. Heating injection drug preparation equipment used for opioid injection may reduce HIV transmission associated with sharing equipment. JAIDS. 2019;81(4):e127.
20. Zinberg N. Drug, set, and setting: the basis for controlled intoxicant use. 1st ed. New Haven/ London: Yale University Press; 1986. 277 p.
21. Ciccarone D, Bourgois P. Explaining the geographical variation of HIV among injection drug users in the United States. Subst Use Misuse. 2003;38(14):2049–63.
22. Saporito RC, Lopez Pineiro MA, Migden MR, Silapunt S. Recognizing skin popping scars: a complication of illicit drug use. Cureus [Internet]. [cited 2020 Feb 15];10(6). Available from: https://www.ncbi.nlm.nih.gov/pmc/articles/PMC6070054/
23. Binswanger IA, Kral AH, Bluthenthal RN, Rybold DJ, Edlin BR. High prevalence of abscesses and cellulitis among community-recruited injection drug users in San Francisco. Clin Infect Dis. 2000;30(3):579–81.

24. Murphy EL, DeVita D, Liu H, Vittinghoff E, Leung P, Ciccarone DH, et al. Risk factors for skin and soft-tissue abscesses among injection drug users: a case-control study. Clin Infect Dis. 2001;33(1):35–40.
25. Peak CM. Wound botulism outbreak among persons who use black tar heroin — San Diego County, California, 2017–2018. MMWR Morb Mortal Wkly Rep [Internet]. 2019 [cited 2020 Feb 15];67. Available from: https://www.cdc.gov/mmwr/volumes/67/wr/mm675152a3.htm
26. Fink DS, Lindsay SP, Slymen DJ, Kral AH, Bluthenthal RN. Abscess and self-treatment among injection drug users at four California syringe exchanges and their surrounding communities. Subst Use Misuse. 2013;48(7):523–31.
27. Monteiro J, Phillips KT, Herman DS, Stewart C, Keosaian J, Anderson BJ, et al. Self-treatment of skin infections by people who inject drugs. Drug Alcohol Depend. 2020;206:107695.
28. Vlahov D, Sullivan M, Astemborski J, Nelson KE. Bacterial infections and skin cleaning prior to injection among intravenous drug users. Public Health Rep. 1992;107(5):595–8.
29. Hutin Y, Hauri A, Chiarello L, Catlin M, Stilwell B, Ghebrehiwet T, et al. Best infection control practices for intradermal, subcutaneous, and intramuscular needle injections. Bull World Health Organ. 2003;81(7):491–500.
30. McKnight C, Des Jarlais DC. Being "hooked up" during a sharp increase in the availability of illicitly manufactured fentanyl: adaptations of drug using practices among people who use drugs (PWUD) in New York City. Int J Drug Policy. 2018;60:82–8.
31. Centers for Disease Control and Prevention. HIV surveillance report, 2017; 29. [Internet]. 2018 Nov [cited 2020 Feb 28]. Available from: http://www.cdc.gov/hiv/library/reports/hiv-surveillance.html
32. Van Handel MM, Rose CE, Hallisey EJ, Kolling JL, Zibbell JE, Lewis B, et al. County-level vulnerability assessment for rapid dissemination of HIV or HCV infections among persons who inject drugs, United States. J Acquir Immune Defic Syndr. 2016;73(3):323–31.
33. Larney S, Peacock A, Leung J, Colledge S, Hickman M, Vickerman P, et al. Global, regional, and country-level coverage of interventions to prevent and manage HIV and hepatitis C among people who inject drugs: a systematic review. Lancet Glob Health. 2017;5(12):e1208–20.
34. Fernandes RM, Cary M, Duarte G, Jesus G, Alarcão J, Torre C, et al. Effectiveness of needle and syringe programmes in people who inject drugs – an overview of systematic reviews. BMC Public Health. 2017;17(1):309.
35. Kasper KJ, Manoharan I, Hallam B, Coleman CE, Koivu SL, Weir MA, et al. A controlled-release oral opioid supports S. aureus survival in injection drug preparation equipment and may increase bacteremia and endocarditis risk. PLoS One. 2019;14(8):e0219777.
36. Grebely J, Matthews GV, Lloyd AR, Dore GJ. Elimination of hepatitis C virus infection among people who inject drugs through treatment as prevention: feasibility and future requirements. Clin Infect Dis. 2013;57(7):1014–20.
37. Ly KN, Hughes EM, Jiles RB, Holmberg SD. Rising mortality associated with hepatitis C virus in the United States, 2003–2013. Clin Infect Dis. 2016;62(10):1287–8.
38. Yehia BR, Schranz AJ, Umscheid CA, Iii VLR. The treatment cascade for chronic hepatitis C virus infection in the United States: a systematic review and meta-analysis. PLoS One. 2014;9(7):e101554.
39. Paintsil E, He H, Peters C, Lindenbach BD, Heimer R. Survival of hepatitis C virus in syringes: implication for transmission among injection drug users. J Infect Dis. 2010;202(7):984–90.
40. Doerrbecker J, Behrendt P, Mateu-Gelabert P, Ciesek S, Riebesehl N, Wilhelm C, et al. Transmission of hepatitis C virus among people who inject drugs: viral stability and association with drug preparation equipment. J Infect Dis. 2013;207(2):281–7.
41. Norton BL, Fleming J, Bachhuber MA, Steinman M, DeLuca J, Cunningham CO, et al. High HCV cure rates for people who use drugs treated with direct acting antiviral therapy at an urban primary care clinic. Int J Drug Policy. 2017;47:196–201.
42. Ghany MG, Morgan TR. Hepatitis C Guidance 2019 Update: American Association for the Study of Liver Diseases–Infectious Diseases Society of America Recommendations for Testing, Managing, and Treating Hepatitis C Virus Infection. Hepatology. 2020;71(2):686–721.

43. Dore GJ, Altice F, Litwin AH, Dalgard O, Gane EJ, Shibolet O, et al. Elbasvir-Grazoprevir to treat hepatitis C virus infection in persons receiving opioid agonist therapy: a randomized trial. Ann Intern Med. 2016;165(9):625–34.
44. Burt RD, Hagan H, Garfein RS, Sabin K, Weinbaum C, Thiede H. Trends in hepatitis B virus, hepatitis C virus, and human immunodeficiency virus prevalence, risk behaviors, and preventive measures among Seattle injection drug users aged 18–30 years, 1994–2004. J Urban Health. 2007;84(3):436–54.
45. Conrad C, Bradley H, Broz D, Buddha S. Community outbreak of HIV infection linked to injection drug use of Oxymorphone — Indiana, 2015. Morb Mortal Wkly Rep MMWR. 2015;64(16):443–4.
46. Peters PJ, Pontones P, Hoover KW, Patel MR, Galang RR, Shields J, et al. HIV infection linked to injection use of Oxymorphone in Indiana, 2014–2015. N Engl J Med. 2016;375(3):229–39.
47. Dasgupta S, Broz D, Tanner M, Patel M, Halleck B, Peters PJ, et al. Changes in reported injection behaviors following the public health response to an HIV outbreak among people who inject drugs: Indiana, 2016. AIDS Behav. 2019;23(12):3257–66.
48. Strathdee SA, Beyrer C. Threading the needle — how to stop the HIV outbreak in rural Indiana. N Engl J Med. 2015;373(5):397–9.
49. Gonsalves GS, Crawford FW. Dynamics of the HIV outbreak and response in Scott County, IN, USA, 2011–15: a modelling study. Lancet HIV. 2018;5(10):e569–77.
50. Wheeler E, Doe Simkins M. Harm reduction programs distribute one million doses of naloxone in 2019 [Internet]. Medium. 2020 [cited 2020 Feb 17]. Available from: https://medium.com/@ejwharmreduction/harm-reduction-programs-distribute-one-million-doses-of-naloxone-in-2019-4884d3535256
51. Coffin PO, Sullivan SD. Cost-effectiveness of distributing naloxone to heroin users for lay overdose reversal. Ann Intern Med. 2013;158(1–9):18.
52. Walley AY, Xuan Z, Hackman HH, Quinn E, Doe-Simkins M, Sorensen-Alawad A, et al. Opioid overdose rates and implementation of overdose education and nasal naloxone distribution in Massachusetts: interrupted time series analysis. BMJ. 2013;346:f174.
53. Dowell D, Haegerich TM, Chou R. CDC guideline for prescribing opioids for chronic pain— United States, 2016. JAMA. 2016;315(15):1624–45.
54. Davis C, Carr D. State legal innovations to encourage naloxone dispensing. J Am Pharm Assoc. 2017;57(2):S180–4.
55. Davis CS, Burris S, Beletsky L, Binswanger I. Co-prescribing naloxone does not increase liability risk. Subst Abuse. 2016;37(4):498–500.
56. Bell A, Bennett AS, Jones TS, Doe-Simkins M, Williams LD. Amount of naloxone used to reverse opioid overdoses outside of medical practice in a city with increasing illicitly manufactured fentanyl in illicit drug supply. Subst Abuse. 2019;40(1):52–5.
57. McClellan C, Lambdin BH, Ali MM, Mutter R, Davis CS, Wheeler E, et al. Opioid-overdose laws association with opioid use and overdose mortality. Addict Behav. 2018;86:90–5.
58. Barratt M, Kowalski M, Maier L, Ritter A. Global review of drug checking services operating in 2017 [Internet]. National Drug and Alcohol Research Centre; 2017 [cited 2020 Feb 9]. Available from: https://ndarc.med.unsw.edu.au/resource/bulletin-no-24-global-review-drug-checking-services-operating-2017
59. O'Donnell J, Halpin J, Mattson C, Goldberger, Bruce. Notes from the field: overdose deaths with Carfentanil and other fentanyl analogs detected — 10 States, July 2016–June 2017. MMWR Morb Mortal Wkly Rep [Internet]. 2018 [cited 2020 Feb 8];67. Available from: https://www.cdc.gov/mmwr/volumes/67/wr/mm6727a4.htm
60. Zibbell JE, Aldridge AP, Cauchon D, DeFiore-Hyrmer J, Conway KP. Association of law enforcement seizures of heroin, fentanyl, and carfentanil with opioid overdose deaths in Ohio, 2014–2017. JAMA Netw Open. 2019;2(11):e1914666.
61. Sherman SG, Park JN, Glick J, McKenzie M, Morales K, Christensen T, Green TC. FORECAST study summary report. [Internet]. Johns Hopkins Bloomberg School of Public Health; Available from: https://americanhealth.jhu.edu/sites/default/files/inline-files/Fentanyl_Executive_Summary_032018.pdf

62. Cowan R. How the narcs created crack. Natl Rev Magazine. 1986;38:26–31.
63. Beletsky L, Davis CS. Today's fentanyl crisis: prohibition's iron law, revisited. Int J Drug Policy. 2017;46:156–9.
64. Fischer B, Oviedo-Joekes E, Blanken P, Haasen C, Rehm J, Schechter MT, et al. Heroin-assisted treatment (HAT) a decade later: a brief update on science and politics. J Urban Health Bull N Y Acad Med. 2007;84(4):552–62.
65. Oviedo-Joekes E, Brissette S, Marsh DC, Lauzon P, Guh D, Anis A, et al. Diacetylmorphine versus methadone for the treatment of opioid addiction. N Engl J Med. 2009;361(8):777–86.
66. Oviedo-Joekes E, Guh D, Brissette S, Marchand K, MacDonald S, Lock K, et al. Hydromorphone compared with diacetylmorphine for long-term opioid dependence: a randomized clinical trial. JAMA Psychiat. 2016;73(5):447–55.
67. Hedrich D. European Report on Drug Consumption Rooms. Lisbon: European Monitoring Centre for Drugs and Drug Addiction (EMCDDA). Published online February 2004.
68. Marshall BDL, Milloy M-J, Wood E, Montaner JSG, Kerr T. Reduction in overdose mortality after the opening of North America's first medically supervised safer injecting facility: a retrospective population-based study. Lancet Lond. 2011;377(9775):1429–37.
69. Burris S, Anderson ED, Davis CS, Beletsky L. Toward healthy drug policy in the United States — the case of safehouse. N Engl J Med. 2019;382:4–5.
70. Kral AH, Davidson PJ. Addressing the Nation's opioid epidemic: lessons from an unsanctioned supervised injection site in the U.S. Am J Prev Med. 2017;53(6):919–22.
71. Davidson PJ, Lopez AM, Kral AH. Using drugs in un/safe spaces: impact of perceived illegality on an underground supervised injecting facility in the United States. Int J Drug Policy. 2018;53:37–44.
72. Irwin A, Jozaghi E, Weir BW, Allen ST, Lindsay A, Sherman SG. Mitigating the heroin crisis in Baltimore, MD, USA: a cost-benefit analysis of a hypothetical supervised injection facility. Harm Reduct J. 2017;14(1):29.
73. Behrends CN, Paone D, Nolan ML, Tuazon E, Murphy SM, Kapadia SN, et al. Estimated impact of supervised injection facilities on overdose fatalities and healthcare costs in New York City. J Subst Abus Treat. 2019;106:79–88.
74. Potier C, Laprévote V, Dubois-Arber F, Cottencin O, Rolland B. Supervised injection services: what has been demonstrated? A systematic literature review. Drug Alcohol Depend. 2014;145:48–68.

Training Medical Students, Residents, and Fellows in Opioid Use Disorder Treatment

11

Kenneth L. Morford, Caroline G. Falker,
and Jeanette M. Tetrault

Introduction

Opioid use disorder (OUD) carries with it substantial morbidity and mortality. This morbidity and mortality is perpetuated by the fact that OUD treatment can be challenging for individuals to access and navigate. Additionally, the stigma surrounding the individual, the disease, and the treatment itself leads to a notable treatment gap between the number of people with OUD and those who receive evidence-based treatment [33]. Medications for OUD (MOUD) are underutilized, particularly methadone and buprenorphine, which have been associated with reduced opioid-related morbidity and mortality [22, 43]. Integrating OUD care into general medical settings provides opportunities to address issues of treatment access and stigma.

The demand for effective and evidence-based OUD treatment clearly outweighs the number of health professionals trained to provide such treatment. Addressing this critical workforce shortage requires increased emphasis on screening, diagnosing, and treating OUD across the continuum of medical education. While the treatment gap calls for widespread change to the public health infrastructure, including integrated treatment models, national data suggest that primary care providers do not perceive MOUD to be more effective than behavioral health approaches for OUD treatment despite conclusive evidence to the contrary.

K. L. Morford · J. M. Tetrault (✉)
Program in Addiction Medicine and Section of General Internal Medicine, Department of Internal Medicine, Yale School of Medicine, New Haven, CT, USA
e-mail: kenneth.morford@yale.edu; jeanette.tetrault@yale.edu

C. G. Falker
Department of Psychiatry, VA Connecticut Healthcare System, West Haven, CT, USA

© Springer Nature Switzerland AG 2021
S. E. Wakeman, J. D. Rich (eds.), *Treating Opioid Use Disorder in General Medical Settings*, https://doi.org/10.1007/978-3-030-80818-1_11

Additionally, these data support the need for added OUD training requirements as many primary care providers express low interest in providing MOUD in their practices [23, 45].

Standard curricula have not comprehensively integrated topics on caring for patients with OUD. However, this is starting to change. Beginning in July 2019, the Accreditation Council for Graduate Medical Education (ACGME) required all graduate medical education programs to incorporate pain management and addiction training into their curricula [1]. Similarly, the American Academy of Medical Colleges (AAMC) has created a series of strategic activities to further enhance collaboration and sharing of best educational practices in response to the opioid overdose crisis.

In this chapter, we describe the evolving landscape of OUD training in medical education and outline a framework for integrating OUD content across different training levels. We also provide examples of curricular interventions and offer key recommendations for successful implementation.

Evolving Landscape of Training in Opioid Use Disorder

Undergraduate Medical Education

Historically, little attention has been given to OUD in undergraduate medical education. In a 1996 survey of all accredited US medical schools, an average of only 12 hours of curricular time across 4 years of medical training was devoted to opioid and other substance use disorders (SUD) [25]. However, in response to the opioid overdose crisis, medical schools across the country have been integrating topics into their curricula related to the prevention and treatment of OUD. According to the Liaison Committee on Medical Education (LCME) 2016–2017 Annual Medical School Questionnaire, 143 of 145 medical schools reported including content on SUD in required coursework and 144 included content on pain management in required courses [19]. In September 2017, the AAMC conducted a survey of Deans of Curricula from LCME-accredited US medical schools assessing four educational domains related to pain and SUD. Of the 102 responding institutions, 87% reported covering all four domains in their curricula and 100% reported addressing at least two domains. The majority of respondents reported incorporating the four domains in required coursework across all 4 years of medical school training.

Although medical schools are increasingly integrating OUD topics into their curricula, there remains variation in the content and teaching modalities being implemented. The literature describes specific teaching on prescription opioid misuse; screening, brief intervention, and referral to treatment (SBIRT); medication treatment with buprenorphine; and overdose response with naloxone administration; among others [6, 8, 38, 46]. Some schools incorporate these topics as part of a pain management curriculum [26], while others include these topics during specific clinical rotations, such as psychiatry, family medicine, and emergency medicine [15, 16, 20, 32]. In addition to traditional didactic lectures, teaching formats may include the use of standardized patients, team-based learning exercises, and online training modules [44].

Efforts are underway to improve the consistency of OUD training across medical school curricula. In Massachusetts, the state's four medical schools partnered with the state government to develop a set of shared core competencies related to safe opioid prescribing and addiction treatment [4]. Other medical schools have also collaborated at the state level to develop cross-institutional core competencies for education on pain, opioids, and addiction [5, 24]. In 2018, the Warren Alpert Medical School of Brown University hosted a national symposium to establish core competencies, identify appropriate teaching modalities, and explore useful assessment models for OUD curricula across medical schools [44].

Graduate Medical Education: Residency Training

In a review of models of resident physician training in SUD, including OUD, less than a third of the 29 OUD training initiatives included education on MOUD, and of those, less than half included application of training content to direct patient care [17]. Psychiatry, Internal Medicine, and Family Medicine are the primary medical specialties that include any type of OUD training for residents [37, 39, 42]. Among these programs, the majority of SUD training focused on behavioral counseling interventions rather than pharmacotherapy, including MOUD [17].

Proposals to address this deficit include requiring residents and core faculty to complete MOUD waiver training, which allows for buprenorphine prescribing [34]. While some educational interventions include content on MOUD, most of these trainings focus on buprenorphine despite efficacy and availability of other MOUD, such as methadone and extended-release naltrexone, as well as other opioid agonist options approved in Canada [10]. Hence, even in residency programs where incorporation of OUD training has been a priority, improvements can be made.

Despite lack of uniform curricula or evaluation tools, residency programs that have implemented OUD training generally report favorable changes in knowledge, attitudes, and confidence regarding OUD treatment [17] and increased postgraduate prescribing of MOUD [21]. Importantly, effective July 1, 2019, the ACGME began to require that all residency programs "provide instruction and experience in pain management if applicable for the specialty including recognition of the signs of addiction" [1]. This requirement directs graduate medical training programs to develop and implement evidence-based educational interventions to teach trainees how to prevent addiction while also treating pain, recognize OUD in early stages, function effectively in systems of care for effective pain relief and OUD, use nonpharmacologic means for the treatment of pain when possible, and participate in clinical trials of nonopioid pain relief customized to the clinical disorders of the populations they serve.

Graduate Medical Education: Fellowship Training

Until recently, the only pathway to becoming an addiction specialist recognized by the American Board of Medical Specialties was through the field of Addiction Psychiatry, which limits fellowship training to individuals who have completed residency training in psychiatry. There are currently 49 Addiction Psychiatry fellowship programs certified by the ACGME. Addiction Medicine, on the other hand, was recognized as a multispecialty field by the American Board of Medical Specialties in 2015. Addiction Medicine fellowship training is open to individuals who have completed residency in any of the 24 primary medical specialties. There are currently 78 Addiction Medicine fellowship programs certified by the ACGME. The ACGME program requirements for both Addiction Psychiatry and Addiction Medicine include adequate training in identification, treatment, and prevention of OUD.

Fellowship training is vital to produce addiction specialists who will continue to drive clinical care, research, and education related to OUD. Despite the existence of ACGME-accredited Addiction Psychiatry and Addiction Medicine fellowship programs, the number of fellowship positions remain inadequate to bridge the OUD treatment gap.

General Approach

Effectively training students, residents, and fellows to identify, treat, and prevent OUD requires a coordinated educational strategy across training levels. We propose an OUD training framework (see Fig. 11.1) where core OUD content and skills are introduced and practiced during medical school, applied and reinforced in various

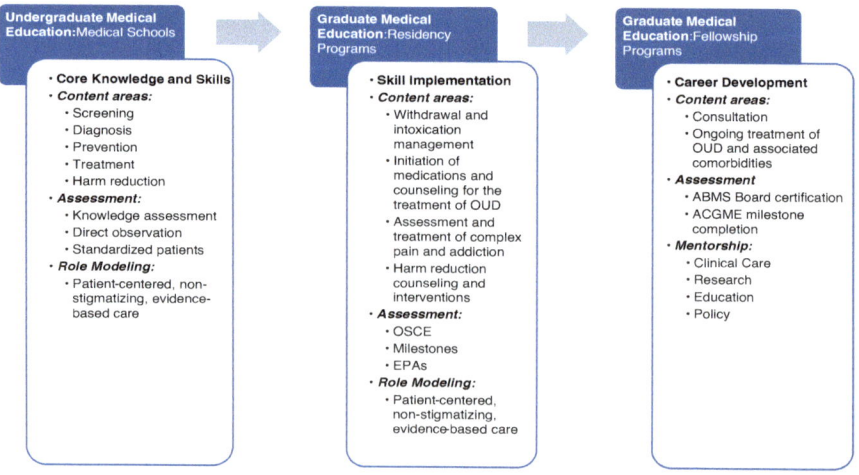

Fig. 11.1 Framework for OUD training across the continuum of medical education

clinical settings during residency, and then championed by targeted trainees pursuing specialized fellowship training to lead OUD educational initiatives and clinical practice. The following section includes examples of teaching modalities and assessment models by training level. While these approaches may be suitable for a range of academic settings, institutions should build on the strengths of their local training environments. Of primary value is the ability for training programs to be adaptable to optimize available resources and respond to the unique needs of their communities.

Undergraduate Medical Education

Undergraduate medical education should prioritize curricula focusing on core OUD knowledge and skills including epidemiology, neurobiology, standardized approaches to screening, assessment and diagnosis, and an overview of treatment options. Prevention of opioid misuse and OUD should also be integrated into the curriculum, as well as harm reduction approaches to optimize safety among patients at risk for overdose, infectious diseases, and other complications of OUD. It is imperative that undergraduate medical educators not only teach but also role-model the use of patient-centered, non-stigmatizing language when delivering lectures, preparing cases for practice-based learning, and teaching in the clinical environment.

This content can be delivered in a variety of ways. Some examples include developing a stand-alone course [30], incorporating OUD content as part of a broader effort to integrate social determinants of health into standard curricula [11, 27, 28], or threading OUD content throughout preclinical and clinical medical school training. Developing and supporting addiction interest groups and involving students in both basic science and clinical research on OUD can help enhance the educational experience for students and help them identify mentors. Other optional, intensive experiences, such as the Betty Ford Summer Institute for Medical Students [7], can help solidify core knowledge and skills delivered in mandatory curricula for select students who show a specific interest in the core content [7].

To assess knowledge and skill acquisition as well as identify areas for improvement, formative assessment is necessary to encourage a dynamic learning process. Brief assessments of OUD content, such as pop quizzes, in-class polling, or one-minute papers, can give a sense of students' level of understanding and also lead to curricular improvement. Use of simulated patient scenarios with role play or nongraded exercises with standardized patients can provide opportunities for students to practice skills prior to implementation in clinical encounters. Flipped-classroom approaches may also be beneficial by allowing students to use class time to ask questions and practice skills. This is especially powerful if the educators have clinical experience caring for patients with OUD, which speaks to the importance of building expertise in OUD among faculty to provide this education. Therefore, we feel that faculty development should dovetail educational interventions.

Graduate Medical Education: Residency Training

The skills introduced during medical school (e.g., OUD prevention, screening, assessment, and treatment) should be implemented and assessed for residents across all medical specialties, but with particular emphasis in Internal Medicine, Primary Care, Family Medicine, Emergency Medicine, and Psychiatry. Key skills that should be integrated into residency training include management of opioid intoxication and withdrawal, initiation of medications and counseling-based approaches for OUD treatment, harm reduction interventions, and assessment and treatment of complex pain and addiction.

Application of the skills necessary to care for patients with OUD can manifest in a variety of ways, depending on the availability of trained faculty and clinical sites. Investing in the development of local "teaching champions" can be vital to delivery of OUD training. Given the important role chief residents play in residency education, training rising chief residents on OUD topics can be an effective model for dissemination of both knowledge and skills into residency training programs [2, 3]. Models that integrate OUD training into the clinical learning environment, which is the primary setting for residency education, have the potential to prepare residents to practice OUD treatment upon graduation. Some programs, notably Psychiatry and Primary Care, have created training opportunities where residents manage patients with OUD in outpatient settings using office-based buprenorphine and/or naltrexone [17, 21, 37, 39, 40]. Additional clinical opportunities exist for residents in hospital-based settings, including primary management of patients with OUD on general medical units and elective rotations on inpatient Addiction Medicine consult services addressing the acute management of hospitalized patients with OUD [14, 36]. If no clinical experiences for OUD treatment exist within residency training programs, rotations can be arranged through community partners, such as local opioid treatment programs. Online modules [13, 31], simulated patient exercises [35] and role play exercises have also been utilized to augment OUD training for residents [17].

Residents can be evaluated using a number of different strategies, including a combination of formative and summative assessments (e.g., quizzes, standardized board exams, objective structured clinical exams [OSCE]) with directly observed clinical practice. As medical education moves toward a competency-based framework, aligning assessment with ACGME milestones is also valuable in residency training. For example, evidence-based screening, diagnosis, and treatment of OUD during routine clinical care and the ACGME common program requirement to provide instruction in pain management and addiction fall within the milestone domains of medical knowledge, patient care, and systems-based practice. Entrustable professional activities (EPAs) represent one method of assessing competency that can be linked to ACGME milestones [18]. EPAs are units of professional practice, defined as tasks or responsibilities to be entrusted to the unsupervised execution by a trainee once they have attained sufficient competence. EPAs are a means to translate competencies into clinical practice and can be used to specifically assess practice, including resident assessment in the field of addiction [9]. It is vital for faculty who supervise residents caring for patients with OUD to role model patient-centered, non-stigmatizing care and assess resident performance in this domain.

Graduate Medical Education: Addiction Specialty Fellowship Training

There are currently two pathways to pursue ACGME-accredited fellowship training in addiction—Addiction Psychiatry and Addiction Medicine [29]. While pursing fellowship in Addiction Psychiatry is limited to physicians who have completed residency training in psychiatry, all physicians who have completed training in any US or Canadian certified residency program are eligible to apply for fellowship in Addiction Medicine, which is considered a subspecialty of Preventive Medicine. These two pathways allow for greater emphasis to rapidly scale up workforce development to address the opioid overdose crisis. Collaboration between fellowship training programs in Addiction Psychiatry and Addiction Medicine is a key step in addressing the OUD education gap [41].

Both addiction fellowship training pathways consist of one year of clinical training. Fellows graduate with skills in assessing and managing individuals with OUD across a range of healthcare settings. Key content areas include inpatient and outpatient consultation and ongoing treatment of patients with OUD and its associated comorbidities. Formative assessment includes direct observation and ACGME milestone assessment. Summative assessment includes passage of the American Board of Medical Specialties Addiction Psychiatry or Addiction Medicine examination.

In addition to core clinical knowledge and skills, fellowship training should provide opportunities for fellows to engage in education, research, and policy initiatives related to OUD. While workforce development should remain the primary focus of fellowship training, creating change agents to address the critical need for systems improvement in OUD treatment should also be a distinct priority.

Key Recommendations

In order to implement effective and comprehensive OUD training across the continuum of medical education, we have developed several key recommendations to integrate OUD content into existing curricula applicable to all training levels.

First, we recommend that training programs perform a needs assessment of existing curricular content and program capacity to identify educational gaps and build on institutional strengths related to OUD care. Programs should be creative and adaptive to meet local needs and address educational gaps through other teaching modalities based on available resources. For example, if relevant clinical experiences are lacking, clinical concepts may be taught using other modalities, such as medical simulation. Ideally, OUD training should be delivered through diverse educational approaches including didactics, skills training, case-based learning, and a variety of clinical experiences.

Second, training programs should prioritize incorporating early longitudinal clinical experiences with patients engaged in OUD treatment. Current clinical training experiences disproportionately expose trainees to patients in times of crisis rather than to patients who have achieved clinical stability with evidence-based care. Trainees should be exposed to the spectrum of addiction care, from the outpatient, chronic disease model to high acuity inpatient management. Giving trainees experience in diverse treatment settings not only provides opportunities to care for individuals with OUD at different stages of the disease process, but also allows trainees to recognize the value and effectiveness of existing interventions to treat OUD.

Third, we recommend that curricula emphasize the role of MOUD as first-line evidence-based treatment for OUD. While behavioral interventions can be an important component of treatment, neglecting to educate trainees in the use of MOUD is problematic. According to the American Society of Addiction Medicine (ASAM) 2020 National Guideline, "the absence of available psychosocial treatment should not preclude or delay pharmacotherapy, with appropriate medication management" [12]. It is imperative that trainees have experiences in settings that promote MOUD in addition to behavioral interventions.

Fourth, OUD training should be interprofessional where feasible. Addressing the OUD treatment gap requires developing a robust and diverse workforce. Providing interprofessional training with other health professionals, including registered and advanced practice nurses, physician assistants, social workers, psychologists, and pharmacists, will breakdown hierarchies, offer a deeper understanding of the unique role each health profession plays in treating OUD, and ultimately prepare trainees to work in effective teams.

Fifth, it is important to strengthen the quality and standardization of competency-based assessments. While clinical experiences for trainees will vary based on the local training environment, efforts to teach and assess core concepts in the treatment of OUD can be universal. Similarly, efforts should be made for annual curriculum evaluation to adapt to the changing landscape of the opioid overdose crisis and respond to both local and national needs.

Finally, we recommend that all educational materials combat stigma by addressing misinformation and misperceptions, incorporating accurate and non-stigmatizing language, and promoting evidence-based treatment. Faculty development is particularly important to ensure that trainees receive appropriate supervision from role models who practice compassionate and nonjudgmental care for patients with OUD.

Conclusions

Integrating OUD training across the continuum of medical education represents a critical step toward developing an effective workforce to address the large treatment gap perpetuating opioid-related morbidity and mortality. Applying a framework to guide core content, assessment, and role modeling across training levels can help standardize and coordinate educational interventions to teach medical students, residents, and fellows how to effectively care for individuals with OUD.

References

1. ACGME Common Program Requirement IV.C.2. 2020. Retrieved from https://www.acgme.org/Portals/0/PFAssets/ProgramRequirements/CPRResidency2020.pdf
2. Alford DP, Bridden C, Jackson AH, Saitz R, Amodeo M, Barnes HN, Samet JH. Promoting substance use education among generalist physicians: an evaluation of the Chief Resident Immersion Training (CRIT) program. J Gen Intern Med. 2009;24(1):40–7. https://doi.org/10.1007/s11606-008-0819-2.
3. Alford DP, Carney BL, Jackson AH, Brett B, Bridden C, Winter M, Samet JH. Promoting addiction medicine teaching through functional mentoring by co-training generalist chief residents with faculty mentors. Subst Abus. 2018;39(3):377–83. https://doi.org/10.1080/08897077.2018.1439799.
4. Antman KH, Berman HA, Flotte TR, Flier J, Dimitri DM, Bharel M. Developing core competencies for the prevention and management of prescription drug misuse: a medical education collaboration in Massachusetts. Acad Med. 2016;91(10):1348–51. https://doi.org/10.1097/acm.0000000000001347.
5. Ashburn MA, Levine RL. Pennsylvania state core competencies for education on opioids and addiction. Pain Med. 2017;18(10):1890–4. https://doi.org/10.1093/pm/pnw348.
6. Babor TF, Higgins-Biddle JC, Higgins PS, Gassman RA, Gould BE. Training medical providers to conduct alcohol screening and brief interventions. Subst Abus. 2004;25(1):17–26. https://doi.org/10.1300/J465v25n01_04.
7. Barron R, Frank E, Gitlow S. Evaluation of an experiential curriculum for addiction education among medical students. J Addict Med. 2012;6(2):131–6. https://doi.org/10.1097/ADM.0b013e3182548abd.
8. Berland N, Fox A, Tofighi B, Hanley K. Opioid overdose prevention training with naloxone, an adjunct to basic life support training for first-year medical students. Subst Abus. 2017;38(2):123–8. https://doi.org/10.1080/08897077.2016.1275925.
9. Boyce P, Spratt C, Davies M, McEvoy P. Using entrustable professional activities to guide curriculum development in psychiatry training. BMC Med Educ. 2011;11:96. https://doi.org/10.1186/1472-6920-11-96.
10. Bruneau J, Ahamad K, Goyer M, Poulin G, Selby P, Fischer B, et al. Management of opioid use disorders: a national clinical practice guideline. CMAJ. 2018;190(9):E247–e257. https://doi.org/10.1503/cmaj.170958.
11. Butkus R, Rapp K, Cooney TG, Engel LS. Envisioning a better U.S. health care system for all: reducing barriers to care and addressing social determinants of health. Ann Intern Med. 2020;172(2 Suppl):S50–s59. https://doi.org/10.7326/m19-2410.
12. Crotty K, Freedman KI, Kampman KM. Executive summary of the focused update of the ASAM national practice guideline for the treatment of opioid use disorder. J Addict Med. 2020;14(2):99–112. https://doi.org/10.1097/adm.0000000000000635.
13. Edens EL, Drew S, Heimer R, Jordan A, Krause R, Powell L, et al. Addiction treatment: clinical skills for healthcare providers [MOOC]. Coursera 2019
14. Englander H, Weimer M, Solotaroff R, Nicolaidis C, Chan B, Velez C, et al. Planning and designing the improving addiction care team (IMPACT) for hospitalized adults with substance use disorder. J Hosp Med. 2017;12(5):339–42. https://doi.org/10.12788/jhm.2736.
15. Feeley RJ, Moore DT, Wilkins K, Fuehrlein B. A focused addiction curriculum and its Impact on student knowledge, attitudes, and confidence in the treatment of patients with substance use. Acad Psychiatry. 2018;42(2):304–8. https://doi.org/10.1007/s40596-017-0771-8.

16. Gano L, Renshaw SE, Hernandez RH, Cronholm PF. Opioid overdose prevention in family medicine clerkships: a CERA study. Fam Med. 2018;50(9):698–701. https://doi.org/10.22454/FamMed.2018.757385.

17. Graddy R, Accurso AJ, Nandiwada DR, Shalaby M, Holt SR. Models of resident physician training in opioid use disorders. Curr Addict Rep. 2019;6:355–64. https://doi.org/10.1007/s40429-019-00271-1.

18. Hart D, Franzen D, Beeson M, Bhat R, Kulkarni M, Thibodeau L, et al. Integration of entrustable professional activities with the milestones for emergency medicine residents. West J Emerg Med. 2019;20(1):35–42. https://doi.org/10.5811/westjem.2018.11.38912.

19. Howley L, Whelan A, Rasouli T. Addressing the opioid epidemic: U.S. medical school curricular approaches. AAMC Analysis in Brief, 18, 2018.

20. Khidir H, Weiner SG. A call for better opioid prescribing training and education. West J Emerg Med. 2016;17(6):686–9. https://doi.org/10.5811/westjem.2016.8.31204.

21. Kunins HV, Sohler NL, Giovanniello A, Thompson D, Cunningham CO. A buprenorphine education and training program for primary care residents: implementation and evaluation. Subst Abus. 2013;34(3):242–7. https://doi.org/10.1080/08897077.2012.752777.

22. Larochelle MR, Bernson D, Land T, Stopka TJ, Wang N, Xuan Z, et al. Medication for opioid use disorder after nonfatal opioid overdose and association with mortality: a cohort study. Ann Intern Med. 2018;169(3):137–45. https://doi.org/10.7326/m17-3107.

23. McGinty EE, Stone EM, Kennedy-Hendricks A, Bachhuber MA, Barry CL. Medication for opioid use disorder: a national survey of primary care physicians. Ann Intern Med. 2020;173(2):160–2. https://doi.org/10.7326/m19-3975.

24. Miller NS. Florida medical schools developing common curriculum for pain and opioid Rx. Orlando Sentinel. 2017. Retrieved from https://www.orlandosentinel.com/health/os-florida-medical-schools-pain-management-group-20170907-story.html

25. Miller NS, Sheppard LM, Colenda CC, Magen J. Why physicians are unprepared to treat patients who have alcohol- and drug-related disorders. Acad Med. 2001;76(5):410–8. https://doi.org/10.1097/00001888-200105000-00007.

26. Morley-Forster PK, Pergolizzi JV, Taylor R Jr, Axford-Gatley RA, Sellers EM. Mitigating the risk of opioid abuse through a balanced undergraduate pain medicine curriculum. J Pain Res. 2013;6:791–801. https://doi.org/10.2147/jpr.S47192.

27. Mullan F. Social mission in health professions education: beyond flexner. JAMA. 2017;318(2):122–3. https://doi.org/10.1001/jama.2017.7286.

28. Muvvala SB, Schwartz ML, Petrakis I, O'Connor PG, Tetrault JM. Stitching a solution to the addiction epidemic: a longitudinal addiction curricular thread across four years of medical training. Subst Abus. 2020;41(4):475–9. https://doi.org/10.1080/08897077.2019.1709606.

29. Nunes EV, Kunz K, Galanter M, O'Connor PG. Addiction psychiatry and addiction medicine: the evolution of addiction physician specialists. Am J Addict. 2020;29(5):390–400. https://doi.org/10.1111/ajad.13068.

30. Oldfield BJ, Tetrault JM, Wilkins KM, Edelman EJ, Capurso NA. Opioid overdose prevention education for medical students: adopting harm reduction into mandatory clerkship curricula. Subst Abus. 2019;41(1):29–34. https://doi.org/10.1080/08897077.2019.1621241.

31. PCSS. Provider Clinical Support System (PCSS).

32. Rasyidi E, Wilkins JN, Danovitch I. Training the next generation of providers in addiction medicine. Psychiatr Clin North Am. 2012;35(2):461–80. https://doi.org/10.1016/j.psc.2012.04.001.

33. SAMHSA. Key substance use and mental health indicators in the United States: Results from the 2019 National Survey on Drug Use and Health (HHS Publication No. PEP20-07-01-001, NSDUH Series H-55). Rockville, MD: Center for Behavioral Health Statistics and Quality, Substance Abuse and Mental Health Services Administration 2020.

34. Sharfstein JM, Olsen Y. Making amends for the opioid epidemic. JAMA. 2019;321(15):1446–7. https://doi.org/10.1001/jama.2019.3505.

35. Stein MR, Arnsten JH, Parish SJ, Kunins HV. Evaluation of a substance use disorder curriculum for internal medicine residents. Subst Abus. 2011;32(4):220–4. https://doi.org/10.1080/08897077.2011.598408.

36. Suhail-Sindhu S, Patel P, Sugarman J, Hansen H. Program for Residency Education, Community Engagement, and Peer Support Training (PRECEPT): connecting psychiatrists to community resources in Harlem, NYC. In: Hansen H, Metzl JM, editors. Structural competency in mental health and medicine: a case-based approach to treating the social determinants of health. Cham: Springer International Publishing; 2019. p. 137–48.

37. Suzuki J, Ellison TV, Connery HS, Surber C, Renner JA. Training in buprenorphine and office-based opioid treatment: a survey of psychiatry residency training programs. Acad Psychiatry. 2016;40(3):498–502. https://doi.org/10.1007/s40596-015-0313-1.

38. Taylor JL, Rapoport AB, Rowley CF, Mukamal KJ, Stead W. An opioid overdose curriculum for medical residents: Impact on naloxone prescribing, knowledge, and attitudes. Subst Abus. 2018;39(3):371–6. https://doi.org/10.1080/08897077.2018.1439800.

39. Tesema L, Marshall J, Hathaway R, Pham C, Clarke C, Bergeron G, et al. Training in office-based opioid treatment with buprenorphine in US residency programs: a national survey of residency program directors. Subst Abus. 2018;39(4):434–40. https://doi.org/10.1080/0889707 7.2018.1449047.

40. Holt SR, Segar N, Cavallo DA, Tetrault JM. The addiction recovery clinic: a novel, primary-care-based approach to teaching addiction medicine. Acad Med. 2017;92(5):680–3. PMID: 28441678.

41. Tetrault JM, Petrakis IL. Partnering with psychiatry to close the education gap: an approach to the addiction epidemic. J Gen Intern Med. 2017;32(12):1387–9. https://doi.org/10.1007/ s11606-017-4140-9.

42. Tong S, Sabo R, Aycock R, Prasad R, Etz R, Kuzel A, Krist A. Assessment of addiction medicine training in family medicine residency programs: a CERA study. Fam Med. 2017;49(7):537–43.

43. Wakeman SE, Larochelle MR, Ameli O, Chaisson CE, McPheeters JT, Crown WH, et al. Comparative effectiveness of different treatment pathways for opioid use disorder. JAMA Netw Open. 2020;3(2):e1920622. https://doi.org/10.1001/jamanetworkopen.2019.20622.

44. Wallace PM, Warrier S, Kahn MJ, Welsh C, Fischer M. Developing an opioid curriculum for medical students: a consensus report from a national symposium. Subst Abus. 2019;41(4):425–31. https://doi.org/10.1080/08897077.2019.1635971.

45. Weimer MB, Tetrault JM, Fiellin DA. Patients with opioid use disorder deserve trained providers. Ann Intern Med. 2019;171(12):931–2. https://doi.org/10.7326/m19-2303.

46. Zerbo E, Traba C, Matthew P, Chen S, Holland BK, Levounis P, et al. DATA 2000 waiver training for medical students: lessons learned from a medical school experience. Subst Abus. 2020;41(4):463–7. https://doi.org/10.1080/08897077.2019.1692323.

Bringing Primary Care to Opioid Treatment Programs

12

Yngvild Olsen and Angela Mason

People with opioid use disorder (OUD) commonly encounter multiple other medical conditions in addition to their addiction. In some instances, the types of substances people use result in medical complications. For example, opioids can affect gonadotropin release, resulting in female menstrual irregularities and male secondary hypogonadism [1]. People with OUD also frequently have other substance use disorders (SUDs), including those related to cocaine, alcohol, and tobacco [2]. In combination with opioids, these other substances put people at risk for cardiovascular disease, premature strokes, myocardial infarction, chronic obstructive pulmonary disease (COPD), and several different types of cancer. At the same time, the way people use opioids confers risks. Injection puts people at risk for abscesses and thrombophlebitis at injection sites. Sharing needles, syringes, or other equipment can result in more distal and systemic infections such as endocarditis, osteomyelitis, hepatitis C, and HIV. Intranasal use of cocaine mixed with opioids may lead to nasal septal perforation and sinusitis.

Infectious complications in people with opioid use disorder have increased significantly over the past two decades, in large part due to the opioid and addiction crisis sweeping the United States [3, 4]. Data from several Appalachian states found a 45% increase in acute hepatitis C infections between 2006 and 2012, with three-quarters of these occurring among people who inject drugs (PWID) [5]. Outbreaks of HIV in Indiana and Massachusetts have occurred in conjunction with more injection opioid use [6, 7]. Rising rates of injection drug use has also contributed to significant increases in the incidence of endocarditis, osteomyelitis, septic arthritis, and epidural abscess in many areas of the country [8].

Not only do these infectious diseases cause acute medical care needs, but patients often continue to require long-term treatment and monitoring as they live with chronic infections, chronic pain, and co-occurring medical and other psychiatric

Y. Olsen (✉) · A. Mason
REACH Health Services, Institutes for Behavior Resources, Inc., Baltimore, MD, USA
e-mail: yolsen@ibrinc.org; amason@ibrinc.org

© Springer Nature Switzerland AG 2021
S. E. Wakeman, J. D. Rich (eds.), *Treating Opioid Use Disorder in General Medical Settings*, https://doi.org/10.1007/978-3-030-80818-1_12

conditions. The Centers for Disease Control and Prevention (CDC) estimates that close to 2.5 million adults in the US live with a chronic hepatitis C infection, with over half of those occurring among people who inject drugs [9]. Close to 200,000 PWID live with HIV [10]. People with OUD are also at risk for the same chronic medical conditions, such as diabetes and hypertension, that afflict those without addiction [1]. To complicate the situation further, large epidemiological studies and systematic reviews find that, annually, over 60% of people with an OUD have a diagnosable, co-occurring mental health condition, such as depression and anxiety disorders [2], with rates two to three times higher than the general population [11]. A sizeable percentage of people with opioid use disorder had their addiction begin with opioids prescribed for chronic, non-cancer pain, a condition which continues to coexist with the OUD [12].

Unfortunately, the presence of an opioid use disorder can complicate effective treatment and care of co-occurring illnesses. Stigma associated with addiction, lack of health insurance coverage, unstable housing, absence of reliable transportation, and multiple competing priorities represent some of the barriers that people with opioid addiction face in trying to access care and manage their overall health. At the same time, systems of care that separate opioid addiction treatment and longitudinal, non-acute services for other illnesses require that patients may need to choose between their OUD treatment and their diabetes or hypertension care, for example. It should come as no surprise then that adherence to medical care, particularly primary care, and effective management of chronic illnesses has historically been low for people with opioid use and other substance use disorders (SUDs) [13, 14]. Instead, people with addiction often end up relying on emergency departments (EDs) for needed medical care when their symptoms become intolerable. Lewer et al., in a recent systematic review of 92 studies of people with non-alcohol, non-nicotine related SUDs, found frequencies of ED utilization between three to ten times that of non-SUD populations [15]. Their review also identified frequency of hospitalizations for people with SUD as two to eight times higher than more general populations.

Associated costs, including for hospitalizations, to the healthcare system have skyrocketed because of the opioid and addiction crisis and the multitude of co-occurring illnesses people with opioid use disorder face. Ronan and Herzig, using data from the Nationwide Inpatient Sample, the largest publicly available, all-payer database of hospital admissions and associated costs in the country, determined that hospitalizations for OUD almost tripled between 2002 and 2012, costing close to $15 billion in 2012 [16]. In their analysis, an associated infection added about $70,000 to the estimated charge per hospitalization. Results from an analysis of 17 state Medicaid programs found that costs associated with medical care due to infections or other co-occurring conditions in addition to OUD increased 363% between 1999 and 2013, even more than the 246% increase in costs related to the OUD itself. In 2013, these Medicaid programs spent a total of $3.18 billion in total OUD-related expenditures [17]. As the age of onset of opioid use disorder has fallen over the past 20 years and severity of the illness has increased, the higher overall disease burden people with opioid addiction live with will result in a long-term increase in both direct and indirect costs to the US health system and economy.

The tremendous personal and societal costs associated with opioid addiction, other substance use disorders, and concurrent chronic medical and mental health conditions have not gone unnoticed. In response, policy makers and healthcare providers alike have increasingly turned to integrated care as a potential solution. Conceptually, combining the medical care and addiction treatment needs of patients with substance use disorders makes logical sense. In practice, the creation of effective models of integrated addiction and medical care is still an evolving process. National events and efforts over the years have significantly furthered the ability for this integration to occur (Fig. 12.1).

With the passage of the Drug Addiction Treatment Act in 2000 and the Food and Drug Administration's (FDA) approval of sublingual buprenorphine/naloxone for the treatment of OUD in 2002, the focus of integrated addiction treatment and other medical care landed on traditional primary care settings. With the expansion of buprenorphine prescribing authority from only physicians to nurse practitioners and physician assistants in the Comprehensive Addiction and Recovery Act (CARA) in 2016, the capacity to effectively treat OUD grew even further. The FDA's approval in 2010 of injectable naltrexone for the treatment of OUD following opioid withdrawal management added to the pharmacological options available to primary care practitioners. To support primary care in taking on these new therapies, state governments and federal agencies collectively have invested hundreds of millions of dollars on prescriber training, technical assistance for healthcare systems and medical practices, grants to support hiring of behavioral health specialists, and health information technology upgrades. Evaluations of integrated care models for opioid use disorder treatment in primary care demonstrate the positive impact of these investments; an increase in the number of practitioners treating opioid use disorder in primary care settings and higher numbers of patients receiving effective therapies [18–20].

However, the ability to treat OUD with effective medications in primary care has not resulted in an end to all barriers to integrated, comprehensive healthcare for people needing these services. Surveys of practitioners with the required "waiver" to prescribe buprenorphine/naloxone consistently find that, on average, they treat fewer patients than their currently allowable limits set by federal law. A study from California found that a third of 467 respondents were not treating any patients for OUD with buprenorphine/naloxone even though they had taken required training and received the necessary certificate to do so [21]. An analysis of prescription monitoring programs from three states severely affected by the opioid crisis

1965	1970	1974	1980s & 1990s	2000 & 2002	2010	2011	2013	2015	2016	2020
• Dole and Nyswander publish landmark study on methadone for OUD	• Comprehensive Drug Abuse Prevention and Control Act lays groundwork for OTPs	• Narcotic Addiction Treatment Act establishes OTPs	• AIDS crisis	• DATA 2000 and FDA approval of buprenorphine for OUD	• FDA approval of naltrexone for OUD	• FDA approval of first DAA for HCV treatment	• Health Home model expansion in OTPs	• CSAT guidelines for OTPs revised	• Comprehensive Addiction and Recovery Act	• Barriers to integrated care in OTPs remain but promising practices persist

Fig. 12.1 Timeline of key national integration events and efforts

identified a mean monthly census of 43 patients cared for by prescribers at 100-patient limit and 14 patients treated by clinicians at the 30-patient limit [22]. While physicians at the highest available limit of 275 patients are more likely to fully utilize their capacity, they represent only 8% of eligible providers [23]. In 2018, 40% of the US counties did not have even one "waivered" provider [23].

While a host of factors influence buprenorphine/naloxone prescribing patterns of "waivered" practitioners [20, 24], negative attitudes about medications for addiction treatment, limited confidence in treating OUD, and enduring stigma toward the illness and the people affected by it continue to create significant barriers [25]. The reality also remains that some patients with moderate to severe opioid use disorder simply may not respond to buprenorphine/naloxone or injectable naltrexone and may require methadone to effectively treat their disease. Drs. Vincent Dole and Marie Nyswander in 1965 initially demonstrated the effectiveness of methadone in reducing heroin use and improving recovery-related outcomes [26]. Since their report, research has built a robust body of evidence for significant reductions in opioid-related morbidity and mortality with methadone treatment [27, 28], less criminal legal system involvement [29, 30], and clinically meaningful improvements in quality of life, employment, and social supports [31–33].

Under current regulatory frameworks, Opioid Treatment Programs (OTPs) are the only setting in the US in which people can access methadone for the treatment of OUD. Established as part of federal legislation in the early 1970s, including the Comprehensive Drug Abuse Prevention and Control Act of 1970 and the subsequent Narcotic Addict Treatment Act of 1974, the focus for decades within OTPs remained on the provision of methadone and counseling services for the treatment of opioid addiction. To the extent medical care was provided, it primarily consisted of the initial comprehensive history and physical examination required by a physician to initiate methadone treatment and any follow-up care specifically related to that medication [34].

With the approval of buprenorphine, some OTPs added that medication to their inventory especially since the strict rules that govern how frequently patients must attend an OTP to receive daily doses of methadone do not all apply to buprenorphine [35]. For example, patients receiving methadone must attend the clinic 6 days per week during the first 90 days of treatment to take their dose under nursing supervision. As patients stabilize, the number of doses they can take home steadily increases, but it can take 2 years in treatment before a patient is eligible to receive a monthly supply of methadone. This same "time in treatment" criterion does not apply to the provision of buprenorphine in an OTP. The strict regulations that govern methadone delivery in OTPs has received criticism over the past few years as being overly rigid and outdated [36]. On the other hand, the frequent contact between healthcare providers and patients possible in this setting, no matter whether methadone or buprenorphine/naloxone is provided, can be beneficial in assisting individuals with complex, multiple health conditions. Evidence shows that the prevalence of multimorbidity, or multiple, simultaneous health conditions, is high in patients receiving care in OTPs. In a 10-year retrospective study of 274 patients attending a primary care–based opioid treatment clinic in Australia [37], 89% fell into the category of multimorbidity and 90% had moderate to severe disease conditions. In comparison to a general patient control population, patients treated with methadone were over seven times more likely to have multimorbidity across two or more domains and almost four times more likely to have multimorbidity over three or more domains. The severity of overall disease was also higher among the patients treated with methadone with 91% of them falling into the moderate or severe categories compared with only 32.5% of the non-SUD control population. This held true across three of four age categories, only converging in the oldest age groups.

While integrating treatment with methadone into primary care settings has occurred in other countries [38, 39], the concept of providing broader medical care and OUD treatment with methadone has been slow to emerge in the US. Some studies have investigated the feasibility of integrating methadone treatment for OUD into primary care [40, 41], but the current regulatory framework makes this logistically and administratively extremely difficult. With the AIDS crisis in the 1980s and early 1990s, interest slowly grew in integrating additional medical care into OTPs instead. Selwyn and colleagues reported on their experience providing on-site medical care for over 900 patients with or at risk for HIV in an OTP in New York City over 2 years during this period [42]. Supported in part by a federal demonstration grant from the National Institutes on Drug Abuse (NIDA) and the Health Resources and Services Administration (HRSA) and after negotiation with the New York State Medicaid program, the OTP provided HIV treatment as needed, integrated tuberculosis therapy, both for active and latent disease, as well as primary care and methadone-related medical services. An evaluation of 476 patients from the program enrolled in a prospective cohort study found that 81% utilized the primary care services offered onsite with an annualized mean number of visits of 6.3. Aside from AIDS-related visits, patients commonly received care for psychiatric illnesses, other substance use disorders, upper respiratory infections and bronchitis, pregnancy, diabetes, and cirrhosis [43].

A clinical research team in Baltimore, Maryland, expanded on the feasibility study done by Selwyn. In a randomized controlled trial of 51 patients, the group compared integrated medical care in an OTP with primary care referral for four common medical conditions: hypertension, latent tuberculosis, HIV, and acute sexually transmitted infections (STIs) [44]. The main primary care referral site was located within walking distance of the OTP, staffed with addiction-knowledgeable practitioners, and the study covered the costs of medical care, including any prescribed medications. The results were striking. Of the patients receiving onsite medical care, 92% attended at least one appointment and adhered to therapeutic recommendations compared with 32% in the referral arm. The average number of visits per patient during the 8-week study was 3.1 for the onsite medical care group compared to 0.4 for the referred patients. A higher number of patients in the onsite medical care group had successful normalization of blood pressure and syphilis treatment, completion of latent tuberculosis evaluation and therapy, and appropriate HIV follow-up and initiation of anti-retroviral medication.

Since these initial demonstrations, other studies have documented the effectiveness on common clinical outcomes of integrating more medical and psychiatric care into OTPs [45–49]. The opioid addiction and overdose crisis over the past two decades and the increasing acceptance of methadone treatment as medical care has heightened the call for OTPs to deliver more comprehensive services to their patients. In revising and updating its OTP regulatory guideline in 2015, the Center for Substance Abuse Treatment (CSAT) at the Substance Abuse and Mental Health Services Administration (SAMHSA) stated that "Increasingly, it is expected that substance abuse [sic] and mental health treatment programs will integrate medical and behavioral health services into their clinical programs in order to address the needs of the whole person receiving treatment services. OTPs may be especially well positioned to do this because they are already required to offer medical and substance use disorder treatment in a single setting [50]." In the same document, CSAT pointedly noted that "It is highly recommended, but not required, that OTP's provide basic primary care onsite. OTP physicians can prescribe medication as appropriate for co-occurring medical and psychiatric disorders [51]."

Despite the increased focus on integrating medical care and other services into OTPs, sometimes referred to as "reverse integration," implementation of this comprehensive care model has been slow in practice. Some have hypothesized that the siloed, historic structure of OTPs has so separated them from the rest of healthcare that there is a cultural or philosophical gap. Research has not borne this out as a primary obstacle [52], but anecdotally, not all OTPs embrace the concept of incorporating primary care and other services into their model. Others have pointed to drastically different financing and reimbursement structures that complicate the sustainability of primary care services in OTPs. However, evidence exists that integrated primary care in an OTP reduces rates of hospital admission and avoidable emergency department visits [53, 54]. This value-added underpins ongoing state- and system-level efforts to broaden and support the scope of services available in OTPs despite the challenges.

The application of the behavioral health home model made available by the Affordable Care Act to Medicaid-enrollees is one example of a system-wide step toward supporting more of a focus on primary care in OTPs [55]. Becoming a Health Home allows OTPs to augment their existing services, building upon and adding to their staff and activities to better serve their patients. The model consists of a multidisciplinary team that includes nurse care managers, physicians and nurse practitioners, substance use counselors, mental health therapists, and administrative staff, all working with patients in a collaborative manner. Clinical approaches incorporated into the health home model combine several evidence-based interventions to engage and motivate patients for broad health-focused behavior change. Techniques include motivational interviewing [56], cognitive behavioral therapy [57], and use of incentives in a modified contingency management model [58].

Patients qualify for health home services by virtue of taking a medication for opioid use disorder and being at risk for another chronic health condition. Based on patient needs, health home team staff connect individuals to various supports and services not available through the OTP, offer health promotion activities, and monitor medical and behavioral health needs. Health Home service categories include comprehensive   care   management,   care   coordination,   health   promotion, comprehensive transitional care, individual and family support, and referral to community and/or social support. OTPs are paid monthly rate per patient if the patient received at least two health home services in the month.

Ultimately, the goal of integrating a Health Home into an OTP is to reduce healthcare costs among individuals with chronic conditions and improve the patient experience of care. The Hilltop Institute, in an evaluation of the first 3 years of Maryland's behavioral health home model [59], which includes OTPs, psychiatric rehabilitation programs (PRPs), and mobile treatment services (MTS), reported that the number of patients enrolled in an OTP-based Health Home increased steadily between inception of the model in 2013 and 2016. By the end of June 2016, OTPs were providing health home services to close to 1200 patients, with all patients across Maryland health homes receiving an average of 5.5–6 services monthly. About 57% of all health home participants met criteria for a very high or high comorbidity level with another 37.5% classified in the moderate comorbidity category. Comprehensive care management, care coordination, and health promotion accounted for the majority of services provided. Emergency department utilization and inpatient hospitalizations among the Maryland health home participants fell significantly the longer participants stayed engaged with these services (Fig. 12.2).

For patients dually enrolled in Medicare and Medicaid, receipt of OTP-based health home services had a particularly positive effect compared to a matched comparison group [60]. In 2015, 25% of these patients experienced at least one inpatient hospital admission compared to 36% in the control group. In addition, there were no 30-day readmissions in this dually enrolled health home group (HHG) in 2015 while 6.8% of the matched comparison group experienced at least one such readmission. That same year, 87.5% of the HHG group had at least one nonbehavioral health-related ambulatory care visit, including to a primary care provider, compared

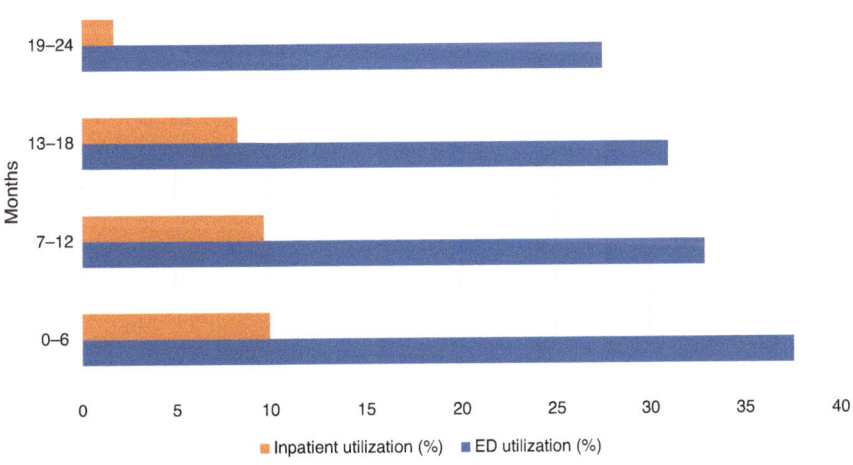

Fig. 12.2 Emergency department and inpatient utilization by length of health home enrollment

to 81.8% of the control group. Importantly, none of the dually enrolled HHG group required a nursing home admission compared to 4.5% of the control group.

The group differences in healthcare utilization for patients receiving OTP-based health home services translated into lower costs. The average hospital inpatient cost in 2015 among the dually Medicare and Medicaid-enrolled HHG was $1820 compared to $5022 in the matched, non-Health Home-enrolled group. The difference was slightly smaller among the remaining group of patients receiving health home services in the OTPs but still, on average, about $1300 lower than the inpatient cost for the matched comparison group. Outpatient costs and the total average cost of healthcare per person was lower among the dually enrolled HHG than for the matched control group [61]. While the report cautions that many of the findings are preliminary and not based on random assignment, it states that there is clearly a demand for health home services. Accrediting bodies, including the Commission on Accreditation of Rehabilitation Facilities' (CARF) or the Joint Commission on Accreditation of Healthcare Organizations (JCAHO), have developed specific accreditation standards for behavioral health homes, lending the model additional credibility.

Anecdotally, the patient experience of care has improved significantly with adoption of health home services [62], including in OTPs. Patients with OUD taking methadone for their illness face significant stigma, often from healthcare professionals. Health Home staff identify and develop relationships with methadone-friendly primary care and mental health providers in their community to decrease the stigma that individuals in treatment face when seeking external healthcare. Health literacy, the degree to which individuals have the capacity to obtain, process, and understand basic health information and services needed to make appropriate health decisions, is another barrier for many patients receiving care in OTPs. The Institute of Medicine/National Academies reports that nearly half the population in the United States has difficulty understanding and using health information [63]. An additional objective of the Health Home is to assist individuals in navigating the healthcare system to equip them with the skills to make fitting healthcare decisions. Health home staff serve as healthcare translators as well, helping to decipher hospital discharge and medication instructions. All the non-judgmental support patients receive from their OTP team builds increased trust, a crucial element to effective healthcare delivery. In turn, patients feel safe accessing other medical and mental health services and focus on their recovery from a different perspective. The communication and care coordination that occurs between OTP health home team members and outside providers also serves an educational purpose, helping disseminate a better understanding of medications for addiction treatment and multidisciplinary approaches to substance use disorder treatment [64].

The advent of curative, oral, direct-acting antiretroviral (DAA) medications for hepatitis C (HCV) has presented another opportunity to integrate additional medical care into OTPs. OTPs can be an ideal setting for people with addiction and hepatitis C to access HCV treatment. Staff at the OTP are familiar with the needs of their patients and if necessary, patients can receive many, if not all, of the DAA medication doses directly observed at the clinic. This directly observed therapy (DOT) model has its roots in the public health approach for treating tuberculosis [65] and evidence for the effectiveness of providing directly administered antiretroviral therapy (DAART) for HIV to achieve HIV RNA suppression in patients enrolled in an OTP. In a nonrandomized, comparative study of 128 HIV-positive matched patients with OUD, most of whom treated with methadone, at month 6, HIV RNA levels were significantly lower in the DAART arm than in the standard care group and in the adherence support group [47]. Nearly 80% of participants enrolled in the DAART initiative achieved suppression of HIV RNA levels to <400 copies/ml compared with about 50% in the comparison groups. The DAART program also led to changes in the culture at the OTP, including greater dialogue among patients and staff about HIV and treatment and greater collaboration between substance use providers and medical staff.

The rate of chronic hepatitis C is extremely high among patients receiving care in OTPs, over 70% in some areas [66]. While many patients in OTPs harbor HCV, in the pre-DAA era, few initiated or completed the treatment process with the rigorous, lengthy regimens of interferon- and ribavirin-based regimens that carried significant side effects [67]. Certainly, the regimen itself presented a barrier for patients but studies from that time period also cite limited access to medical evaluations and concerns about adherence as significant barriers, despite evidence to the contrary [67, 68].

The introduction of well-tolerated, simple regimens using DAA medications removed the treatment itself as a rationale for withholding hepatitis C cure to people who inject drugs (PWID). However, some providers continue to exclude people with SUDs when considering candidacy for DAA therapy due to concerns about treatment adherence. Evidence disputes this assumption. Several studies show that adherence to the new regimens is high among PWID, including HCV-infected patients receiving care in OTPs. Furthermore, because the available medications are so effective, sustained cure rates among people with OUD is also high. In a series of three large, international, randomized trials of ledipasvir/sofosbuvir, commonly called the ION studies, 97% of individuals with OUD taking methadone or buprenorphine completed HCV therapy compared to 98% of those without OUD. There were no differences in adherence rates. Similarly, the proportion of patients in both groups who achieved sustained cure (measured as SVR12, or Sustained Virologic Response at 12 weeks following completion of DAA therapy) was high; 94% in the treated OUD group vs 97% in the control group ($p = 0.28$) [69]. The C-EDGE CO-STAR study, a randomized, placebo-controlled, double-blind trial of over 300 methadone or buprenorphine-treated OUD patients conducted across 12 countries, was pivotal in proving that patients in OTPs showed high medication adherence and efficacy with elbasvir/grazoprevir. Adherence was extremely high and 94% of the patients treated with the DAA medications achieved SVR12, the measure of HCV cure. Of note, almost 60% of study participants had at least one positive drug test for cocaine, amphetamines, benzodiazepines, cannabis, and/or other opioids at baseline and at points throughout the 12-week course of their DAA treatment [70]. In additional trials using sofosbuvir/velpatasvir [71], SVR12 was achieved in 96% of patients taking methadone or buprenorphine and 98% of patients without an SUD. No clinically significant medication interactions occurred and no dose adjustments of either opioid agonist medication was needed. Cohort studies demonstrate that adherence and HCV cure rates remain high among this population even in community settings outside of strict research protocols [72–74].

A crucial piece of increasing initiation of DAA treatment among PWID is education about hepatitis C and the possibility of cure. Education is needed to ensure patients understand that continued drug use is not a contraindication to HCV treatment and has not been associated with treatment failure. In a validated survey study of 124 HCV-infected patients from two OTPs in Baltimore [75], 60% had seen a clinician who could treat HCV, but only 40% had therapy recommended to them. Of these, 20% had started or completed DAA treatment. Of the 68 participants providing open-ended comments, 51% reported that having additional information about HCV and its treatment with DAA would facilitate treatment among PWID. In this study, 72% of patients had awareness of the potential risk of reinfection post-HCV cure.

While reinfection is certainly a possibility, a review of several studies shows that reinfection rates are low, even among PWID [76]. This may be due to partial protective immunity or harm reduction practices that are known to reduce HCV transmission risk [77]. Health home staff in OTPs and peer recovery specialists play key roles here as they provide education regarding safer sex practices, referrals to syringe service programs, and harm reduction education on reducing the sharing of drug equipment. Having Health Home services in place can also assist with providing pretreatment education on HCV transmission, risk factors for fibrosis progression, HCV treatment options, side effects, and reinfection risk. Health home staff can also encourage participation in HCV care including group treatment. Group treatment of HCV is an option that allows patients to openly discuss adherence and adverse effects and receive mutual supports, including the assistance of peer recovery specialists. SVR rates of individuals randomized to a directly observed treatment (DOT) arm in the PREVAIL studies show 98% cure versus 90% for self-administration and 96% for group treatment [78]. Involvement of the multidisciplinary team with increased treatment linkage improved SVR rates independently of any other variables.

Unfortunately, stigma remains a large barrier for people with SUDs seeking healthcare for HCV treatment [79]. Several health insurance companies have varying requirements regarding abstinence, ranging from 1 to 12 months in order to obtain prior authorization for DAA. Due to the high costs of DAA medications, many state Medicaid programs restrict coverage of treatment to people with more advanced stages of liver fibrosis which negatively impacts progress through the care continuum and can send the message that HCV treatment is not a health priority. People with OUD and other SUDs have interactions with law enforcement that land them in prison and jails where access to addiction care and HCV treatment is limited. Many people with OUD avoid traditional healthcare settings for fear of being judged, verbally abused, or otherwise treated poorly. However, the American Association for the Study of Liver Diseases (AASLD) and the Infectious Diseases

Society of America (IDSA) both recommend that HCV treatment be considered for all individuals, regardless of their illicit drug use or treatment for OUD [80]. Their guideline on hepatitis C testing, management, and treatment concludes that there "is no data to support the utility of pretreatment screening for illicit drug or alcohol use in identifying a population more likely to successfully complete HCV therapy, and these requirements should be abandoned [81]." Based on all the evidence, the World Health Organization considers HCV treatment for all HCV-infected individuals, including people who inject drugs (PWID), as prevention and an imperative public health approach to reach the elimination goals of 90% diagnosed, 80% treated, and 65% reduction in mortality by 2030 [82]. Integrating universal screening for and treatment of chronic HCV in OTPs will go a long way toward helping meet these goals.

Integrated substance use disorder and primary care services can improve patients' physical and mental health, increase the likelihood that patients with HIV and HCV will receive antiretroviral therapy, and decrease hospitalization rates, inpatient days, and emergency department utilization. Integrating SUD services with medical care can importantly lead to significant healthcare cost savings for patients with conditions related to substance use. As healthcare systems, payers, and policymakers look to identify effective models of integrated care, a "reverse integration" strategy involving OTPs should not be overlooked. OTPs in the US provide care to over 350,000 people with OUD [83]. The incorporation of medical services into these substance use treatment programs offers a valuable and proven approach to providing effective, holistic care to a vulnerable patient population with historically low levels of engagement with preventive and routine healthcare. For many patients, the ability to access primary care through their OTPs can mean all the difference in their journeys towards better health.

References

1. Saitz R. Medical and surgical complications of addiction. In: Miller SC, Fiellin DA, Rosenthal RN, Saitz R, editors. The ASAM principles of addiction medicine. ASAM; 2019. p. 1128.
2. Jones CM, McCance-Katz EF. Co-occurring substance use and mental disorders among adults with opioid use disorder. Drug Alcohol Depend. 2019;197:78–82. https://doi.org/10.1016/j.drugalcdep.2018.12.030.
3. Zibbell JE, Asher AK, Patel RC, et al. Increases in acute hepatitis C virus infection related to a growing opioid epidemic and associated injection drug use, United States, 2004 to 2014. Am J Public Health. 2018;108(2):175–81. https://doi.org/10.2105/AJPH.2017.304132.
4. Kadri AM, Wilner B, Hernandez AV, Nakhoul G, Chahine J, Griffin B, et al. Geographic trends, patient characteristics, and outcomes of infective endocarditis associated with drug abuse in the United States from 2002 to 2016. J Am Heart Assoc. 2019;8:e012969. https://doi.org/10.1161/JAHA.119.012969.
5. Zibbell JE, Iqbal K, Patel RC, et al. Increases in hepatitis C virus infection related to injection drug use among persons aged ≤30 years – Kentucky, Tennessee, Virginia, and West Virginia, 2006–2012. MMWR Morb Mortal Wkly Rep. 2015;64(17):453–8.
6. Peters PJ, Pontones P, Hoover KW, et al. HIV infection linked to injection use of oxymorphone in Indiana, 2014–2015. N Engl J Med. 2016;375(3):229–39. https://doi.org/10.1056/NEJMoa1515195.

7. Alpren C, Dawson EL, John B, et al. Opioid use fueling HIV transmission in an urban setting: an outbreak of HIV infection among people who inject drugs-Massachusetts, 2015-2018. Am J Public Health. 2020;110(1):37–44. https://doi.org/10.2105/AJPH.2019.305366.
8. Fleischauer AT, Ruhl L, Rhea S, Barnes E. Hospitalizations for endocarditis and associated health care costs among persons with diagnosed drug dependence – North Carolina, 2010–2015. MMWR Morb Mortal Wkly Rep. 2017;66(22):569–73. https://doi.org/10.15585/mmwr.mm6622a1.
9. Centers for disease control and prevention: hepatitis C questions and answers for health professionals. https://www.cdc.gov/hepatitis/hcv/hcvfaq.htm#Ref01 2020. Accessed 1 Jun 2020.
10. Centers for disease control and prevention: HIV and people who inject drugs. https://www.cdc.gov/hiv/group/hiv-idu.html 2020. Accessed 27 Feb 2020.
11. Goldner EM, Lusted A, Roerecke M, Rehm J, Fischer B. Prevalence of Axis-1 psychiatric (with focus on depression and anxiety) disorder and symptomatology among non-medical prescription opioid users in substance use treatment: systematic review and meta-analyses. Addict Behav. 2014;39(3):520–31. https://doi.org/10.1016/j.addbeh.2013.11.022.
12. Cicero TJ, Ellis MS, Surratt HL, Kurtz SP. The changing face of heroin use in the United States: a retrospective analysis of the past 50 years. JAMA Psychiat. 2014;71(7):821–6. https://doi.org/10.1001/jamapsychiatry.2014.366.
13. Riley ED, Wu AW, Junge B, Marx M, Strathdee SA, Vlahov D. Health services utilization by injection drug users participating in a needle exchange program. Am J Drug Alcohol Abuse. 2002;28(3):497–511. https://doi.org/10.1081/ada-120006738.
14. Artenie AA, Jutras-Aswad D, Roy É, et al. Visits to primary care physicians among persons who inject drugs at high risk of hepatitis C virus infection: room for improvement. J Viral Hepat. 2015;22(10):792–9. https://doi.org/10.1111/jvh.12393.
15. Lewer D, Freer J, King E, et al. Frequency of health-care utilization by adults who use illicit drugs: a systematic review and meta-analysis. Addiction. 2020;115(6):1011–23. https://doi.org/10.1111/add.14892.
16. Ronan MV, Herzig SJ. Hospitalizations related to opioid abuse/dependence and associated serious infections increased sharply, 2002–12. Health Aff (Millwood). 2016;35(5):832–7. https://doi.org/10.1377/hlthaff.2015.1424.
17. Leslie DL, Ba DM, Agbese E, Xing X, Guodong L. The economic burden of the opioid epidemic on states: the case of medicaid. Am J Manag Care. 2019;25:S0. https://www.ajmc.com/journals/supplement/2019/deaths-dollars-diverted-resources-opioid-epidemic/the-economic-burden-opioid-epidemic-on-states-case-of-medicaid. Accessed 7 Jun 2020.
18. Stein BD, Gordon AJ, Sorbero M, Dick AW, Schuster J, Farmer C. The impact of buprenorphine on treatment of opioid dependence in a Medicaid population: recent service utilization trends in the use of buprenorphine and methadone. Drug Alcohol Depend. 2012;123(1–3):72–8. https://doi.org/10.1016/j.drugalcdep.2011.10.016.
19. LaBelle CT, Han SC, Bergeron A, Samet JH. Office-Based Opioid Treatment with Buprenorphine (OBOT-B): statewide implementation of the Massachusetts collaborative care model in community health centers. J Subst Abus Treat. 2016;60:6–13. https://doi.org/10.1016/j.jsat.2015.06.010.
20. Stein BD, Pacula RL, Gordon AJ, et al. Where is buprenorphine dispensed to treat opioid use disorders? The role of private offices, opioid treatment programs, and substance abuse treatment facilities in urban and rural counties. Milbank Q. 2015;93(3):561–83. https://doi.org/10.1111/1468-0009.12137.
21. UCLA Integrated Substance Abuse Programs. Waivered prescriber support initiative: training needs survey summary report 2019. http://uclaisap.org/MATPrescriberSupport/docs/SOR-Waivered%20Prescriber%20Support_SurveyReport30oct2019-FINALA.pdf. Accessed 7 Jun 2020.
22. Thomas CP, Doyle E, Kreiner PW, et al. Prescribing patterns of buprenorphine waivered physicians. Drug Alcohol Depend. 2017;181:213–8. https://doi.org/10.1016/j.drugalcdep.2017.10.002.
23. U.S. Department of Health and Human Services. Office of inspector general. geographic disparities affect access to buprenorphine services for opioid use disorder 2020;

January:OEI-12-17-0024. https://oig.hhs.gov/oei/reports/oei-12-17-00240.pdf. Accessed 7 Jun 2020.

24. Andraka-Christou B, Capone MJ. A qualitative study comparing physician-reported barriers to treating addiction using buprenorphine and extended-release naltrexone in U.S. office-based practices. Int J Drug Policy. 2018;54:9–17. https://doi.org/10.1016/j.drugpo.2017.11.021.

25. Louie DL, Assefa MT, McGovern MP. Attitudes of primary care physicians toward prescribing buprenorphine: a narrative review. BMC Fam Pract. 2019;20(1):157. https://doi.org/10.1186/s12875-019-1047-z.

26. Dole VP, Nyswander M. A Medical treatment for diacetylmorphine (heroin) addiction. A clinical trial with methadone hydrochloride. JAMA. 1965;193:646–50. https://doi.org/10.1001/jama.1965.03090080008002.

27. Mattick RP, Breen C, Kimber J, Davoli M. Methadone maintenance therapy versus no opioid replacement therapy for opioid dependence. Cochrane Database Syst Rev. 2009;2009(3):CD002209. https://doi.org/10.1002/14651858.CD002209.pub2.

28. Wakeman SE, Larochelle MR, Ameli O, et al. Comparative effectiveness of different treatment pathways for opioid use disorder. JAMA Netw Open. 2020;3(2):e1920622. https://doi.org/10.1001/jamanetworkopen.2019.20622.

29. Hubbard RL, Craddock SG, Anderson J. Overview of 5-year follow-up outcomes in the drug abuse treatment outcome studies (DATOS). J Subst Abus Treat. 2003;25(3):125–34. https://doi.org/10.1016/s0740-5472(03)00130-2.

30. National Academies of Sciences, Engineering, and Medicine. Medications for opioid use disorder save lives. Washington, DC: The National Academies Press; 2019. https://doi.org/10.17226/25310. Accessed 30 Jan 2020.

31. Fullerton CA, Kim M, Thomas CP, et al. Medication-assisted treatment with methadone: assessing the evidence. Psychiatr Serv. 2014;65(2):146–57. https://doi.org/10.1176/appi.ps.201300235.

32. Chou YC, Shih SF, Tsai WD, Li CS, Xu K, Lee TS. Improvement of quality of life in methadone treatment patients in northern Taiwan: a follow-up study. BMC Psychiatry. 2013;13:190. https://doi.org/10.1186/1471-244X-13-190.

33. Sun HM, Li XY, Chow EP, et al. Methadone maintenance treatment programme reduces criminal activity and improves social well-being of drug users in China: a systematic review and meta-analysis. BMJ Open. 2015;5(1):e005997. https://doi.org/10.1136/bmjopen-2014-005997.

34. Institute of Medicine (US) Committee on Federal Regulation of Methadone Treatment. In: Rettig RA, Yarmolinsky A, editors. Federal regulation of methadone treatment. Washington, DC: National Academies Press; 1995.

35. Department of Health and Human Services. Federal register. Opioid drugs in maintenance and detoxification treatment of opiate addiction; proposed modification of dispensing restrictions for buprenorphine and buprenorphine combinations as used in approved opioid treatment medications. December 6, 2012. https://www.federalregister.gov/documents/2012/12/06/2012-29417/opioid-drugs-in-maintenance-and-detoxification-treatment-of-opiate-addiction-proposed-modification. Accessed 30 Jan 2020.

36. Samet JH, Botticelli M, Bharel M. Methadone in primary care – one small step for congress, one giant leap for addiction treatment. N Engl J Med. 2018;379(1):7–8. https://doi.org/10.1056/NEJMp1803982.

37. Arnold-Reed DE, Brett T, Troeung L, O'Neill J, Backhouse R, Bulsara MK. Multimorbidity in patients enrolled in a community-based methadone maintenance treatment programme delivered through primary care. J Comorb. 2014;4:46–54. https://doi.org/10.15256/joc.2014.4.42.

38. Morozova O, Dvoriak S, Pykalo I, Altice FL. Primary healthcare-based integrated care with opioid agonist treatment: first experience from Ukraine. Drug Alcohol Depend. 2017;173:132–8. https://doi.org/10.1016/j.drugalcdep.2016.12.025.

39. Ordean A, Kahan M, Graves L, Abrahams R, Boyajian T. Integrated care for pregnant women on methadone maintenance treatment: Canadian primary care cohort study. Can Fam Physician. 2013;59(10):e462–9.

40. Novick DM, Salsitz EA, Joseph H, Kreek MJ. Methadone medical maintenance: an early 21st-century perspective. J Addict Dis. 2015;34(2–3):226–37. https://doi.org/10.1080/1055088
7.2015.1059225.
41. Novick DM, Joseph H, Salsitz EA, et al. Outcomes of treatment of socially rehabilitated methadone maintenance patients in physicians' offices (medical maintenance): follow-up at three and a half to nine and a fourth years. J Gen Intern Med. 1994;9(3):127–30. https://doi.org/10.1007/BF02600025.
42. Selwyn PA, Feingold AR, Iezza A, et al. Primary care for patients with human immunodeficiency virus (HIV) infection in a methadone maintenance treatment program. Ann Intern Med. 1989;111(9):761–3. https://doi.org/10.7326/0003-4819-111-9-761.
43. Selwyn PA, Budner NS, Wasserman WC, Arno PS. Utilization of on-site primary care services by HIV-seropositive and seronegative drug users in a methadone maintenance program. Public Health Rep. 1993;108(4):492–500.
44. Umbricht-Schneiter A, Ginn DH, Pabst KM, Bigelow GE. Providing medical care to methadone clinic patients: referral vs on-site care. Am J Public Health. 1994;84(2):207–10. https://doi.org/10.2105/ajph.84.2.207.
45. Gourevitch MN, Wasserman W, Panero MS, Selwyn PA. Successful adherence to observed prophylaxis and treatment of tuberculosis among drug users in a methadone program. J Addict Dis. 1996;15(1):93–104. https://doi.org/10.1300/J069v15n01_07.
46. Batki SL, Gruber VA, Bradley JM, Bradley M, Delucchi K. A controlled trial of methadone treatment combined with directly observed isoniazid for tuberculosis prevention in injection drug users. Drug Alcohol Depend. 2002;66(3):283–93. https://doi.org/10.1016/s0376-8716(01)00208-3.
47. Lucas GM, Weidle PJ, Hader S, Moore RD. Directly administered antiretroviral therapy in an urban methadone maintenance clinic: a nonrandomized comparative study. Clin Infect Dis. 2004;38(Suppl 5):S409–13. https://doi.org/10.1086/421405.
48. Berkman ND, Wechsberg WM. Access to treatment-related and support services in methadone treatment programs. J Subst Abus Treat. 2007;32(1):97–104. https://doi.org/10.1016/j.jsat.2006.07.004.
49. Brooner RK, Kidorf MS, King VL, et al. Managing psychiatric comorbidity within versus outside of methadone treatment settings: a randomized and controlled evaluation. Addiction. 2013;108(11):1942–51. https://doi.org/10.1111/add.12269.
50. Substance Abuse and Mental Health Services Administration. Federal guidelines for opioid treatment programs. HHS publication no. (SMA) PEP15-FEDGUIDEOTP. Substance Abuse and Mental Health Services Administration: Rockville; 2015.
51. Substance Abuse and Mental Health Services Administration. Federal Guidelines for Opioid Treatment Programs. HHS Publication No. (SMA) PEP15-FEDGUIDEOTP. Rockville: Substance Abuse and Mental Health Services Administration; 2015. p. 43.
52. Friedmann PD, Alexander JA, D'Aunno TA. Organizational correlates of access to primary care and mental health services in drug abuse treatment units. J Subst Abus Treat. 1999;16(1):71–80. https://doi.org/10.1016/s0740-5472(98)00018-x.
53. Friedmann PD, Hendrickson JC, Gerstein DR, Zhang Z, Stein MD. Do mechanisms that link addiction treatment patients to primary care influence subsequent utilization of emergency and hospital care? Med Care. 2006;44(1):8–15. https://doi.org/10.1097/01.mlr.0000188913.50489.77.
54. Gourevitch MN, Chatterji P, Deb N, Schoenbaum EE, Turner BJ. On-site medical care in methadone maintenance: associations with health care use and expenditures. J Subst Abus Treat. 2007;32(2):143–51. https://doi.org/10.1016/j.jsat.2006.07.008.
55. Maryland Medicaid Health Homes. 2015. https://mmcp.health.maryland.gov/SiteAssets/SitePages/Healthy%20Homes/Maryland%20Medicaid%20Health%20Homes-%201%20pager%2011.13.15.pdf. Accessed 27 Jan 2020.
56. Rubak S, Sandbaek A, Lauritzen T, Christensen B. Motivational interviewing: a systematic review and meta-analysis. Br J Gen Pract. 2005;55(513):305–12.

57. Magill M, Ray L, Kiluk B, et al. A meta-analysis of cognitive-behavioral therapy for alcohol or other drug use disorders: treatment efficacy by contrast condition. J Consult Clin Psychol. 2019;87(12):1093–105. https://doi.org/10.1037/ccp0000447.
58. Rash CJ, Stitzer M, Weinstock J. Contingency management: new directions and remaining challenges for an evidence-based intervention. J Subst Abus Treat. 2017;72:10–8. https://doi.org/10.1016/j.jsat.2016.09.008.
59. The Hilltop Institute. 2016 health home evaluation report. June 14, 2017. https://mmcp.health.maryland.gov/SiteAssets/SitePages/Health%20Home%20Program%20Evaluation%20and%20Outcomes/health_home_2016_evaluation_report.pdf. Accessed 20 May 2020.
60. The Hilltop Institute. 2016 health home evaluation report. June 14, 2017. https://mmcp.health.maryland.gov/SiteAssets/SitePages/Health%20Home%20Program%20Evaluation%20and%20Outcomes/health_home_2016_evaluation_report.pdf. P. 23–28. Accessed 20 May 2020.
61. The Hilltop Institute. 2016 health home evaluation report. June 14, 2017. https://mmcp.health.maryland.gov/SiteAssets/SitePages/Health%20Home%20Program%20Evaluation%20and%20Outcomes/health_home_2016_evaluation_report.pdf. P. 31–32 and 35. Accessed 7 Jun 2020.
62. U.S. Department of Health and Human Services. Assistant secretary for planning and evaluation. office of disability, aging, and long-term care policy. Evaluation of the medicaid health home option for beneficiaries with chronic conditions: evaluation of outcomes of selected health home program, annual report – year five. May 2017. https://aspe.hhs.gov/system/files/pdf/258871/HHOption5.pdf. Accessed 27 Jan 2020.
63. Institute of Medicine (US) Committee on Health Literacy. In: Nielsen-Bohlman L, Panzer AM, Kindig DA, editors. Health literacy: a prescription to end confusion. Washington, DC: National Academies Press (US); 2004. p. 1. https://doi.org/10.17226/10883.
64. Personal communications with clinicians at Institutes for Behavior Resources, Inc/REACH Health Services, Baltimore, MD and Absolute Care, Baltimore, MD. 2013–2020.
65. Chaulk CP, Kazandjian VA. Directly observed therapy for treatment completion of pulmonary tuberculosis: consensus statement of the public health tuberculosis guidelines panel [published correction appears in JAMA 1998 Jul 8;280(2):134]. JAMA. 1998;279(12):943–8. https://doi.org/10.1001/jama.279.12.943.
66. Fareed A, Musselman D, Byrd-Sellers J, et al. On-site basic health screening and brief health counseling of chronic medical conditions for veterans in methadone maintenance treatment. J Addict Med. 2010;4(3):160–6. https://doi.org/10.1097/ADM.0b013e3181b6f4e5.
67. Batki SL, Canfield KM, Smyth E, Ploutz-Snyder R, Levine RA. Hepatitis C treatment eligibility and comorbid medical illness in methadone maintenance (MMT) and non-MMT patients: a case-control study. J Addict Dis. 2010;29(3):359–69. https://doi.org/10.1080/10550887.2010.489449.
68. Sylvestre DL, Litwin AH, Clements BJ, Gourevitch MN. The impact of barriers to hepatitis C virus treatment in recovering heroin users maintained on methadone. J Subst Abus Treat. 2005;29(3):159–65. https://doi.org/10.1016/j.jsat.2005.06.002.
69. Grebely J, Mauss S, Brown A, et al. Efficacy and safety of ledipasvir/sofosbuvir with and without ribavirin in patients with chronic HCV genotype 1 infection receiving opioid substitution therapy: analysis of phase 3 ION trials. Clin Infect Dis. 2016;63(11):1405–11. https://doi.org/10.1093/cid/ciw580.
70. Dore GJ, Altice F, Litwin AH, et al. Elbasvir-grazoprevir to treat hepatitis C virus infection in persons receiving opioid agonist therapy: a randomized trial. Ann Intern Med. 2016;165(9):625–34. https://doi.org/10.7326/M16-0816.
71. Grebely J, Dore GJ, Zeuzem S, et al. Efficacy and safety of sofosbuvir/velpatasvir in patients with chronic hepatitis C virus infection receiving opioid substitution therapy: analysis of phase 3 ASTRAL trials. Clin Infect Dis. 2016;63(11):1479–81. https://doi.org/10.1093/cid/ciw579.
72. Litwin AH, Agyemang L, Akiyama M, Heo M, Wong J, Soloway J, et al. High rates of sustained virological response in people who inject drug treated with all-oral direct acting

antiviral regimens 2016. https://na.eventscloud.com/file_uploads/ec626d74ab97207d900ddc9 3eeb18144_166_AlainLitwin.pdf. Accessed 7 Jun 2020.
73. Butner JL, Gupta N, Fabian C, Henry S, Shi JM, Tetrault JM. Onsite treatment of HCV infection with direct acting antivirals within an opioid treatment program. J Subst Abus Treat. 2017;75:49–53. https://doi.org/10.1016/j.jsat.2016.12.014.
74. Norton BL, Fleming J, Bachhuber MA, et al. High HCV cure rates for people who use drugs treated with direct acting antiviral therapy at an urban primary care clinic. Int J Drug Policy. 2017;47:196–201. https://doi.org/10.1016/j.drugpo.2017.07.021.
75. Falade-Nwulia O, Irvin R, Merkow A, et al. Barriers and facilitators of hepatitis C treatment uptake among people who inject drugs enrolled in opioid treatment programs in Baltimore. J Subst Abus Treat. 2019;100:45–51. https://doi.org/10.1016/j.jsat.2019.01.021.
76. Weir A, McLeod A, Innes H, et al. Hepatitis C reinfection following treatment induced viral clearance among people who have injected drugs. Drug Alcohol Depend. 2016;165:53–60. https://doi.org/10.1016/j.drugalcdep.2016.05.012.
77. Rossi C, Butt ZA, Wong S, et al. Hepatitis C virus reinfection after successful treatment with direct-acting antiviral therapy in a large population-based cohort. J Hepatol. 2018;69(5):1007–14. https://doi.org/10.1016/j.jhep.2018.07.025.
78. Akiyama MJ, Norton BL, Arnsten JH, Agyemang L, Heo M, Litwin AH. Intensive models of hepatitis C care for people who inject drugs receiving opioid agonist therapy: a randomized controlled trial. Ann Intern Med. 2019;170(9):594–603. https://doi.org/10.7326/M18-1715.
79. Grebely J, Dore GJ, Morin S, Rockstroh JK, Klein MB. Elimination of HCV as a public health concern among people who inject drugs by 2030 – what will it take to get there? J Int AIDS Soc. 2017;20(1):22146. https://doi.org/10.7448/IAS.20.1.22146.
80. Ghany MG. Morgan TR; AASLD-IDSA hepatitis C guidance panel. Hepatitis C guidance 2019 update: American association for the study of liver diseases-infectious diseases society of America recommendations for testing, managing, and treating hepatitis C virus infection. Hepatology. 2020;71(2):686–721. https://doi.org/10.1002/hep.31060.
81. The American association for the study of liver diseases and the infectious diseases society of America. HCV guidance: recommendations for testing, managing, and treating hepatitis C. Last updated 2019, p. 7. www.hcvguidelines.org. Accessed 27 May 2020.
82. World Health Organization. Combating hepatitis B and C to reach elimination by 2030. https://apps.who.int/iris/bitstream/handle/10665/206453/WHO_HIV_2016.04_eng.pdf;jsessionid =F934E4918D492E935FCE9C069C428EB7?sequence=1. Accessed 27 Jan 2020.
83. Alderks CE. Trends in the use of methadone, buprenorphine, and extended-release naltrexone at substance abuse treatment facilities: 2003–2015 (update). The CBHSQ report: August 22, 2017. Rockville: Center for Behavioral Health Statistics and Quality, Substance Abuse and Mental Health Services Administration; 2017. https://www.samhsa.gov/data/sites/default/files/report_3192/ShortReport-3192.pdf. Accessed 7 Jun 2020.

Incorporating a Race Equity Framework into Opioid Use Disorder Treatment

13

Ayana Jordan, Caridad Ponce Martinez, and Jessica Isom

Race is a sociopolitical construct, given the false weight of biological relevance in the United States (U.S.) and around the world. The consequences of this misapplication of racial significance are far-reaching. Racial categories are determined by a combination of physical traits, language, geographic ancestry, religion, and a number of other cultural factors, rather than biology. Still, socially defined racial categories are predictive of a number of health outcomes [1]. This results from the biological consequences of membership within a marginalized racial category, causing racial inequality [2]. This phenomenon develops through the selective exposure of marginalized racial groups to high-risk environmental stress-producing biological sequelae [2]. It's therefore imperative to underscore that racism, not race, is inherently what places racial/ethnic minorities with an opioid use disorder (OUD) at risk for experiencing poor health outcomes. Many times, the emphasis is incorrectly placed on the person's racial group, the social interpretation of how one looks (what we call race) as opposed to racism, a system of structuring opportunity and assigning value, which preferentially advantages one group of people and systematically disadvantages others [3]. In this chapter, we explain how social dominance hierarchy [4], the connection between race and associated health outcomes, can help to achieve racial equity among racial/ethnic minorities with OUD.

Social dominance theory provides a framework for understanding how resources, including health status, are distributed among socially constructed groups inclusive

A. Jordan (✉)
Department of Psychiatry, Yale University School of Medicine, New Haven, CT, USA
e-mail: ayana.jordan@yale.edu

C. P. Martinez
Department of Psychiatry, University of Massachusetts Medical School, Worcester, MA, USA
e-mail: caridad.poncemartinez@umassmemorial.org

J. Isom
Codman Square Health Center/Boston Medical Center, Dorchester, MA, USA

© Springer Nature Switzerland AG 2021
S. E. Wakeman, J. D. Rich (eds.), *Treating Opioid Use Disorder in General Medical Settings*, https://doi.org/10.1007/978-3-030-80818-1_13

of biological factors (age) and arbitrary categories (race). The dominant groups (usually White) possess a disproportionately large share of high-value items with positive social value and conversely the subordinate groups (racial/ethnic minorities) share a disproportionately large share of low-value items with negative social value. In the context of OUD, high-value items might include greater access to medication for opioid use disorder (MOUD) and the overwhelmingly positive framing of individual narratives on substance use disorders (SUDs) in the media. In contrast, low-value items might include restricted access to MOUD or none at all, accompanied by a tendency to criminalize the use of opioids within subordinate groups, readily seen in the War on Drugs targeting Black and Latino communities [5]. For the purpose of this chapter, we will refer to dominant groups as those that are socially assigned the categories of White and middle- to high-income class and subordinate groups that are socially assigned the categories of non-White (racial/ethnic minority) and low-income class. It is important to recognize these social hierarchies as a key step in disrupting their influence on OUD diagnosis, treatment and related health consequences.

Social dominance theory is also useful for understanding how hierarchies are maintained. The ability to stratify health metrics by race, including access to care and the quality of care received, is a manifestation of structural and interpersonal racism supported by explicit and implicit hierarchical racial beliefs [6]. Stated simply, a socially assigned racial and class category can evoke a predictable narrative of experiences, in this case seeking and being granted treatment for OUD from the health care system (see case example at the close of the chapter). These experiences can be located within interpersonal interactions and larger structural dynamics. In the treatment of OUD, those at the front lines are providing substance use treatment explicitly grounded in egalitarian principles, yet, the disparities in the approach to OUD across race and class remains the same. To understand this discordance, we must systematically interrogate the societal race and class assumptions which support beliefs and actions that perpetuate disparities. This process is best supported by the use of a racial equity framework.

Racial equity is achieved when socially assigned racial categories are no longer strong predictors of outcomes with regards to diagnosis, treatment, and health outcomes for persons with OUD. As outlined above, these differences are supported by a socially determined racial hierarchy that has no biological basis, yet results in real biological consequences. A racial equity framework explicitly inserts race and power into the decision-making process, thereby illuminating opportunities to make different choices in support of equity goals. These decisions are sometimes referred to as "choice points," representing key branch points that can move an outcome toward or away from racial equity. The use of a racial framework promotes active engagement of stakeholders, often a key component missing in the decision-making processes impacting racial/ethnic minorities with OUD. This framework also offers a distinct, specific, and adequate focus on disparities and inequities producing intentional decisions that move us toward equity rather than the status quo. Incorporating a race equity framework helps to identify measurable goals and outcomes, relevant strategies for removal of barriers, and a systematic assessment of the decisional

Table 13.1 Stages of equity and empowerment lens

1. Assessment of organizational capacity for equity work
2. Description of current direction and strategies
3. Identification of inequities and injustices in the current issue
4. Reflection and understanding of strengths and challenges
5. Enhancement of what is leading to equity and empowerment
6. Elimination of strategies and root causes leading to inequities and injustice
7. Celebrate success and improvements

Adapted from [7]

impact of racial/ethnic groups with OUD that have been marginalized in current treatment systems. An example of one such framework, outlining steps for equity and empowerment [7] is seen in Table 13.1.

Prevalence of OUD Among Racial/Ethnic Minorities and Importance of Opioid Preferences

In addition to understanding how race and power contribute to worsening outcomes for racial/ethnic minorities with OUD, the systematic exclusion of racial/ethnic minority experiences from national media coverage, academic, and research institutions must be examined [8]. With an overwhelming focus on rates of opioid use among White populations, the opioid overdose crisis has been deemed a public health emergency [8], ignoring a predominately Black population during the 1960s and 1970s who were largely criminalized as a result of their opioid use [8, 9]. Given limited attention to non-White populations with OUD, there has been discrepancies in reporting the rates of opioid use among racial and ethnic minorities [10]. While the rates of opioid overdose deaths remain highest among White populations, there has been a drastic increase in death rates among Black and Latino populations, largely fueled by illicitly-manufactured fentanyl [11]. Researchers found that between 2011 and 2016, fentanyl death rates among Black people increased 140.6% annually, with an increase of 118.3% annually in the Latino population [11]. Further, there are eight states and the District of Columbia where opioid overdose rates are greater among Black populations than among White populations, however this is not covered in the mainstream media [9, 12]. From 1999 to 2015, the Substance Abuse and Mental Health Services Administration (SAMHSA) looked at the racial breakdown of opioid overdose rates and found that Native populations, during certain years, had higher death rates from opioids compared with White people. Given this information has been excluded from the larger context when discussing the opioid crisis, many physicians, clinicians, and researchers are misinformed of the impact opioids have on racial/ethnic minority communities. This may provide insight into why people from this demographic are not properly being assessed or provided treatment recommendations for opioid use, thereby unintentionally perpetuating the disparities many racial/ethnic minorities with OUD face.

Another important consideration when discussing racial/ethnic minorities with OUD includes opioid preference and other substances of misuse. For example, in contrast to White communities, many racial/ethnic minority communities are more likely to use heroin as their primary opioid of use, as opposed to the use of nonmedical prescription opioids [13]. This may be influenced by cultural acceptability, ease, and increased availability of heroin in minority neighborhoods, and also cost, as heroin is markedly cheaper than nonmedical prescription opioids [14]. It's also important to note that many Black and Latino people in particular intentionally or unintentionally use opioids (fentanyl) mixed with cocaine. Cocaine is an illicit drug that kills more Black and Latino people than opioids, and is the second cause of death among illicit substances for all people [8]. Fentanyl mixed with cocaine is thought to be the major driver of the rapid deaths seen from opioids among Black and Latino populations [9, 11].

Given the types of opioids that are used in these demographics, predominantly heroin, the route of use becomes vital in managing risk, including harm reduction strategies. For example, injection use of heroin, drastically increases the risk of HIV, Hepatitis B and C, and serious bacterial infections. Making sure these communities have free access to sterile injection equipment and safe places to use, such as supervised consumption spaces, is paramount in decreasing death rates. This is of particular importance in racial/ethnic communities, where many are living in poverty [15], with decreased access to treatment facilities for MOUD [10], and higher attrition rates from treatment [16]. We can learn from global examples that supervised consumptions sites are key to decreasing rates of infectious diseases and death, in addition to crime [17].

Common Medical Comorbidities of OUD and the Disparities Among Racial/Ethnic Minorities

Racial/ethnic minorities with OUD experience worse health outcomes when compared to White people. Psychiatric and medical comorbidities are common among people with OUD, including HIV/AIDs and viral hepatitis [18]. Racial/ethnic minorities are more likely to experience negative drug-related consequences, including higher rates of Hepatitis C and HIV, when compared to White individuals with OUD [19–23]. There is also a disparity that exists in the number of patients from racial/ethnic minorities that are tested for HIV/AIDs and viral hepatitis (Hepatitis A, B, and C) [18] and an even larger gap with initiation in treatment, despite an availability of a cure for Hepatitis C [24]. Since racial/ethnic minorities are less likely to engage in substance use treatment, which typically involves HIV and hepatitis antibody testing at admission, or a referral for antibody testing- [18], there is a higher likelihood of undetected infection progressing to advanced disease, disability leading to unemployment, and premature death. Deliberate attention to timely initiation, engagement, and adherence to culturally informed care remains paramount to taking care of racial/ethnic minorities with OUD. An overview of considerations that must take place when treating patients from this demographic is discussed in great detail in the assessment and treatment section of this chapter. Finally, in addition to the most common medical comorbidities discussed, racial/

ethnic minorities are more likely to be arrested or incarcerated, homeless, or unemployed as a result of their opioid use [8].

Vulnerabilities in the Social Determinants of Health

Persons with OUD experience the social and psychological consequences of illicit drug use, highlighting the importance of adequate diagnosis and treatment. These consequences can reinforce the pattern of drug use, including recurrence rates, and are thus rightly characterized as social determinants of OUD. When applied more broadly to health, social determinants of health are defined as the conditions in which individuals live, learn, work, and grow [25]. Exposures to disproportionately high vulnerabilities in the social determinants such as low socioeconomic (SES), poor quality education, unemployment, and food insecurity will result in adverse health consequences. These adverse exposures are highest among racialized minorities, rural populations, and individuals with low SES status. Approaches to the opioid use disorder and overdose crisis must include a focus on addressing social determinants as major contributors to high-risk behaviors and health status in persons with OUD. Recognizing that the social determinants are associated with status in the social hierarchy, specific attention should be paid to the compounding effects of adverse exposures when working with patients who are racial minorities, in rural settings, or of low SES status.

About 65% of all individuals experiencing incarceration meet criteria for a substance use disorder (SUD) and the use of opioids are linked with higher rates of recidivism [26]. Opioid use has been shown to correlate with involvement in the legal system with at least 20% of persons with OUD experiencing arrests, incarceration, probation, or parole [26]. There is an overwhelming overrepresentation of Black people in the carceral system for drug-related crimes resulting from the war on drugs [10]. People released from jails or prisons are at a very high risk of mortality from opioid overdoses relative to the general population [27]. Patients of racial/ethnic minority populations are more likely to enter SUD treatment via involvement in the legal system [28], where sentencing time can be reduced or eliminated if court recommendations for SUD treatment are followed. Some patients view this as coercion, which is not a collaborative or empowering process. Being involved in the carceral system and navigating a high degree of burden in the social determinants can determine access to post-release MOUD and psychosocial interventions for racial/ethnic minorities, thereby reinforcing the need to highlight and address intersectional vulnerabilities within marginalized groups.

In addition to overrepresentation in the carceral system, racial/ethnic minorities with OUD are at high risk for experiencing homelessness [29]. People experiencing homelessness are also at higher rates of opioid overdoses [30]. A study in New Haven found that nearly 25% of persons experiencing homelessness attributed their status to drug use, where longer periods of homelessness were associated with a higher prevalence of substance use [31]. Both adults with current OUD and past OUD experience lower rates of employment [32]. The vulnerabilities in these social determinants are greatest among racial/ethnic minorities, which may reinforce drug use, worsen psychiatric comorbidities, increase exposures to poverty and, if unaddressed, disrupt efforts to connect persons with OUD to treatment [33].

Cultural Considerations in the Assessment and Treatment of Racial/Ethnic Minorities with OUD

To incorporate race, power, medical comorbidities, and the social determinants, the ideal assessment of a patient with OUD from a racial/ethnic minority population goes beyond the traditional SUD evaluation to include an understanding of one's personal and societal circumstance. A comprehensive evaluation must consider the factors that have contributed to the OUD, and a full appreciation of the dynamics that can interfere with access to treatment, thereby interfering with the likelihood of recovery. For this section, we will focus on Black and Latino patients as the principal racial/ethnic minority populations in the US, but some of this information may be applicable to other racial/ethnic minority groups. Black and Latino individuals have been shown to disproportionately bear the negative consequences of substance use, yet they are less likely to access treatment and be retained in treatment [34, 35]. However, when available services for SUDs are adequate in number and quality, racial/ethnic minority patients have positive outcomes for reduced substance use and improved functioning [22, 35].

Racial/ethnic minority populations with SUDs experience greater cultural barriers to accessing treatment [16]. Language can be an obstacle in treatment access for Latino patients who do not speak English [28]. An inability to communicate effectively with clinical providers may affect adherence with treatment recommendations, retention in treatment, and satisfaction with services. One important consideration is that availability of interpreters alone may not be sufficient, as poor literacy skills, including health literacy, could also be a barrier to communication [36]. From a cultural perspective, patients may not feel that there is a need for treatment, especially when they remain able to fulfill their obligations and are "functional" [37] or if their pattern of use or even specific substance of use is more socially acceptable within their cultural and/or racial group. Treatment engagement may improve in these situations by incorporating harm reduction strategies, rather than exclusively focusing on abstinence models.

For Latino patients, in particular, it is important to recognize the heterogeneity of the population in terms of ethnic, linguistic, and nationality backgrounds. This may result in different patterns of use, drug of choice, and acceptance of treatment interventions [35]. This heterogeneity is further compounded by the differences in the degree of acculturation into American society experienced [38]. Immigrants who came to the U.S. as adults are likely to maintain cultural norms of their countries or societies of origin. However, loss of family and societal ties can result in stress that contributes to substance use. Therefore, cultural identity takes precedence over general racial identity (e.g., a Puerto Rican person living in New York has a different identity to that of a Mexican national living in the Los Angeles area, yet both are Latino), and may better guide the distinct interventions for OUD in a particular geographical location [16, 35, 39]. A good suggestion is to further refine treatment interventions for racial/ethnic minorities with OUD, by better understanding the variation across different identity groups within a certain racial or ethnic group.

As stated earlier, paying close attention to the social determinants can affect access and retention in OUD treatment. These include, but are not limited to, cost, homelessness and residential instability, unemployment, access to childcare, and transportation problems, among others [16, 36]. As a result of structural racism, Latino and Black people are overrepresented in the Medicaid population, where there may be regional disparities in whether SUD treatment facilities accept Medicaid [28]. As a result of immigration or citizenship status of themselves or their family members, patients may be fearful of accessing treatment [36]. Careful consideration of these factors during assessment and treatment planning is key to developing culturally informed treatment strategies.

Even when people from racial/ethnic minority populations access treatment for OUD, one critical factor that may be missing in their assessment is consideration of comorbid psychiatric disorders. Numerous studies have found that people from racial/ethnic minority populations are less likely to receive treatment for co-occurring psychiatric illness [35], which can have a significant impact on the likelihood of recovery from either disorder. Assessment of trauma may often be overlooked, with patients being reluctant to disclose or even acknowledge prior traumatic experiences. Yet the prevalence of trauma is high due to higher levels of psychosocial stressors in racial/ethnic minority populations [16]. This can be of particular relevance when violence is often witnessed and/or experienced as part of the environment in which drug procurement and use occurs. Finally, as we learned in the beginning of this chapter, an assessment of the vulnerabilities that a patient from a racial/ethnic minority background faces cannot be complete without consideration of racism, which is a chronic stressor for racial/ethnic minority communities [28] and a form of insidious trauma.

The areas described previously (social determinants, including that of trauma and racism) must be obtained in a medical and psychiatric interview. They allow a better understanding of a patient's resources and risk factors on an individual and community basis that could contribute to and maintain the existence of an OUD. An assessment of a patient's structural vulnerability allows exploration of socioeconomic and demographic attributes such as citizenship and socioeconomic status, in combination with less tangible statuses attributed to a group, such as credibility and assumed intelligence. One proposed strategy in the evaluation of racial/ethnic minority patients with OUD is to utilize the structural vulnerability tool, defined as a clinical assessment tool that allows structural vulnerability to be operationalized by identifying power relationships and hierarchies that could exacerbate an individual patient's health problems. This assessment tool (Table 13.2) can be used clinically for screening and helps in the development of a comprehensive treatment plan for patients [40].

Table 13.2 Structural Vulnerability Assessment Tool

Domain	Screening questions
Financial Security	Do you have enough money to live comfortably – pay rent, get food, pay utilities, telephone?
Residence	Do you have a safe, stable place to sleep and store your possessions?
Risk environments	Do the places where you spend your time each day feel safe and healthy?
Food access	Do you have adequate nutrition and access to healthy food?
Social network	Do you have friends, family, or other people who help you when you need it?
Legal status	Do you have any legal problems?
Education	Can you read?
Discrimination	Have you experienced discrimination (being treated differently)? Do some service providers (including me) make you feel unwelcome or make it hard for you to access treatment?

Adapted from [40]

While recognizing that these are complex issues that cannot be all addressed in a single clinic visit, lack of recognition could lead to continued negative health outcomes. Clinicians may partner with community resources to address some of these issues with the goal of reducing patients' structural vulnerability.

Deliberate attention to the cultural norms and treatment preferences of patients from racial/ethnic minority communities must be integrated into care if treatment disparities for OUD are to be eliminated. Closing the gap in treatment initiation, engagement, and adherence [41, 42] among racial/ethnic minorities is not just aspirational, but also achievable if a race equity framework is employed. A key part of the treatment approach is to recognize and acknowledge to racial/ethnic minority patients that they have indeed been left out of the larger conversation of the current opioid overdose crisis, which is centered in whiteness [43] (a system or set of structures that results in White privilege) [44]. By doing so, there is an honest acknowledgment that indeed racial/ethnic minorities have been detrimentally affected in the past by opioids, namely heroin [8], while also emphasizing the toll that the current crisis has had on racial/ethnic minorities who are not receiving MOUD [8, 41]. An example of how a provider might begin this reparative work includes: *"I know there has been so much focus on the use of opioids and treatment because of how it's been affecting White communities ... I just want you to know that I realize people of color have been dealing with the effects of opioids like heroin for years, without the same emphasis. I am so sorry and this is not fair, but I am going to work with you to get you the help you need, and give you and people that look like you the attention they deserve. Your life and recovery matters to me."* Treatment must include a frame that strategically centers conversation on the value of people's lives from racial/ethnic minority communities, and the importance of MOUD, given the exponential rates of overdose rates among Black and Latino populations, largely due to illicitly manufactured fentanyl [45].

Researchers and medical providers must also understand a lack of cultural representation in treatment settings can negatively impact adherence leading to higher attrition rates. For instance, when there is a lack of signage or providers from similar racial/ethnic backgrounds in the treatment setting, this can impact how one thinks about treatment, unduly alienate, or even determine if treatment should continue. Among Black and Latino patients, there is a higher dissatisfaction with treatment [28], given the absence of cultural representation. Culturally relevant and responsive treatment takes into account the cultural, linguistic, and socioenvironmental context of the patients being served, and is better aligned with patient priorities [28], thereby increasing patient satisfaction and retention.

It is important for treatment programs to move beyond a superficial engagement of cultural proficiency, for example, by focusing only on providing Spanish interpreters to a primarily Spanish-speaking population, yet failing to understand the impact of living in a violent neighborhood with limited access to ancillary services. Research and understanding of the local target population is essential for the development of sensitive interventions in the treatment of SUDs among racial/ethnic minority populations [38]. However, culturally sensitive and culturally informed treatment must not exclude evidenced-based treatment. Low-income populations including racial/ethnic minorities are subject to receiving lower-quality treatment or treatment with less evidence-based options (e.g., decreased access to MOUD and increased focus on treatment based on moral principles) [28, 46]. We propose that the delivery of MOUD can change to adapt to the cultural context of racial/ethnic minority populations, but the treatment being offered should be equal in quality to that offered to majority White groups.

Addressing the root causes of inequity would likely increase treatment initiation and engagement for racialized minorities. At present, there are disparities in the enrollment and completion of substance use programs in the US. There is research identifying a higher rate of treatment drop out for racial minority groups in some metropolitan areas, with decreased first time engagement for all substance use disorders [47] and specifically low rates for OUD [39]. Use of a race equity framework could inform an examination of the institutional relevance of data showing differences in the referral patterns, discharge diagnosis, and length of stay in substance use treatment for racialized minorities with a focus on intervention design [48]. For example, there is ample evidence supporting the utility of culturally informed substance use treatment services as a barrier reduction strategy for racial minority groups.

Avoiding a "one size fits all" treatment approach to OUD is paramount in effectively disrupting racial inequities. One of the antidotes, culturally sensitive services, offers validation of cultural identities and creates a respectful treatment atmosphere that will promote engagement in other areas of care. Cultural sensitivity in OUD treatment, as described by Resnicow et al., involves being responsive to the ethnic/cultural characteristics, experiences, norms, values, behavioral patterns, and beliefs of a target population of a treatment program [38]. This approach can include surface structure interventions, which match the intervention materials to the characteristics of a target population, and/or deep structure interventions which incorporate the cultural, historical, environmental, social, and psychological forces that influence a target health behavior, within a defined population. The effectiveness of programs in regards to post-intervention substance use rates has been shown to increase with culturally sensitive treatment approaches [49]. Recognizing the importance of culturally informed services, federal agencies have developed targeted cultural competency resources [50] to improve the quality of care delivered to racialized minorities as well as treatment improvement protocols [51].

The structural vulnerability tool described earlier may identify specific needs of the targeted community in need of treatment for OUD. This may require immediate attention to certain vulnerabilities that would impact access to treatment or retention in treatment [40]. For example, an unemployed Black patient without identified sources of support who lives in a neighborhood without access to public transportation will not be able to visit a methadone clinic regularly for treatment of his OUD. A successful treatment plan will require either problem-solving access to the clinic or considering a different treatment plan to target the OUD.

Social services that could be linked with OUD treatment include job training and placement, stable housing, child and family services, transportation, community-based care following incarceration, gang-prevention services, access to other medical services (chronic or infectious diseases), and mental health treatment [36]. The need to consider structural vulnerabilities and referral or provision of these services in the treatment of OUD could be perceived as cumbersome to the clinicians, who may already have limitations on time and resources. However, lack of recognition of these problems and integration into a comprehensive treatment plan is likely to maintain the current pattern of decreased engagement and retention in treatment. From a practical standpoint, addressing a patient's context as part of OUD treatment will likely require a team approach, which can exist within a clinic or using community resources. This can be aided by use of a health information system which can share information about protective and risk factors for an individual among a multidisciplinary group of clinical providers [35]. Other innovative interventions can be utilized to facilitate access to treatment and overcome logistical challenges, and may include telemedicine, web-based treatment, and text messaging, among others [37].

One consideration is that cultural values of racial/ethnic minority populations can be marshalled as strengths or protective factors in the treatment of OUD. In Black people, these cultural values include spiritualism, respect for verbal communication skills and commitment to family; and for Latino people, respect for elders, importance of family, and the value of self-worth [38]. Effective treatment for racial/ethnic minorities with OUD must not occur in a vacuum, if it is to be effective. Treatment should be evidence based, responsive to the patient's individual and structural vulnerabilities, and acceptable to the individual's unique circumstances and values. True cultural competence can increase awareness in clinical systems and allow for the development of rapport with the population we serve, which is crucial for effective treatment.

An example of a race equity framework in action is discussed in the case example below.

Case Example

Betzaida, a 48-year-old woman from the Dominican Republic with OUD residing in rural North Carolina, has presented to the area's Federally Qualified Health Center (FQHC) urgent care with concern for an injection drug use (IDU)–associated infection. She reports onset of a rash with streaks 2 days prior and a subjective fever. The physician offers antibiotics and astutely inquiries about recent IDU. Betzaida confirms injecting heroin on a regular basis. She is given a referral pamphlet for the SUD team and offered an intake with the methadone clinic. Betzaida requests a pamphlet in Spanish, which is not available in the clinic. She asks whether there are evening hours for the clinic. As she leaves the urgent care, she is observed eying the security guard closely. Two weeks later, Betzaida returns to the urgent care clinic with a chief complaint of malodorous vaginal discharge. She reports recent unprotected sex, as a result of sexual assault in an area shelter. Due to her escalating heroin use, she lost her job and apartment 6 months ago. She describes a depressed mood and passive thoughts of not caring if she wakes up in the morning. Betzaida also reports significant shame regarding her ongoing IDU and the problems it is causing for her life. She updates the physician on missing the intake appointment at the methadone clinic and asks to be offered another date. She expresses concerns for "getting in trouble," if she attends the appointment and points to the security guard. She is reassured that the services are not offered in connection with law enforcement and is given another appointment for the following day. Betzaida arrives to her intake appointment 2 hours late citing issues with public transportation. She meets with an intake coordinator who presents the information on methadone in a rushed manner supplemented by written materials. The images on the patient education materials, similar to the pamphlet, do not appear similar to Betzaida or her family members. She again struggles to read the text written in English and denies having questions about the medication when asked. While in the waiting room prior to her meeting with the physician who will prescribe methadone, Betzaida decides she is not ready for methadone initiation and quickly exits the building.

Case Discussion

The patient discussed above with OUD may develop an interest in treatment rooted in the social, psychological, or medical consequences of substance use. Each of these care entry points represents an opportunity for moving closer to or away from equity. Applying a race equity framework, the communications team might choose a pamphlet that is culturally sensitive in its imagery and linguistically appropriate for the patient demographics. Another choice point can be incorporating the use of the structural vulnerability tool into the referral process to ensure patients are assessed for vulnerabilities in legal status, as well as risks in the built environment and discrimination. The methadone clinic might apply a race equity framework in its attempt to understand how patients similar to

Betzaida experience the waiting room, intake process, and encounters with staff. This can include use the of the Equity and Empowerment lens to support an examination of the current system and possible contributions to inequities such as lack of treatment engagement. All of these choice points in the decision-making process for structuring treatment with MOUD are ripe opportunities for enhancing what is leading to equity and for eliminating what is not.

References

1. White K, Lawrence JA, Tchangalova N, Huang SJ, Cummings JL. Socially-assigned race and health: a scoping review with global implications for population health equity. Int J Equity Health. 2020;19(1):25.
2. Gravlee CC. How race becomes biology: embodiment of social inequality. Am J Phys Anthropol. 2009;139(1):47–57.
3. Jones CP. Levels of racism: a theoretic framework and a gardener's tale. Am J Public Health. 2000;90(8):1212.
4. Sidanius J, Pratto F. Social dominance: an intergroup theory of social hierarchy and oppression. Cambridge University Press; 2001.
5. Jensen EL, Gerber J, Mosher C. Social consequences of the war on drugs: the legacy of failed policy. Crim Justice Policy Rev. 2004;15(1):100–21.
6. Williams DR, Lawrence JA, Davis BA. Racism and health: evidence and needed research. Annu Rev Public Health. 2019;40:105–25.
7. The Equity and Empowerment Lens Worksheet is adapted from Equity and Empowerment Lens 2012. Multnomah County Office of Diversity and Equity. https://multco.us/file/31833/download. Accessed 22 Feb 2020.
8. James K, Jordan A. The opioid crisis in Black Communities. J Law Med Ethics. 2018;46(2):404–21.
9. Schmitz Bechteler S, Kane-Willis K. Whitewashed: the African American opioid epidemic. Chicago: The Chicago Urban League. Research and Policy Center; 2017.
10. Santoro TN, Santoro JD. Racial bias in the US opioid epidemic: a review of the history of systemic bias and implications for care. Cureus. 2018;10(12):e3733.
11. Hedegaard H, Bastian BA, Trinidad JP, Spencer M, Warner M. Drugs most frequently involved in drug overdose deaths: United States, 2011–2016. National Vital Statistics Reports; vol 67 no 9. Hyattsville: National Center for Health Statistics, 2018.
12. Garfield R, Damico A, Orgera K. The coverage gap: Uninsured poor adults in states that do not expand Medicaid. Kaiser Family Foundation, 2016.
13. Pouget ER, Fong C, Rosenblum A. Racial/ethnic differences in prevalence trends for heroin use and non-medical use of prescription opioids among entrants to opioid treatment programs, 2005–2016. Subst Use Misuse. 2018;53(2):290–300.
14. Dasgupta N, Freifeld C, Brownstein JS, Menone CM, Surratt HL, Poppish L, et al. Crowdsourcing black market prices for prescription opioids. J Med Internet Res. 2013;15(8):e178.
15. Chow JC-C, Jaffee K, Snowden L. Racial/ethnic disparities in the use of mental health services in poverty areas. Am J Public Health. 2003;93(5):792–7.
16. Mennis J, Stahler GJ. Racial and ethnic disparities in outpatient substance use disorder treatment episode completion for different substances. J Subst Abus Treat. 2016;63:25–33.
17. Hathaway AD, Tousaw KI. Harm reduction headway and continuing resistance: insights from safe injection in the city of Vancouver. Int J Drug Policy. 2008;19(1):11–6.
18. SAMHSA. Common Comorbidities [Internet] 2019. Available from: https://www.samhsa.gov/medication-assisted-treatment/treatment/common-comorbidities.

19. Acevedo A, Garnick DW, Lee MT, Horgan CM, Ritter G, Panas L, et al. Racial and ethnic differences in substance abuse treatment initiation and engagement. J Ethn Subst Abus. 2012;11(1):1–21.
20. Galvan FH, Caetano R. Alcohol use and related problems among ethnic minorities in the United States. Alcohol Res Health: the journal of the National Institute on Alcohol Abuse and Alcoholism. 2003;27(1):87–94.
21. Mojtabai R, Olfson M, Sampson NA, Jin R, Druss B, Wang PS, et al. Barriers to mental health treatment: results from the National Comorbidity Survey Replication. Psychol Med. 2011;41(8):1751–61.
22. Schmidt L, Greenfield T, Mulia N. Unequal treatment: racial and ethnic disparities in alcoholism treatment services. Alcohol Res Health. 2006;29(1):49–54.
23. Office of the Surgeon General (US); Center for Mental Health Services (US); National Institute of Mental Health (US). Mental health: culture, race, and ethnicity: a supplement to mental health: a report of the surgeon general. Rockville: Substance Abuse and Mental Health Services Administration (US); 2001 Aug. Available from: https://www.ncbi.nlm.nih.gov/books/NBK44243/.
24. Panel AIHG. Hepatitis C guidance: AASLD-IDSA recommendations for testing, managing, and treating adults infected with hepatitis C virus. Hepatology. 2015;62(3):932–54.
25. Healthy people 2020. Washington, DC: US Department of Health and Human Services, Office of Disease Prevention and Health Promotion, 2018, Oct.
26. Winkelman TN, Chang VW, Binswanger IA. Health, polysubstance use, and criminal justice involvement among adults with varying levels of opioid use. JAMA Netw Open. 2018;1(3):e180558-e.
27. Joudrey PJ, Khan MR, Wang EA, Scheidell JD, Edelman EJ, McInnes DK, et al. A conceptual model for understanding post-release opioid-related overdose risk. Addict Sci Clin Pract. 2019;14(1):17.
28. Sprague Martinez L, Walter AW, Acevedo A, Lopez LM, Lundgren L. Context matters: health disparities in substance use disorders and treatment. J Soc Work Pract Addict. 2018;18(1):84–98.
29. Iheanacho T, Stefanovics E, Rosenheck R. Opioid use disorder and homelessness in the Veterans Health Administration: the challenge of multimorbidity. J Opioid Manag. 2018;14(3):171–82.
30. Yamamoto A, Needleman J, Gelberg L, Kominski G, Shoptaw S, Tsugawa Y. Association between homelessness and opioid overdose and opioid-related hospital admissions/emergency department visits. Soc Sci Med. 2019;242:112585.
31. Spinner GF, Leaf PJ. Homelessness and drug abuse in New Haven. Psychiatr Serv. 1992;43(2):166–8.
32. Rhee TG, Rosenheck RA. Association of current and past opioid use disorders with health-related quality of life and employment among US adults. Drug Alcohol Depend. 2019;199:122–8.
33. Dasgupta N, Beletsky L, Ciccarone D. Opioid crisis: no easy fix to its social and economic determinants. Am J Public Health. 2018;108:182–6.
34. Alegría M, Page JB, Hansen H, Cauce AM, Robles R, Blanco C, et al. Improving drug treatment services for Hispanics: research gaps and scientific opportunities. Drug Alcohol Depend. 2006;84:S76–84.
35. Guerrero EG, Marsh JC, Khachikian T, Amaro H, Vega WA. Disparities in Latino substance use, service use, and treatment: implications for culturally and evidence-based interventions under health care reform. Drug Alcohol Depend. 2013;133(3):805–13.
36. Alegria M, Page JB, Hansen H, Cauce AM, Robles R, Blanco C, et al. Improving drug treatment services for Hispanics: research gaps and scientific opportunities. Drug Alcohol Depend. 2006;84(Suppl 1):S76–84.
37. Pinedo M, Zemore S, Rogers S. Understanding barriers to specialty substance abuse treatment among Latinos. J Subst Abus Treat. 2018;94:1–8.
38. Resnicow K, Soler R, Braithwaite RL, Ahluwalia JS, Butler J. Cultural sensitivity in substance use prevention. J Community Psychol. 2000;28(3):271–90.

39. Stahler GJ, Mennis J. Treatment outcome disparities for opioid users: are there racial and ethnic differences in treatment completion across large US metropolitan areas? Drug Alcohol Depend. 2018;190:170–8.
40. Bourgois P, Holmes SM, Sue K, Quesada J. Structural vulnerability: operationalizing the concept to address health disparities in clinical care. Acad Med: journal of the Association of American Medical Colleges. 2017;92(3):299.
41. Lagisetty PA, Ross R, Bohnert A. Buprenorphine treatment divide by race/ethnicity and payment. JAMA Psychiat. 2019;76(9):979–81.
42. Mennis J, Stahler G. Racial and ethnic disparities in outpatient substance use disorder treatment episode completion for different substances. J Subst Abus Treat. 2016;63:25–33.
43. Spanierman LB, Soble JR. Understanding whiteness: previous approaches and possible directions in the study of White racial attitudes and identity. In: Handbook of multicultural counseling. 3rd ed. Thousand Oaks: Sage Publications, Inc; 2010. p. 283–99.
44. Kendall F. Understanding White privilege: creating pathways to authentic relationships across race. New York: Routledge; 2012.
45. Spencer MR, Warner M, Bastian BA, Trinidad JP, Hedegaard H. Drug overdose deaths involving fentanyl, 2011–2016. National Vital Statistics Reports; vol 68 no 3. Hyattsville: National Center for Health Statistics, 2019.
46. Guerrero EG, Garner BR, Cook B, Kong Y. Does the implementation of evidence-based and culturally competent practices reduce disparities in addiction treatment outcomes? Addict Behav. 2017;73:119–23.
47. Guerrero EG, Marsh JC, Duan L, Oh C, Perron B, Lee B. Disparities in completion of substance abuse treatment between and within racial and ethnic groups. Health Serv Res. 2013;48(4):1450–67.
48. Delphin-Rittmon ME, Flanagan EH, Andres-Hyman R, Ortiz J, Amer MM, Davidson L. Racial-ethnic differences in access, diagnosis, and outcomes in public-sector inpatient mental health treatment. Psychol Serv. 2015;12(2):158.
49. Steinka-Fry KT, Tanner-Smith EE, Dakof GA, Henderson C. Culturally sensitive substance use treatment for racial/ethnic minority youth: a meta-analytic review. J Subst Abus Treat. 2017;75:22–37.
50. Substance Abuse and Mental Health Services Administration. Improving cultural competence. Treatment Improvement Protocol (TIP) Series No. 59. HHS Publication No. (SMA) 14–4849. Rockville, MD: Substance Abuse and Mental Health Services Administration, 2014.
51. Substance Abuse and Mental Health Services Administration. Behavioral health services for American Indians and Alaska natives. Treatment Improvement Protocol (TIP) Series 61. HHS Publication No. (SMA) 18-5070EXSUMM. Rockville: Substance Abuse and Mental Health Services Administration, 2018. .

Caring for Pregnant and Parenting Women with Opioid Use Disorder

14

Mishka Terplan, Caitlin E. Martin, Ashish Premkumar, and Elizabeth E. Krans

Introduction

Pregnancy is a unique stage of the life course. Generally speaking, it is a time of increased access to care and healthcare utilization. In contrast, the postpartum period (the year following delivery) is a time of decreased access to care. Opioid use disorder (OUD) is a chronic disease and, as with other chronic conditions (such as hypertension or diabetes), both maternal and newborn outcomes are greatly improved with treatment. Although OUD is often first diagnosed during pregnancy, no one develops the disease of addiction de novo during the gestational period [1].

Opioid use is far less common in pregnancy than nicotine, alcohol, or cannabis use. Estimates of OUD during pregnancy vary by data source. National Survey on Drug Use and Health (NSDUH) data estimate that there are at least 20,000 pregnancies with OUD annually in the US [2, 3]. Kern-Goldberger et al., applying a cross-sectional analytic approach to the Nationwide Inpatient Sample (NIS) from 1998 to 2014, estimated almost 80,000 antepartum hospitalizations occurred for management of OUD [4]. Wen et al., applying the same analytic approach to the NIS,

M. Terplan (✉)
Friends Research Institute, Baltimore, MD, USA
e-mail: mterplan@friendsresearch.org

C. E. Martin
Obstetrics and Gynecology, Virginia Commonwealth University, Richmond, VA, USA
e-mail: Caitlin.Martin@vcuhealth.org

A. Premkumar
Obstetrics and Gynecology, Northwestern University, Chicago, IL, USA
e-mail: ashish.premkumar@northwestern.edu

E. E. Krans
Obstetrics and Gynecology, University of Pittsburgh, Pittsburgh, PA, USA
e-mail: kransee@upmc.edu

© Springer Nature Switzerland AG 2021
S. E. Wakeman, J. D. Rich (eds.), *Treating Opioid Use Disorder in General Medical Settings*, https://doi.org/10.1007/978-3-030-80818-1_14

estimated almost 67,000 women between 2010 and 2014 were affected by OUD postpartum [5].

Infants exposed to opioids in utero may develop signs and symptoms of opioid withdrawal after birth. Neonatal abstinence syndrome (NAS) (also termed "neonatal opioid withdrawal syndrome" or NOWS) affects almost 20,000 neonates yearly and contributes significantly to rising costs of neonatal care [2, 6, 7]. Populations whose infants may develop NAS include people chronically treated with opioid medications who do not have OUD, people with untreated OUD, and people receiving medications for OUD (MOUD).

OUD, specifically untreated OUD, has been associated with maternal and neonatal complications, such as fetal growth restriction, preterm birth, and the acquisition and vertical transmission of Hepatitis C virus and HIV. In contrast, birth outcomes among women with treated OUD are quite similar to that of the general population. The opioid overdose crisis has profoundly affected pregnancy as overdose is one of the leading causes of maternal mortality in the US [8–10], primarily in the postpartum period [11–15].

Screening

Pregnancy is an essential time for behavioral health assessments, in part because most people have access to health insurance. Universal screening for substance use is recommended ideally with a validated instrument [16]. Ondersma et al. directly compared the following screening instruments in pregnancy: the Substance Use Risk Profile-Pregnancy (SURP-P), CRAFFT, 5Ps, Wayne Indirect Drug Use Screener (WIDUS), and the National Institute on Drug Abuse (NIDA) Quick Screen. All performed with similar efficacy though none had both high sensitivity and high specificity [17]. Regardless of which instrument is used, a positive screen should be followed by diagnostic assessment and initiation of or referral to treatment. Urine drug testing (or other biological measurement) is not an appropriate substitute for screening and should never be obtained without patient consent.

Treatment

Medication for OUD (MOUD) is the recommended, evidence-based treatment for the management of OUD during pregnancy and is supported by consensus of professional organizations and government agencies, including the Substance Abuse and Mental Health Services Administration (SAMHSA), the American Society of Addiction Medicine (ASAM), and the American College of Obstetrics and Gynecology (ACOG) [16, 18, 19]. MOUD during pregnancy improves maternal health outcomes by reducing the risk of recurrence, overdose, and morbidity from infectious diseases such as HIV and HCV [20]. In an evaluation over 6000 pregnant women with OUD in Massachusetts, MOUD use was associated with lower rates of overdose both during pregnancy and for 1-year postpartum [10]. MOUD use during pregnancy also improves neonatal health outcomes by stabilizing the intrauterine environment and minimizing the fetal stress response from the cyclic pattern of withdrawal associated with untreated OUD [21, 22].

In contrast, medically assisted withdrawal or "detoxification" is not recommended in pregnancy due to high rates of recurrence (48–74%) and overdose [23]. A systematic review of medically assisted withdrawal during pregnancy found low detoxification completion rates, high rates of illicit drug use, OUD recurrence, and limited outcome data after delivery across 15 detoxification studies [23]. Thus, MOUD use during pregnancy is associated with superior health outcomes compared to medically assisted withdrawal and outweighs any potential increase in outcomes associated with in utero opioid exposure such as NAS.

Methadone and buprenorphine are both safe and effective in pregnancy. Both bind to the mu-opioid receptor, thereby controlling withdrawal symptoms and cravings when provided at adequate dosages and both provide an effective opioid receptor blockade [24]. Although prospective trials are underway evaluating the safety and efficacy of naltrexone during pregnancy, data remain insufficient, and naltrexone is currently not recommended for use during pregnancy [25, 26].

Historically, methadone was the most extensively used MOUD and has been considered the "gold standard" for the treatment of OUD during pregnancy [20]. Published data extend from the 1970s and demonstrate improved prenatal care utilization, term delivery of normal weight infants, and a greater rate of infants discharged to maternal care with methadone versus no medication [27].

Methadone inductions during pregnancy can occur in either the inpatient or outpatient setting, depending on local resources [28]. Based on current regulations in the United States, once a therapeutic dose is achieved, patients continue to receive medication daily through a licensed outpatient treatment facility. Methadone clinics should take the unique challenges parenting people face accessing medical treatment (e.g., childcare, transportation, etc.) into consideration when determining availability of take-home doses, especially given the more frequent dose adjustments needed during pregnancy [29]. Due to physiologic changes that occur during pregnancy including blood volume expansion and changes in drug metabolism and clearance primarily through induction of CYP450 enzymes, methadone dosages may need to be increased, or split in the second and third trimesters to mitigate signs and symptoms of opioid withdrawal [30]. Importantly, methadone has significant pharmacokinetic interactions with many other medications (i.e., antiretroviral agents) and can prolong the QT interval, especially at high doses (>100 mg per day) [31]. Thus, a thorough concomitant medication review and electrocardiogram is recommended prior to methadone induction. Research focused on the effects of methadone dose on neonatal outcomes including a systematic review and meta-analysis have not been able to establish a relationship between methadone dose and the development of NAS [20, 32–37]. As such, methadone dosing should not be minimized during pregnancy in an effort to decrease the incidence or severity of NAS.

In 2002, the Food and Drug Administration approved buprenorphine, a partial *mu* agonist, for the treatment of OUD. Subsequent randomized controlled trials have established buprenorphine's safety and efficacy in pregnancy [38–41]. In 2010, a multicenter randomized controlled trial comparing buprenorphine with methadone among 175 mother–infant dyads demonstrated that infants exposed to buprenorphine had a shorter treatment duration for NAS, required less morphine and had a shorter hospital stay (10.0 vs. 17.5 days; $p < 0.05$) than infants exposed to methadone [42]. In a recent meta-analysis of 12 studies comparing infants whose mothers received methadone versus buprenorphine, buprenorphine-exposed infants had a lower risk of treatment for NAS, a shorter hospital length of stay, a higher mean gestational age at delivery, and a greater birth weight and head circumference compared to methadone-exposed infants [43].

Due to an enhanced safety profile from partial agonist activity, buprenorphine inductions and ongoing maintenance prescribing can be conducted in office-based settings which has led to the increased utilization during pregnancy [8]. While buprenorphine monotherapy predominantly has been used in pregnancy, the combination product (buprenorphine/naloxone) has been increasingly used due to limited access to monotherapy in many parts of the US. Further, the safety and efficacy profiles of buprenorphine/naloxone appear to be equivalent to the monotherapy as several small cohort studies and a recent systematic review with meta-analysis have not demonstrated any adverse maternal or neonatal outcomes following the use of the combination product in pregnancy [44–46]. The physiological changes that occur during pregnancy may require split dosing or dose increases for buprenorphine in the second and third trimester to mitigate opioid withdrawal symptoms [47, 48]. In a pharmacokinetic evaluation of buprenorphine concentrations following different mechanisms of dosing during pregnancy, three-times daily and four-times daily dosing were often required to sustain buprenorphine plasma concentrations above 1 ng/ml, the threshold necessary to prevent opioid withdrawal symptoms [49].

Both buprenorphine and methadone are safe and effective in pregnancy. However, transitioning from one to the other is not recommended unless clinically indicated [20, 50]. Treatment adherence may be greater for methadone [51] as are drug interactions. Although the likelihood of NAS is similar between the two medications, medication for NAS, and length of stay is shorter for buprenorphine. Ultimately, medication decisions should be a shared decision-making process between each patient and their provider taking into account previous treatment experiences, patient preference, available treatment program options, and resource availability [16].

Treatment Barriers

Pregnancy is a unique opportunity to engage people in comprehensive preventative healthcare services due to expanded Medicaid-eligibility criteria, healthcare access prioritization, and enhanced maternal investment in neonatal health outcomes. Consequentially, treatment is often first initiated during pregnancy [52]. However, despite increased healthcare access, only half of people with OUD receive MOUD during pregnancy [53–55], a proportion that has remained relatively unchanged over the past 20 years [8, 54, 55].

Multiple patient-, provider- and system-level barriers to MOUD utilization exist. Stigma and misinformation associated with medications for OUD, a lack of trained providers, and insurance authorization requirements prevent access to MOUD [56, 57]. Further, women are more likely than men to be unemployed, have limited financial resources, increased financial stressors (i.e., childcare) and suffer from financial abuse by partners which may adversely affect OUD treatment utilization rates [58–60]. Disparities in MOUD utilization are also impacted by racism and geographic location. Among Medicaid-enrolled pregnant people with OUD, Black and Latina women are significantly less likely to use MOUD compared to White women suggesting racial and ethnic disparities in MOUD use [8]. Barriers to MOUD use during pregnancy are also significantly greater in rural versus urban geographic areas. In an evaluation of outpatient buprenorphine providers in four rural, Appalachian states, only 53% accepted pregnant people [61]. Stigma is especially powerful in rural areas where social and kinship networks are especially close [62, 63] and fear of judgment, prosecution, and child welfare involvement prevents many people from self-disclosure during pregnancy and OUD treatment engagement [64, 65].

Punitive policies related to substance use in pregnancy have increased over the past two decades [66], and states with punitive policies have higher rates of NAS [67]. Hence, state regulations necessitating child protective service reporting due to substance exposure that does not discriminate between MOUD and nonprescribed substances promote further stigmatization of, and thus barrier to use of, MOUD during pregnancy [68].

Due to limited treatment provider availability, alternative healthcare models and non-addiction medicine providers can play a critical role in initiating MOUD [69]. Between 2014 and 2016, the medical specialties of buprenorphine prescribers for over 4000 pregnant people with OUD enrolled in Pennsylvania Medicaid were described [70]. Of 569 prescribing providers, 63.1% were primary care physicians, 17.8% were psychiatrists or behavioral health providers, 5.1% were obstetrician/gynecologists, and 4.6% were emergency medicine providers [70]. When specialty was stratified by rural versus urban practice setting, emergency medicine providers were a significantly greater proportion of prescribing providers in rural versus urban areas [70]. Remotely supported provider training initiatives, such as Project ECHO (Extension for Community Healthcare Outcomes), and telemedicine have also been shown to be effective in expanding MOUD access to pregnant people in rural and underserved areas [71–73].

Comprehensive treatment for OUD extends beyond medication and includes screening and management of other medical and psychosocial comorbidities. All pregnant people with OUD should be screened for Hepatitis C virus (HCV) and HIV [74], co-occurring psychiatric disorders (e.g., depression, anxiety) [75, 76], and intimate partner violence (IPV) and trauma [77]. Behavioral health interventions such group or individual counseling and cognitive behavioral therapy (CBT) can be effective adjuncts to medication especially among patients with OUD from prescription opioids, although MOUD should not be withheld if patients are not interested in adjunctive psychosocial treatment [78]. Because people with OUD often have multiple medical and psychosocial comorbidities that can negatively impact treatment engagement, a clinical checklist can help providers confirm that each component of care has been provided and that referral mechanisms are in place for people with positive screens. Table 14.1 provides an example clinical checklist for common medical and psychosocial comorbidities among people with OUD from pregnancy through delivery and postpartum.

Labor and Delivery

Preparing for labor and delivery can be a stressful component of the peripartum transition. Pregnant people with OUD identify concerns about potential upcoming challenges with pain control, stigmatizing interactions with healthcare providers, and fear of child welfare involvement postpartum [79]. Conversely, labor and delivery providers also express concern that they are not prepared to care properly for this patient population [80]. Therefore, a clear plan for how to manage people with OUD through the process of labor and delivery, including those receiving MOUD, should be arranged during pregnancy, agreed upon by all members of the clinical care team, and documented appropriately.

Pain is frequently comorbid with addiction, and neurobiologically there is substantial overlap between these two conditions, [81] especially among women [82]. Individuals with comorbid pain conditions differ in pain coping efficacy and strategies. Pain, such as that associated with delivery, is stressful for all individuals. For people with OUD, the interplay between an added stressor, such as pain, with addiction and recovery may contribute to the heightened vulnerability to substance use and overdose in the peripartum period. Addiction has been classified as a multistage disease each involving different neurocircuitries. Preoccupation/anticipation is a stage driven by the prefrontal cortex that is linked to drug-seeking behaviors and disease recurrence or substance use after a period of abstinence [83]. Pain disorders also have an anticipation stage, which can be characterized by negative emotional constructs such as anxiety and catastrophizing [84]. The anticipation aspect of pain modulates pain perception [85], and is associated with worse pain outcomes, [86] opioid cravings, [87] more frequent opioid use, [88] and is present more often for women than men [89]. Therefore, an evaluation of the patient's confidence and competence to cope with pain should be included in the making of the care plan. This can be done in many ways, such as simply asking the patient, *"Think back to the last time you had pain, how did it make you feel?"* or using a tool such as the Pain Catastrophizing Scale (PCS) [84] or the Pain Anxiety Symptom Scale (PASS-20) [90]. If the patient is then noted to have poor coping, integration of behavioral health strategies focused on healthy coping with anticipation of the pain with labor and delivery could be implemented during pregnancy. Such interventions have shown promise to improve outcomes of people with chronic pain [91], undergoing surgery [92], and receiving methadone for OUD [93].

Patients receiving MOUD (methadone or buprenorphine) should continue it at the same total daily dose throughout labor and delivery [94]. MOUD should be

Table 14.1 Clinical checklist for pregnant women with opioid use disorder

	Clinical pathway	Tools
Initial prenatal visit/first trimester		
Opioid use disorder	Assess for opioid pharmacotherapy use (e.g., methadone, buprenorphine) and engagement in behavioral health therapy Obtain appropriate consent to communicate with treatment provider Monitor dose and engagement with treatment provider Discuss with patient expectations regarding pharmacotherapy and OUD treatment during pregnancy and postpartum	DSM 5 diagnostic criteria SAMHSA patient handout http://store.samhsa.gov/system/files/sma 18-5071fst.pdf
Overdose prevention	Provide naloxone prescriptions and instructions	Harm Reduction Coalition Manuals and Best Practice Documents: https://harmreduction.org/issues/overdose-prevention/tools-best-practices/manuals-best practice/
Second/third trimester		
Peripartum pain management	Continue pharmacotherapy through labor and delivery Consider OB anesthesia consultation visit Formulate and document peripartum pain management plan with anesthesia, labor, and delivery staff, obstetric and addiction provider Discuss pain management plan with patient	SAMHS Clinical Guidance for Treating Pregnant and Parenting Women with Opioid Use Disorder
Neonatal withdrawal (NAS)	Discuss NAS expectations with family Consider prenatal consultation with pediatrics/neonatology	SAMHSA patient handout http://store.samhsa.gov/system/files/sma 18-5071fs3.pdf
Breastfeeding	Discuss benefits of breastfeeding with patient, including positive effects on NAS	SAMHSA patient handout: http://store.samhsa.gov/system/files/sma 18-5071fs4.pdf
Family planning	Contraception counseling and postpartum method choice	Bededer.org
Child welfare	Discuss with patient expectations regarding involvement of child protective services	SAMHSA patient handout: https://store.samhsa.gov/system/files/sma 18-5071fs1.pdf
Postpartum		
Opioid use disorder	Coordinate early and frequent follow-up with both OB and addiction providers Continue pharmacotherapy at same dose	SAMHSA Clinical Guidance for Treating Pregnant and Parenting Women with Opioid Use Disorder

(continued)

Table 14.1 (continued)

	Clinical pathway	Tools
Ongoing assessment and management of comorbidities		
Tobacco use	Smoking cessation counseling Pharmacotherapy (e.g., nicotine replacement) if indicated and desired	5 As (Ask, Advise, Assess, Assist, Arrange)
Psychiatric disorders	Screen for depression and other behavioral health conditions Referral to behavioral health provider or psychiatry	Edinburgh Postnatal Depression Scale (EPDS); Patient Health Questionnaire 9 (PHQ-9)
Infectious disease	Screen for HIV and HCV during the initial prenatal visit and third trimester if injection/intranasal drug use continues HCV-infected patients should be referred to hepatology and receive immunizations for hepatitis A and B HIV-infected patients should be referred to infectious disease	HCV and HIV antibody for initial screening If HCV antibody (+). HCV genotype, viral load, liver transaminases
Intimate partner violence (IPV) Trauma	Screen during the initial prenatal care visit and periodically as needed Screening during initial visit and periodically as needed	Abuse Assessment Screen (AAS) HITS Screening Assessment Trauma Assessment for Adults (TAA) Posttraumatic Stress Disorder (PT5D) Symptom Scale

Abbreviations: HCV hepatitis C virus, *HIV* human immunodeficiency virus, *OB* obstetric, *OUD* opioid use disorder

Previously published Clin Perinatol 46 (2019) 833–847 https://doi.org/10.1016/j.clp.2019.08.013

understood as treatment for the chronic condition of addiction and not as providing any analgesia. In fact, analgesic requirements are often greater for people with OUD, especially following a cesarean delivery. Analgesic requirements, however, do not differ by MOUD. In a retrospective cohort comparing 185 women receiving methadone to 88 receiving buprenorphine all undergoing cesarean delivery, there were no significant differences in preoperative, intraoperative, or postoperative opioid requirements [95]. Tapering of MOUD prior to delivery is potentially harmful and is not recommended.

Epidural regional anesthesia is standard for both vaginal and cesarean deliveries, and should be available for all people with OUD. MOUD does not influence epidural effectiveness or safety. In general, pain management for labor, delivery, and postpartum should be multimodal in intervention and both person centered and recovery oriented in expression (Table 14.2). Pregnant and parenting people commonly report past negative experiences interacting with the health system, many related to stigmatizing interactions with staff and providers [68]. Therefore, labor and delivery staff and health systems should promote education in addiction and its treatment and utilize recovery-oriented and person-centered language [96].

Although professional society recommendations are clear (1) that urine drug testing is not an appropriate assessment for substance use and use disorder; and (2) that a positive drug test does not constitute evidence of child abuse or neglect, urine

Table 14.2 Recommended peripartum analgesic options for women with opioid use disorder

	Vaginal delivery	Cesarean delivery
Preoperative/labor	Continue MOUD at same total daily dose	Continue MOUD at same total daily dose
	Anesthesia consult in third trimester	Anesthesia consult in third trimester
	Pain plan reviewed and agreed upon by all providers (OB, Addiction, Anesthesia, Nursing)	Pain plan reviewed and agreed upon by all providers (OB, Addiction, Anesthesia, Nursing)
	Discuss pain plan with patient[a]	Discuss pain plan with patient[a]
	Document pain plan in medical record	Document pain plan in medical record
Intrapartum/ Intraoperative	Continue MOUD at same total daily dose	Continue MOUD at same total daily dose
	Neuraxial anesthesia (epidural)	Neuraxial anesthesia (combined spinal epidural)
	Consider nitrous oxide	Consider TAP block
Postoperative/ Postpartum	Continue MOUD at same total daily dose	Continue MOUD at same total daily dose[b]
	PRN or scheduled NSAIDs (IV Ketorolac or PO ibuprofen)	Scheduled IV NSAIDs (Ketorolac) for 24–48 hours > scheduled PO NSAIDs (ibuprofen)
	PRN PO acetaminophen	Scheduled po acetaminophen
		Consider epidural removal at 24 hours post-operatively[c]
	Local analgesia (ice, lidocaine cream, sitz baths)	Local analgesia (lidocaine patches)
		PRN po opioids (will likely need higher doses and more frequent dosing)[d]
	Restart any nonopioid pain medications for comorbid chronic pain disorders (e.g., gabapentin)	Restart any non-opioid pain medications for comorbid chronic pain disorders (e.g., gabapentin)
Discharge	MOUD prescription as needed[e]	MOUD prescription as needed[e]
	Naloxone prescription	Naloxone prescription
	Prescription filled for nonopioid medications utilized during inpatient admission	Prescription filled for all nonopioid medications utilized during inpatient admission
		Opioid prescription based on needs of patient on day of discharge until OB follow-up (≤7 days)

(continued)

Table 14.2 (continued)

	Vaginal delivery	Cesarean delivery
	Patient informed of all follow-up appointments (OB, Addiction)	Patient informed of all follow-up appointments (OB, Addiction)
	Discuss recovery-oriented techniques with patient (close follow-up with addiction provider, phone number for urgent needs)	Discuss recovery-oriented techniques with patient (close follow-up with addiction provider, phone number for urgent needs), family member management of opioid pills with lock box, at follow-up visits inform of plan for pill counts

[a]Addiction provider should also discuss plan for recovery-oriented strategies (see table) after discharge if discharged with opioid pain medications

[b]For buprenorphine, can consider split dosing (every 6–8 hours) for additional analgesia

[c]Patients should be administered po opioids at the time of epidural removal so patients have adequate pain relief as the local anesthesia subsequently weans down

[d]For patients who need an opioid PCA for adequate pain control, make sure to discontinue PO opioids while on PCA and that there is no basal component

[e]For patients on buprenorphine, prescriptions should be filled at discharge pharmacy to bridge patient to appointment with addiction provider. For patients on methadone, coordination with clinic before delivery should be arranged for take home doses, administration of methadone in hospital if patient rooming in with infant during observation, or transportation arranged for patient to go to clinic

drug testing is common on labor and delivery and positive urine drug test results are often reported by birthing hospitals to child welfare agencies, with higher instances of testing and reporting for Black families. These "test and report" policies, which can result in child removal, not only undermine public health efforts to address addiction as a health condition, but also violate the autonomy of pregnant people and their newborns. Therefore, informed consent including a discussion of indication for testing and possible outcomes must be obtained prior to urine drug testing at the time of birth [16]. If a pregnant person does not consent to a drug test, it should not be performed. The right of refusal is a central to medical ethics, should be respected, and not seen as evidence of substance use. If drug testing is performed, ASAM guidance should be followed: All presumptive positive test results should be follow by definitive testing prior to changes in clinical management [97] which would include child welfare notification.

Throughout the peripartum period, a multidisciplinary team approach is central to providing care for the mother–infant dyad. Figure 14.1 outlines the clinical domains which are central to the care of pregnant people with OUD. Optimal clinical care involves coordination across providers through "warm handoffs" as illustrated in Fig. 14.2.

Postpartum – The Fourth Trimester

The postpartum period is defined as the year following the end of the pregnancy and is associated with increased, medical, social, and psychological stressors. The term "Fourth Trimester" is used to represent this critical transition and make it more

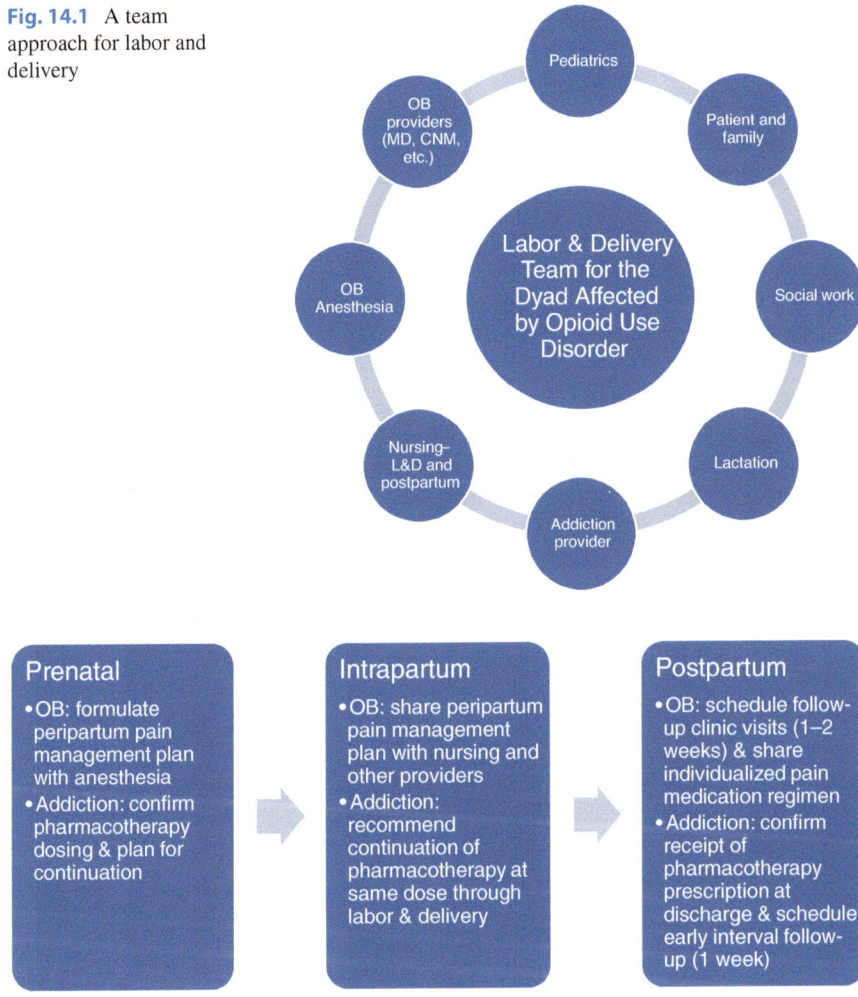

Fig. 14.1 A team approach for labor and delivery

Fig. 14.2 "Warm handoffs" through labor and delivery

inclusive of pregnancy [98]. Mood changes are common [99] and insurance coverage transitions from pregnancy- to income-based eligibility often results in a realignment of healthcare coverage or "churn" [100] for many people without employment-based coverage. People with OUD have additional vulnerabilities specific to addiction and recovery, including child custody, stigma, and legal issues [15]. While MOUD continuation rates after delivery are poor, [101] methadone dose has been associated with better postpartum treatment retention [102].

Overdose is one of the leading causes of maternal mortality in the US, with the majority occurring after delivery [103]. In Utah, more women died from drug-induced deaths between 2005 and 2014 than any other causes, with 80% occurring after the traditional 6-week postpartum window and 77% involving opioids. The majority (58%) of the women who died from a drug-induced cause did not attend a postpartum visit, and only 26% were linked to mental health services although 77%

had a known mental health condition [12]. MOUD continuation is protective of overdose and overdose death postpartum [10]. Earlier engagement in medication during pregnancy may confer greater protection in the postpartum, especially in states that have expanded Medicaid coverage by decreasing income eligibility thresholds [104].

Co-occurring mood disorders are associated with both poorer treatment outcomes in pregnancy [105] and increased overdose risk postpartum [104]. In contrast, integrating mental health assessment and treatment into prenatal care improves outcomes [106]. Therefore, depression screening via a validated instrument such as the Edinburgh Postnatal Depression Scale [107] complemented by a patient–provider discussion about mood should be routine adopted during pregnancy and, especially, postpartum.

Evidence-based guidelines regarding MOUD dose changes postpartum do not exist and, generally speaking, dosage adjustments should be individualized [108]. Among 101 postpartum patients receiving methadone, the average decrease in methadone 12 weeks postpartum was 3.7 mg (95% CI 1.1–6.3 mg) and oversedation was rare (6 participants) [109]. O'Connor et al. reported retrospectively on 151 women prescribed buprenorphine at delivery maintained in treatment postpartum; at 6 months, 51% were on the same dose, 16% a higher dose, and 33% a lower dose than at delivery. Delivery dose was not associated with treatment retention, but the association with postpartum dose changes were not evaluated [106]. In nonpregnant populations, higher buprenorphine doses are associated with improved treatment outcomes [110]. Routine postpartum decreases in methadone or buprenorphine should not be implemented. Instead, people should be assessed for signs and symptoms of both over (e.g., sedation) and under (e.g., cravings) treatment in order to effectively individualize any dose changes after delivery.

Contraceptive access should be a routine part of postpartum care. Provision of person-centered family planning services to people with OUD is not only a reproductive right, but also a strategy to better support recovery [111]. Postpartum contraceptive uptake is low among women with OUD [112]. Only 18% of pregnant people with OUD who wanted long-acting contraception received it postpartum, highlighting gaps in care delivery following delivery [113]. ACOG recommends that all people who desire immediate long-acting reversible contraception (LARC) placement after delivery should receive it before hospital discharge [114]. For people with OUD, this should be no exception.

Public Health and Public Policy

While the primary public health and media attention in the current wave of the opioid overdose epidemic is focused on non-Hispanic White people, living in rural areas, and of middle-to-high socioeconomic status, the historical effects of illicit substance use are primarily felt among low-income, urban, and marginalized populations, predominantly of minoritized racial/ethnic background [9, 115–120]. The current era of decriminalization of drug use is driven to a large extent by the whiteness of the initial phase of the crisis [121]. In contrast to general drug policy, public policy for pregnant people who use drugs has become more punitive over the past two decades [122, 123]. These punitive policies are driven, in part, by an increase in child welfare reporting requirements which are not associated with decreases in substance use during pregnancy at the population level but are associated with a 25% to 33% increased odds of NAS as well as a decreased likelihood of treatment engagement [67, 124].

Child welfare involvement and the potential loss of custody are major and legitimate concerns for pregnant people with OUD, [68] especially for Black, Indigenous, and Latinx people. Racial inequities in child welfare notification and report are well documented [125] and persist even following implementation of universal drug testing at the time of delivery [126], which reflects racial discrimination within clinical care as well as structural racism within the child welfare system where Black and American Indian children are twice as likely to be removed as White children [127]. There is currently an epidemic of foster care placements, driven primarily by child welfare involvement for concerns related to parental substance use [128]. The effect of foster care includes permanent separation, which can lead to long-standing trauma for both children and their mothers [129, 130].

Providers who care for pregnant and parenting people with OUD need to be aware of state statutes regarding reporting but should balance reports with their ethical obligation to the patient and her family. Policies that further stigmatize people with substance use disorders need to be revised to reflect our contemporary understanding of addiction as a chronic disease with a neurobiological basis, not a moral failing or a marker of unfit parenting, such as those policies classifying prenatal substance use as child abuse/neglect and requiring equivalent levels of child welfare reporting for MOUD and non-prescribed substances. Further, we should all work to align public policy with public health and evidence-based practice, grounded in respect and dignity, especially for pregnant and parenting people with SUD.

References

1. Medicine ASoA. Public Policy Statement on Substance Use, Misuse, and Use Disorders During and Following Pregnancy, with an Emphasis on Opioids. 2017. https://www.asam.org/docs/default-source/public-policy-statements/substance-use-misuse-and-use-disorders-during-and-following-pregnancy.pdf?sfvrsn=644978c2_4. Accessed 20 March 2020.
2. Patrick SW, Davis MM, Lehman CU, Cooper WO. Increasing incidence and geographic distribution of neonatal abstinence syndrome: United States 2009-2012. J Perinatol. 2015;35(8):650–5.
3. Substance Abuse and Mental Health Services Administration (SAMHSA). Results From the 2015 National Survey on Drug Use and Health: Detailed Tables. 2016.; https://www.samhsa.gov/data/sites/default/files/NSDUH-DetTabs-2015/NSDUH-DetTabs-2015/NSDUH-DetTabs-2015.pdf.
4. Kern-Goldberger AR, Huang Y, Polin M, et al. Opioid use disorder during antepartum and postpartum hospitalizations. Am J Perinatol. 2019. [ePub ahead of print].
5. Wen T, Batista N, Wright JD, et al. Postpartum readmissions among women with opioid use disorder. Am J Obstet Gynecol MFM. 2019;1(1):89–98.

6. Patrick SW, Dudley J, Martin PR, et al. Prescription opioid epidemic and infant outcomes. Pediatrics. 2015;135(5):842–50.

7. Patrick SW, Schumacher RE, Benneyworth BD, Krans EE, McAllister JM, Davis MM. Neonatal abstinence syndrome and associated health care expenditures: United States, 2000-2009. JAMA. 2012;307(18):1934–40.

8. Ecker JL, Abuhamad A, Hill W, et al. Substance use disorders in pregnancy: clinical, ethical, and research imperatives of the opioid epidemic: a report of a joint workshop of the Society for Maternal-Fetal Medicine, American College of Obstetricians and Gynecologists, and American Society of Addiction Medicine. Am J Obstet Gynecol. 2019;221(1):B5–28.

9. Reddy UM, Davis JM, Ren Z, et al. Opioid use in pregnancy, neonatal abstinence syndrome, and childhood outcomes: executive summary of a joint workshop by the Eunice Kennedy Shriver National Institute of Child Health and Human Development, American College of Obstetricians and Gynecologists, American Academy of Pediatrics, Society for Maternal-Fetal Medicine, Centers for Disease Control and Prevention, and the March of Dimes Foundation. Obstet Gynecol. 2017;130(1):10–28.

10. Schiff DM, Nielsen T, Terplan M, et al. Fatal and nonfatal overdose among pregnant and postpartum women in Massachusetts. Obstet Gynecol. 2018;132(2):466–74.

11. Goldman-Mellor S, Margerison CE. Maternal drug-related death and suicide are leading causes of postpartum death in California. Am J Obstet Gynecol. 2019;221(5):489. e481-489.e489.

12. Smid MC, Stone NM, Baksh L, et al. Pregnancy-associated death in Utah: contribution of drug-induced deaths. Obstet Gynecol. 2019;133(6):1131–40.

13. Koch AR, Geller SE. Addressing maternal deaths due to violence: the Illinois experience. Am J Obstet Gynecol. 2017;217(5):556.e551–556.e556.

14. Illinois Perinatal Quality Collaborative (ILPQC). Mothers and Newborns affected by Opioids (MNO)-OB Initiative. 2019; http://ilpqc.org/?q=MNO-OB.

15. Metz TD, Rovner P, Hoffman MC, Allshouse AA, Beckwith KM, Binswanger IA. Maternal deaths from suicide and overdose in Colorado, 2004–2012. Obstet Gynecol. 2016;128(6):1233–40.

16. Committee Opinion No. 711: opioid use and opioid use disorder in pregnancy. Obstet Gynecol. 2017;130(2):e81–94.

17. Ondersma SJ, Chang G, Blake-Lamb T, et al. Accuracy of five self-report screening instruments for substance use in pregnancy. Addiction. 2019;114(9):1683–93.

18. Kampman K, Jarvis M. American Society of Addiction Medicine (ASAM) national practice guideline for the use of medications in the treatment of addiction involving opioid use. J Addict Med. 2015;9(5):358.

19. Klaman SL, Isaacs K, Leopold A, et al. Treating women who are pregnant and parenting for opioid use disorder and the concurrent care of their infants and children: literature review to support national guidance. J Addict Med. 2017;11(3):178.

20. Mascola MA, Borders AE, Terplan M, Practice CO, Med ASA. Opioid use and opioid use disorder in pregnancy. Obstet Gynecol. 2017;130(2):E81–94.

21. Zuspan FP, Gumpel JA, Mejia-Zelaya A, Madden J, Davis R. Fetal stress from methadone withdrawal. Am J Obstet Gynecol. 1975;122(1):43–6.

22. McCarthy JJ, Leamon MH, Finnegan LP, Fassbender C. Opioid dependence and pregnancy: minimizing stress on the fetal brain. Am J Obstet Gynecol. 2017;216(3):226–31.

23. Terplan M, Laird HJ, Hand DJ, et al. Opioid detoxification during pregnancy: a systematic review. Obstet Gynecol. 2018;131(5):803–14.

24. Dole VP, Nyswander M. The treatment of heroin addiction. JAMA. 1966;195(11):972.

25. Kelty E, Hulse G. A retrospective cohort study of birth outcomes in neonates exposed to naltrexone in utero: a comparison with methadone-, buprenorphine- and non-opioid-exposed neonates. Drugs. 2017;77(11):1211–9.

26. Wachman EM, Saia K, Miller M, et al. Naltrexone treatment for pregnant women with opioid use disorder compared with matched buprenorphine control subjects. Clin Ther. 2019;41(9):1681–9.

27. Harper RG, Solish GI, Purow HM, Sang E, Panepinto WC. The effect of a methadone treatment program upon pregnant heroin addicts and their newborn infants. Pediatrics. 1974;54(3):300–5.
28. Baxter LE Sr, Campbell A, Deshields M, et al. Safe methadone induction and stabilization: report of an expert panel. J Addict Med. 2013;7(6):377–86.
29. McCarthy JJ, Jones HE, Terplan M, Rudolf VP, von Klimo MC. Changing outdated methadone regulations that harm pregnant patients. J Addict Med. 2020;15:93.
30. McCarthy JJ, Vasti EJ, Leamon MH, Graas J, Ward C, Fassbender C. The use of serum methadone/metabolite ratios to monitor changing perinatal pharmacokinetics. J Addict Med. 2018;12(3):241–6.
31. Fareed A, Casarella J, Amar R, Vayalapalli S, Drexler K. Methadone maintenance dosing guideline for opioid dependence, a literature review. J Addict Dis. 2010;29(1):1–14.
32. Dashe JS, Sheffield JS, Olscher DA, Todd SJ, Jackson GL, Wendel GD. Relationship between maternal methadone dosage and neonatal withdrawal. Obstet Gynecol. 2002;100(6):1244–9.
33. Berghella V, Lim PJ, Hill MK, Cherpes J, Chennat J, Kaltenbach K. Maternal methadone dose and neonatal withdrawal. Am J Obstet Gynecol. 2003;189(2):312–7.
34. Cleary BJ, Eogan M, O'Connell MP, et al. Methadone and perinatal outcomes: a prospective cohort study. Addiction. 2012;107(8):1482–92.
35. Jones HE, Jansson LM, O'Grady KE, Kaltenbach K. The relationship between maternal methadone dose at delivery and neonatal outcome: methodological and design considerations. Neurotoxicol Teratol. 2013;39:110–5.
36. Pizarro D, Habli M, Grier M, Bombrys A, Sibai B, Livingston J. Higher maternal doses of methadone does not increase neonatal abstinence syndrome. J Subst Abus Treat. 2011;40(3):295–8.
37. Cleary BJ, Donnelly J, Strawbridge J, et al. Methadone dose and neonatal abstinence syndrome-systematic review and meta-analysis. Addiction. 2010;105(12):2071–84.
38. Metz V, Jagsch R, Ebner N, et al. Impact of treatment approach on maternal and neonatal outcome in pregnant opioid-maintained women. Hum Psychopharmacol Clin Exp. 2011;26(6):412–21.
39. Kakko J, Heilig M, Sarman I. Buprenorphine and methadone treatment of opiate dependence during pregnancy: comparison of fetal growth and neonatal outcomes in two consecutive case series. Drug Alcohol Depend. 2008;96(1–2):69–78.
40. Fischer G, Ortner R, Rohrmeister K, et al. Methadone versus buprenorphine in pregnant addicts: a double-blind, double-dummy comparison study. Addiction. 2006;101(2):275–81.
41. Lacroix I, Berrebi A, Garipuy D, et al. Buprenorphine versus methadone in pregnant opioid-dependent women: a prospective multicenter study. Eur J Clin Pharmacol. 2011;67(10):1053–9.
42. Jones HE, Kaltenbach K, Heil SH, et al. Neonatal abstinence syndrome after methadone or buprenorphine exposure. N Engl J Med. 2010;363(24):2320–31.
43. Brogly SB, Saia KA, Walley AY, Du HM, Sebastiani P. Prenatal buprenorphine versus methadone exposure and neonatal outcomes: systematic review and meta-analysis. Am J Epidemiol. 2014;180(7):673–86.
44. Debelak K, Morrone WR, O'Grady KE, Jones HE. Buprenorphine + naloxone in the treatment of opioid dependence during pregnancy-initial patient care and outcome data. Am J Addict. 2013;22(3):252–4.
45. Lund IO, Fischer G, Welle-Strand GK, et al. A comparison of buprenorphine + naloxone to buprenorphine and methadone in the treatment of opioid dependence during pregnancy: maternal and neonatal outcomes. Subst Abuse: Res Treat. 2013;7:61–74.
46. Wiegand SL, Stringer EM, Stuebe AM, Jones H, Seashore C, Thorp J. Buprenorphine and naloxone compared with methadone treatment in pregnancy. Obstet Gynecol. 2015;125(2):363–8.
47. Shiu JR, Ensom MH. Dosing and monitoring of methadone in pregnancy: literature review. Can J Hosp Pharm. 2012;65(5):380–6.

48. Bastian JR, Chen H, Zhang H, Rothenberger S, Tarter R, English D, Venkataramanan R, Caritis SN. Dose-adjusted plasma concentrations of sublingual buprenorphine are lower during than after pregnancy. Am J Obstet Gynecol. 2017;216(1):64.e1–64.e7.
49. Caritis SN, Bastian JR, Zhang H, et al. An evidence-based recommendation to increase the dosing frequency of buprenorphine during pregnancy. Am J Obstet Gynecol. 2017;217(4):459 e451–459 e456.
50. Krans EE, Campopiano M, Cleveland LM, Goodman DJ, Kilday D, Kendig S, Leffert LR, Main EK, Mitchell KT, O'Gurek DT, D'Oria R, McDaniel D, Terplan M. National partnership for maternal safety: consensus bundle on obstetric care for women with opioid use disorder. Obstet Gynecol. 2019;134(2):365–75.
51. Jones HE, Finnegan LP, Kaltenbach K. Methadone and buprenorphine for the management of opioid dependence in pregnancy. Drugs. 2012;72(6):747–57.
52. Terplan M, Garrett J, Hartmann K. Gestational age at enrollment and continued substance use among pregnant women in drug treatment. J Addict Dis. 2009;28(2):103–12.
53. Krans EE, Kim JY, James AE, Kelley D, Jarlenski MP. Medication-assisted treatment utilization among pregnant women with opioid use disorder. Obstet Gynecol. 2019;133(5):943–51.
54. Bachhuber MA, Mehta PK, Faherty LJ, Saloner B. Medicaid coverage of methadone maintenance and the use of opioid agonist therapy among pregnant women in specialty treatment. Med Care. 2017;55(12):985–90.
55. Short VL, Hand DJ, MacAfee L, Abatemarco DJ, Terplan M. Trends and disparities in receipt of pharmacotherapy among pregnant women in publicly funded treatment programs for opioid use disorder in the United States. J Subst Abus Treat. 2018;89:67–74.
56. Knudsen HK, Abraham AJ, Roman PM. Adoption and implementation of medications in addiction treatment programs. J Addict Med. 2011;5(1):21–7.
57. Clark RE, Baxter JD. Responses of state Medicaid programs to buprenorphine diversion: doing more harm than good? JAMA Intern Med. 2013;173(17):1571–2.
58. Bawor M, Dennis BB, Varenbut M, et al. Sex differences in substance use, health, and social functioning among opioid users receiving methadone treatment: a multicenter cohort study. Biol Sex Differ. 2015;6:21.
59. Levine AR, Lundahl LH, Ledgerwood DM, Lisieski M, Rhodes GL, Greenwald MK. Gender-specific predictors of retention and opioid abstinence during methadone maintenance treatment. J Subst Abus Treat. 2015;54:37–43.
60. Pallatino C, Chang JC, Krans EE. The intersection of intimate partner violence and substance use among women with opioid use disorder. Subst Abus. 2019;42:1–8.
61. Patrick SW, Buntin MB, Martin PR, et al. Barriers to accessing treatment for pregnant women with opioid use disorder in Appalachian states. Subst Abus. 2019;40(3):356–62.
62. Keyes KM, Cerda M, Brady JE, Havens JR, Galea S. Understanding the rural-urban differences in nonmedical prescription opioid use and abuse in the United States. Am J Public Health. 2014;104(2):e52–9.
63. Jackson A, Shannon L. Barriers to receiving substance abuse treatment among rural pregnant women in Kentucky. Matern Child Health J. 2012;16(9):1762–70.
64. Lander LR, Marshalek P, Yitayew M, Ford D, Sullivan CR, Gurka KK. Rural healthcare disparities: challenges and solutions for the pregnant opioid-dependent population. W V Med J. 2013;109(4):22–7.
65. Kremer ME, Arora KS. Clinical, ethical, and legal considerations in pregnant women with opioid abuse. Obstet Gynecol. 2015;126(3):474–8.
66. Faherty LJ, Stein BD, Terplan M. Consensus guidelines and state policies: the gap between principle and practice at the intersection of substance use and pregnancy. Am J Obstetr Gynecol MFM. 2020;2:100137.
67. Faherty LJ, Kranz AM, Russell-Fritch J, Patrick SW, Cantor J, Stein BD. Association of punitive and reporting state policies related to substance use in pregnancy with rates of neonatal abstinence syndrome. JAMA Netw Open. 2019;2(11):–e1914078.

68. Frazer Z, McConnell K, Jansson LM. Treatment for substance use disorders in pregnant women: motivators and barriers. Drug Alcohol Depend. 2019;205:107652.
69. Jones HE, Deppen K, Hudak ML, et al. Clinical care for opioid-using pregnant and postpartum women: the role of obstetric providers. Am J Obstet Gynecol. 2014;210(4):302–10.
70. Hollander M, Jarlenski MP, Kim JY, James AE, Kelley D, Krans EE. Medical specialty of buprenorphine prescribers for pregnant women with opioid use disorder. Am J Obstet Gynecol. 2019;220:502.
71. Komaromy M, Duhigg D, Metcalf A, et al. Project ECHO (extension for community health-care outcomes): a new model for educating primary care providers about treatment of substance use disorders. Subst Abus. 2016;37(1):20–4.
72. Katzman JG, Galloway K, Olivas C, et al. Expanding health care access through education: dissemination and implementation of the ECHO model. Mil Med. 2016;181(3):227–35.
73. Hager B, Hasselberg M, Arzubi E, et al. Leveraging behavioral health expertise: practices and potential of the project ECHO approach to virtually integrating care in underserved areas. Psychiatr Serv. 2018;69(4):366–9.
74. Krans EE, Zickmund SL, Rustgi VK, Park SY, Dunn SL, Schwarz EB. Screening and evaluation of hepatitis C virus infection in pregnant women on opioid maintenance therapy: a retrospective cohort study. Subst Abus. 2016;37(1):88–95.
75. Tuten M, Heil SH, O'Grady KE, Fitzsimons H, Chisolm MS, Jones HE. The impact of mood disorders on the delivery and neonatal outcomes of methadone-maintained pregnant patients. Am J Drug Alcohol Abuse. 2009;35(5):358–63.
76. ACOG Committee Opinion No. 757: screening for perinatal depression. Obstet Gynecol. 2018;132(5):e208–12.
77. McLafferty LP, Becker M, Dresner N, et al. Guidelines for the management of pregnant women with substance use disorders. Psychosomatics. 2016;57(2):115–30.
78. Carroll KM, Weiss RD. The role of behavioral interventions in buprenorphine maintenance treatment: a review. Am J Psychiatry. 2017;174(8):738–47.
79. O'Rourke-Suchoff D, Sobel L, Holland E, Perkins R, Saia K, Bell S. The labor and birth experience of women with opioid use disorder: a qualitative study. Women Birth : Journal of the Australian College of Midwives. 2020;33:592.
80. Ko JY, Tong VT, Haight SC, et al. Obstetrician-gynecologists' practices and attitudes on substance use screening during pregnancy. J Perinatol. 2020;40(3):422–32.
81. Leknes S, Tracey I. A common neurobiology for pain and pleasure. Nat Rev Neurosci. 2008;9(4):314–20.
82. Hser YI, Mooney LJ, Saxon AJ, Miotto K, Bell DS, Huang D. Chronic pain among patients with opioid use disorder: results from electronic health records data. J Subst Abus Treat. 2017;77:26–30.
83. Koob GF, Volkow ND. Neurobiology of addiction: a neurocircuitry analysis. Lancet Psychiatry. 2016;3(8):760–73.
84. Sullivan M. The pain catastrophizing scale: development and validation. Psychol Assess. 1995;7(4):524–32.
85. Shih YW, Tsai HY, Lin FS, et al. Effects of positive and negative expectations on human pain perception engage separate but interrelated and dependently regulated cerebral mechanisms. J Neurosci. 2019;39(7):1261–74.
86. Martin CE, Johnson E, Wechter ME, Leserman J, Zolnoun DA. Catastrophizing: a predictor of persistent pain among women with endometriosis at 1 year. Hum Reprod. 2011;26(11):3078–84.
87. Martel MO, Jamison RN, Wasan AD, Edwards RR. The association between catastrophizing and craving in patients with chronic pain prescribed opioid therapy: a preliminary analysis. Pain Med (Malden, Mass). 2014;15(10):1757–64.
88. Finan PH, Carroll CP, Moscou-Jackson G, et al. Daily opioid use fluctuates as a function of pain, catastrophizing, and affect in patients with sickle cell disease: an electronic daily diary analysis. J Pain. 2018;19(1):46–56.

89. Sharifzadeh Y, Kao MC, Sturgeon JA, Rico TJ, Mackey S, Darnall BD. Pain catastrophizing moderates relationships between pain intensity and opioid prescription: nonlinear sex differences revealed using a learning health system. Anesthesiology. 2017;127(1):136–46.

90. McCracken LM, Dhingra L. A short version of the Pain Anxiety Symptoms Scale (PASS-20): preliminary development and validity. Pain Res Manag. 2002;7(1):45–50.

91. Darnall BD, Sturgeon JA, Kao MC, Hah JM, Mackey SC. From catastrophizing to recovery: a pilot study of a single-session treatment for pain catastrophizing. J Pain Res. 2014;7:219–26.

92. Nicholls JL, Azam MA, Burns LC, et al. Psychological treatments for the management of postsurgical pain: a systematic review of randomized controlled trials. Patient Relat Outcome Meas. 2018;9:49–64.

93. Barry DT, Beitel M, Cutter CJ, et al. An evaluation of the feasibility, acceptability, and preliminary efficacy of cognitive-behavioral therapy for opioid use disorder and chronic pain. Drug Alcohol Depend. 2019;194:460–7.

94. SAMHSA. Clinical guidance for treating pregnant and parenting women with opioid use disorder and their infants. HHS Publication No. (SMA) 18–5054. Rockville: Substance Abuse and Mental Health Services Administration; 2018.

95. Vilkins AL, Bagley SM, Hahn KA, et al. Comparison of post-cesarean section opioid analgesic requirements in women with opioid use disorder treated with methadone or buprenorphine. J Addict Med. 2017;11(5):397–401.

96. Zgierska AE, Miller MM, Rabago DP, et al. Language matters: it is time we change how we talk about addiction and its treatment. J Addict Med. 2020;15:10.

97. Jarvis M, Williams J, Hurford M, et al. Appropriate use of drug testing in clinical addiction medicine. J Addict Med. 2017;11(3):163–73.

98. Tully KP, Stuebe AM, Verbiest SB. The fourth trimester: a critical transition period with unmet maternal health needs. Am J Obstet Gynecol. 2017;217(1):37–41.

99. Barthel D, Kriston L, Barkmann C, et al. Longitudinal course of ante- and postpartum generalized anxiety symptoms and associated factors in West-African women from Ghana and Cote d'Ivoire. J Affect Disord. 2016;197:125–33.

100. Daw JR, Hatfield LA, Swartz K, Sommers BD. Women in the United States experience high rates of coverage 'Churn' in months before and after childbirth. Health Affairs (Project Hope). 2017;36(4):598–606.

101. Wilder C, Lewis D, Winhusen T. Medication assisted treatment discontinuation in pregnant and postpartum women with opioid use disorder. Drug Alcohol Depend. 2015;149:225–31.

102. Wilder CM, Hosta D, Winhusen T. Association of methadone dose with substance use and treatment retention in pregnant and postpartum women with opioid use disorder. J Subst Abus Treat. 2017;80:33–6.

103. Gemmill A, Kiang MV, Alexander MJ. Trends in pregnancy-associated mortality involving opioids in the United States, 2007-2016. Am J Obstet Gynecol. 2019;220(1):115–6.

104. Nielsen T, Bernson D, Terplan M, et al. Maternal and infant characteristics associated with maternal opioid overdose in the year following delivery. Addiction. 2019;115:291.

105. Fitzsimons HE, Tuten M, Vaidya V, Jones HE. Mood disorders affect drug treatment success of drug-dependent pregnant women. J Subst Abus Treat. 2007;32(1):19–25.

106. O'Connor AB, Uhler B, O'Brien LM, Knuppel K. Predictors of treatment retention in postpartum women prescribed buprenorphine during pregnancy. J Subst Abus Treat. 2018;86:26–9.

107. Smith-Nielsen J, Matthey S, Lange T, Vaever MS. Validation of the Edinburgh Postnatal Depression Scale against both DSM-5 and ICD-10 diagnostic criteria for depression. BMC Psychiatry. 2018;18(1):393.

108. Bogen DL, Perel JM, Helsel JC, et al. Pharmacologic evidence to support clinical decision making for peripartum methadone treatment. Psychopharmacology. 2013;225(2):441–51.

109. Pace CA, Kaminetzky LB, Winter M, et al. Postpartum changes in methadone maintenance dose. J Subst Abus Treat. 2014;47(3):229–32.

110. Mattick RP, Breen C, Kimber J, Davoli M. Buprenorphine maintenance versus placebo or methadone maintenance for opioid dependence. Cochrane Database Syst Rev. 2014(2):Cd002207.

111. Wright TE. Integrating reproductive health services into opioid treatment facilities: a missed opportunity to prevent opioid-exposed pregnancies and improve the health of women who use drugs. J Addict Med. 2019;13(6):420–1.
112. Krans EE, Kim JY, James AE 3rd, Kelley DK, Jarlenski M. Postpartum contraceptive use and interpregnancy interval among women with opioid use disorder. Drug Alcohol Depend. 2018;185:207–13.
113. Kotha A, Chen BA, Lewis L, Dunn S, Himes KP, Krans EE. Prenatal intent and postpartum receipt of long-acting reversible contraception among women receiving medication-assisted treatment for opioid use disorder. Contraception. 2019;99(1):36–41.
114. ACOG. Committee Opinion No. 670: immediate postpartum long-acting reversible contraception. Obstet Gynecol. 2016;128(2):e32–7.
115. Hughes PH. Behind the wall of respect: community experiments in heroin addiction control. Chicago: University of Chicago Press; 1977.
116. Bourgois P. In search of respect: selling crack in El Barrio. 2nd ed. New York: Cambridge University Press; 2003.
117. Bourgois P, Schonberg J. Righteous Dopefiend. Berkeley: University of California Press; 2009.
118. Spillane J. The making of an underground market: drug selling in Chicago, 1900-1940. J Soc Hist. 1998;32(1):27–47.
119. Hughes PH, Barker NW, Crawford GA, Jaffe JH. The natural history of a heroin epidemic. Am J Public Health. 1972;62(7):995–1001.
120. Patrick SW, Faherty LJ, Dick AW, Scott TA, Dudley J, Stein BD. Association among county-level economic factors, clinician supply, metropolitan or rural location, and neonatal abstinence syndrome. JAMA. 2019;321(4):385–93.
121. Netherland J, Hansen H. White opioids: pharmaceutical race and the war on drugs that wasn't. BioSocieties. 2017;12(2):217–38.
122. Roberts SCM, Mericle AA, Subbaraman MS, et al. State policies targeting alcohol use during pregnancy and alcohol use among pregnant women 1985-2016: evidence from the behavioral risk factor surveillance system. Womens Health Issues. 2019;29(3):213–21.
123. Thomas S, Treffers R, Berglas NF, Drabble L, Roberts SCM. Drug use during pregnancy policies in the United States from 1970 to 2016. Contemp Drug Probl. 2018;45(4):441–59.
124. Kozhimannil KB, Dowd WN, Ali MM, Novak P, Chen J. Substance use disorder treatment admissions and state-level prenatal substance use policies: evidence from a national treatment database. Addict Behav. 2019;90:272–7.
125. Chasnoff IJ, Landress HJ, Barrett ME. The prevalence of illicit-drug or alcohol use during pregnancy and discrepancies in mandatory reporting in Pinellas County, Florida. N Engl J Med. 1990;322(17):1202–6.
126. Roberts SC, Nuru-Jeter A. Universal screening for alcohol and drug use and racial disparities in child protective services reporting. J Behav Health Serv Res. 2012;39(1):3–16.
127. Wildeman C, Emanuel N. Cumulative risks of foster care placement by age 18 for US children, 2000–2011. PLoS One. 2014;9(3):e92785.
128. Meinhofer A, Anglero-Diaz Y. Trends in Foster Care entry among children removed from their homes because of parental drug use, 2000 to 2017. JAMA Pediatr. 2019; [ePub ahead of print].
129. Knight KR. Addicted. pregnant. poor. Durham: Duke University Press; 2015.
130. Falletta L, Hamilton K, Fischbein R, Aultman J, Kinney B, Kenne D. Perceptions of child protective services among pregnant or recently pregnant, opioid-using women in substance abuse treatment. Child Abuse Negl. 2018;79:125–35.

Care for Opioid Use Disorder in Medical Settings: Lived Experiences

15

Zachary Siegel and Maia Szalavitz

Zach's Story

I remember the first time my friends and I used a powerful opioid together. We were 17 years old and we each snorted a small line of oxycodone that we had bought from a friend. Like the majority of people who begin misusing prescriptions, the drugs we used had not been prescribed for us; we were seeking euphoria. I remember looking over at my friends being glued to the couch, barely able to keep their eyes open. We all did roughly the same amount, and rather than nodding out, I felt warm, energized, and chatty, a far cry from my usual anxious self. My unique psychology and physiology reacted to opioids differently. For me, opioids melted tension and, most importantly, muted cacophonous thoughts of harsh self-criticism and judgment. They simply made me feel comfortable inside myself, so I kept on using them.

After years of regular use, I eventually crossed the Rubicon into full-blown addiction. Without opioids I experienced mind-numbing insomnia, deep canyons of depression, and intense physical anguish. Pursuing education, relationships, and experiencing joy and meaning in life became impossible while chained to a 4- to 6-hour timetable, oscillating between warm euphoria and a fevered sickness. My world as a 22-year-old addicted to opioids was small and lonely. I only left my apartment on Chicago's North Side to secure the heroin I needed to avoid nightmarish symptoms and dread. By this point, in 2011, prescription opioids had become prohibitively expensive and scarce; heroin, sold as a mystery powder on the street, was my only option.

My parents lived in a nearby suburb and when they finally saw me at my worst, I confessed that I was addicted, miserable, and exhausted. Feeding an opioid

Z. Siegel (✉)
Health in Justice Action Lab, Northeastern University School of Law, Boston, MA, USA
e-mail: z.siegel@northeastern.edu

M. Szalavitz
New York, NY, USA

© Springer Nature Switzerland AG 2021
S. E. Wakeman, J. D. Rich (eds.), *Treating Opioid Use Disorder in General Medical Settings*, https://doi.org/10.1007/978-3-030-80818-1_15

addiction requires more energy than any full-time job I could think of – a logistical juggle unlike anything else I've ever achieved. As the saying goes, I was sick and tired of being sick and tired. Fortunately, my mother had worked as an operating room nurse for decades and knew her share of doctors who had become addicted to the anesthesia they administered. She heard stories about opioid addiction and knew it was serious. In addition to my mom's medical knowledge, which helped her respond rationally and compassionately, I was also helped by my father's resources as a successful business executive. I also benefited from the passage of the Affordable Care Act. In 2010, when the ACA passed, I was 21 years old, a dependent on my father's excellent insurance plan, which would cover addiction treatment. In America, all of these structural advantages meant that I would receive the best available treatment. So we thought.

Immediately after telling my parents about my addiction, they sprang into action. Within 2 days, I was admitted into a behavioral health hospital outside of Chicago for "detox." Fortunately, I had managed to avoid abscesses, blood-borne illnesses, and other serious complications that stem from injection drug use in not-so-sterile conditions. This was thanks to having access to new and unused syringes, yet another privilege from which few others in my shoes benefit. An early study of HIV transmission found that having diabetes was protective in people who inject drugs: Of course, it was not the metabolic disease that was beneficial, but the legal access to sterile needles [1].

In "detox," I was prescribed buprenorphine/naloxone and quetiapine for sleep. After meeting with a psychiatrist, I was also prescribed citalopram for depression and anxiety. For young people with severe opioid use disorder (OUD) like mine, past year mental health issues – commonly depression, anxiety disorders, and ADHD – affect more than 60% [2]. Childhood trauma is another major risk factor: People who have more adverse childhood experiences like neglect, sexual and physical abuse, homelessness, and parental loss, have a markedly higher risk of opioid misuse compared to those without childhood trauma [3].

After 4 days of medication, regular meals, and some fitful nights of sleep, the question looming over me became: What happens now? This was my first experience in any medical setting for addiction and I was clueless. Medically supervised withdrawal management, after all, is only temporary. Soon I'd be released into the same alienating world I'd been so desperate to escape. I began to ask other patients what their plans were. Where were they going? To my surprise, out of a dozen other patients, I was one of the only ones with no prior treatment attempts. It struck me when one older man said he'd lost count of how many treatments he tried over the years. Almost everyone had been to this same exact inpatient facility before. I felt nervous about my own prospects – would I wind up on the same years-long carousel? How many times would I have to come back here, in total shame and agony?

Asking about next steps, a staff member at the hospital handed me a packet listing nearby treatment centers. Some were 28-day, residential inpatient programs and others were intensive outpatient programs (IOP) that I could attend during the day. I had no idea which route to take. Since my parents wanted me to stay at their place instead of returning to my own apartment in Chicago, it didn't seem necessary to spend considerable amounts of money to live inside a facility for a month. So, I started looking at IOPs, which seemed cheaper and less disruptive. Staff also encouraged me to look for local Alcoholics Anonymous (AA) meetings to attend once I was discharged. Until my last day in the program, I'd only seen AA meetings in the media, books, and movies. Three men visiting the inpatient facility sat in the lounge among us patients and read "How it Works" from the *Big Book of Alcoholics Anonymous*. "Remember that we deal with alcohol – cunning, baffling, powerful! Without help it is too much for us. But there is One who has all power – that One is God. May you find Him now!" This language felt alien to me. The AA members discussed how steps and meetings work and urged us to get a sponsor: Someone who could walk us through the steps laid out in the *Big Book*. They also emphasized prayer and the spiritual benefits of service, such as helping others who struggle. Each of them noted how many years it had been since their last drink. Being 21 years old, I had little drinking experience to speak of. I sat there thinking to myself maybe if people can quit drinking for good, then I could quit using opioids.

To end the meeting, everyone stood up, held hands, and recited The Lord's Prayer. Raised Jewish, I had never heard that prayer, because it is a Christian prayer. I seemed to be the only person in the room who didn't know the words by heart. After hearing the religious connotations in "How it Works" and looking at the 12-Step posters on the wall in the lounge, I found that over half of the steps either include the word "God" or make a reference to God as a "higher power" or "Him."

Prior to this experience, I had never thought of my addiction in any spiritual or religious context. I preferred what seemed like a more plausible physiological and psychological understanding. I was told to keep an open mind, but I doubted that I'd keep up with the 12-Steps after leaving the facility. I expressed these doubts to the staff and my fellow patients. The most common response was that it was impossible for me to recover on my own. My primary concern when leaving the program was whether or not I was leaving with a prescription for the one thing that kept me from wanting to inject heroin: buprenorphine. Indeed, I was discharged with a month-long prescription, 12 milligrams per day, which satiated my cravings for opioids and made me feel – for the first time since I could remember – normal. The circuitous track of self-degrading and endlessly critical thoughts quieted down. More than just normal, buprenorphine even made me feel comfortable.

Leaving with a steady prescription of buprenorphine was a relief. I wasn't afraid of using heroin because truly, I didn't want to and thanks to the buprenorphine, my body didn't need it. The depression and restlessness lifted. Still, I had the sense that relying on a drug like buprenorphine wasn't enough, that I needed to do more in order to truly *recover*. After all the movies and reality TV shows about addiction I watched, and all the drug memoirs I read, I figured I should go to "rehab." I chose an outpatient program from the list of facilities given to me called Gateway Foundation. It was one of the only ones that specifically mentioned young people, which, judging from the AA meeting I found hard to relate to, seemed like a plus. I could drive there every morning and be home by evening. It was in "rehab" where the medication prescribed to me for OUD treatment became contentious.

Gateway was located on a secluded lakeside campus. It was May, and it felt like I was at my first day at summer camp. I saw basketball courts, a big gymnasium, and old white lodges where groups and counseling sessions took place. There was also residential housing, and I quickly learned that I was one of the only people enrolled in the program who was not living on campus. I also learned that the vast majority of people staying at Gateway were either transitioning out of a correctional setting or were court-mandated to be there. Asking around, almost everyone had numerous charges pending against them, ranging from simple possession to possession with intent to distribute to driving under the influence. They would receive a reduced punishment upon successful completion of the program. I once again saw how lucky I had been. Not only did I manage to avoid blood-borne illnesses, but also managed to avoid criminal charges, despite breaking the law every single day for 5 years. Clearly, having white skin and coming from an affluent family are significant advantages in just about every aspect of American life, especially when it comes to suffering the harms of our racist drug policies.

I wasn't sure what to expect from Gateway. I thought, like my medically supervised withdrawal treatment, that "rehab" would occur within more of a medical or clinical setting, not at what felt like a summer camp. I spent the majority of the morning doing an intake where I was asked a series of questions about my substance use history. I then met my "group," about a dozen guys sitting in a circle that was moderated by a soft-spoken but strict counselor. I had a difficult time following the language. Though I understood the individual words and terms, like "self-will" and "character defects," I felt like I was missing their context in the group's dialogue. Looking around the room, I just kept reading the same poster I saw in the inpatient facility with the 12-Steps on the wall. After group therapy, we all ate inside an echoey cafeteria. Lots of people smoked cigarettes afterward. After lunch, everyone went to the gym to play basketball. Never big on sports, I just walked around the court in circles, chatting with others, listening to their war stories and the times they got arrested, and how long they have left in the program. Instead of people asking, "What are you in for?" The question I was asked most often was, "What's your DOC?" (drug of choice). While heroin was indeed popular, it seemed that criminal charges, not substance use, is what landed most young people at Gateway.

The rest of the day entailed more groups and educational lectures. Because it was my first day, I only had to briefly introduce myself to the group. Mostly, I listened. A lot of my peers discussed prayer and thanked God. I also noticed that before people spoke, they first said, "My name is so and so, and I'm an addict, or alcoholic," and then they would proceed to what they wanted to say. When I introduced myself or said something without that qualifier, people looked at me like I was doing something wrong. The day of groups, therapy, and lectures would end at around 4 o'clock.

In the United States, in 2012, the vast majority of addiction treatment was faith-based, unlike treatment for any other medical or psychiatric condition. And this hasn't changed much: When my coauthor, Maia Szalavitz, put out a call to the leading experts on addiction in America recently, no one could name 10 treatment centers that do not emphasize the 12-Steps. Additionally, a recent evaluation of therapies offered in residential addiction treatment programs found that 92% reported offering 12-step programming [4].

On my way home from that first day, thinking about the conversations I had and everything I saw, I knew I would not go back to Gateway. It wasn't that the staff were rude, or that I didn't fit in. I sort of always feel like I don't fit in. I just didn't see how playing basketball between hours of group therapy was going to help me. Driving home, thinking about the day, multiple aspects of the program felt peculiar. My peers discussed something they called the "hot seat," an event that every person in the program participates in before they leave. A person sits in a chair in front of their peers, who are instructed to hurl criticisms about that person's character and behavior. I thought to myself: A megaphone of insults and criticisms occurs within my own head every day. Why would I want others confirming all the worst beliefs I have about myself? Research has shown conclusively that this type of confrontational and humiliating therapy can do lasting harm, and yet, it, too, is widespread and few people who have had contact with the system have no experience with it [5, 6].

On my way home, I also thought about a peculiar exchange during the intake process. When I was asked what medications I was on, I said buprenorphine. Asked how much I was on, I said 12 milligrams. The intake counselor gasped. "That's way too high," she said, after quizzing me about whether I feel euphoria or ever "nod out" from this dose. I told her that I just felt normal. "We're going to have to get that lower," she said. I didn't understand how an intake counselor had the clinical training to evaluate what medications and what dose I should be on. (Later on, I'd learn that there are few academic requirements to work in the industry and interact with patients.) Buprenorphine was also the only thing keeping me from using heroin. Basketball, group therapy, and prayer couldn't possibly achieve the same effect.

After making my decision to not attend Gateway Foundation, I was informed by a friend that Hazelden might be a better fit. I could take the train to Chicago every morning and once again be home with my parents by evening while I adjusted to life without using heroin every day. In retrospect, I was clearly a *highly* motivated patient. On buprenorphine, I managed to not use heroin for several days in a row. My parents commented that I was looking healthy. My face had expression and color again. They told me I was acting more like my old self again. Since I had always had a knack for writing and found pleasure in journaling, I started to read and write again. It felt wonderful. In the plainest terms, the will to live my life and the ability to feel joy had come back after years of anhedonia. Sure, I had cravings for the warm euphoria, and the occasional dream about using, or trying to use and being thwarted, but I knew that so long as I took buprenorphine, using an opioid like heroin would be pointless given buprenorphine's high affinity at the mu-receptor. But still, I felt like conventional wisdom dictated that I should attend "rehab."

After a few days of phone calls, I took the train down to Hazelden's intensive outpatient program located in Chicago for a consultation and in-take. Once again, I said I was on buprenorphine, to which the intake counselor responded, "We don't do that here." In order to enroll in the outpatient program – which entailed group therapy, lectures, lunch, and more group therapy – I had to sign a "contract" stating that

I planned to taper my dose of buprenorphine down to zero. Once again, the medication I was doing so well on was made to seem like something bad. The message was clear: I wasn't doing "recovery" the right way. Both Gateway and Hazelden, facilities with good reputations that were recommended by the hospital and covered by insurance, were explicitly telling me to get off effective medication treatment.

Moreover, I had been told Hazelden was the best place to go, that they knew what they were doing: it had literally been the originator of the model of treatment most widely used in American rehab, the "Minnesota Model." With two different and highly acclaimed facilities telling me the same thing, I thought maybe they're right? Perhaps taking an opioid agonist every day *is* trading one addiction for another. I had no idea that research data showed that there are only two treatments proven to cut the death rate from opioid addiction – one of the highest in all of medicine – by 50% or more and that buprenorphine was one of them. I didn't know that the so-called "experts" had for decades simply ignored the research. (In 2012, Hazelden finally capitulated and became more open to buprenorphine, but they still describe it as "only an adjunct" to 12-step-based recovery programming.)

I wanted to enroll in Hazelden. My parents wanted me to, as well. Hazelden gave me a reference for a psychiatrist nearby to discuss a buprenorphine taper plan. I met with the psychiatrist, who was board certified in addiction medicine, and he said he had successfully weaned people off of buprenorphine before. The jump from 12 milligrams to 8 milligrams was quick and painless. We then started to drop my dose by 2 milligrams every month.

What happens next should come as no surprise to those who know the research. I graduated from the program. I started taking college classes to finish my bachelor's. But, of course, when I made the jump from 2 mg to 0, I started using heroin again. When the taper was completed, I felt anxious and depressed again. I dreaded going to sleep every night. I couldn't concentrate in class. The very feelings that had driven me to use opioids in the first place came rushing back. So, I did what I knew worked to relieve pain. I was afraid to ask for help. I didn't know how to ask a doctor for buprenorphine without feeling like I was "drug seeking." Fearing an overdose, I started out buying small amounts of heroin to snort. However, that soon escalated. My tolerance grew much faster than I anticipated and very rapidly, I was back to injecting. I was back to feeling the agony, shame, and embarrassment I felt on my first day of seeking treatment that I so dreaded.

America's Treatment System Landscape

Thus far, this book has examined the best therapies and medications for the treatment of OUD within medical settings. This chapter, written by two journalists who have researched and reported extensively about public health policy and the science of substance use disorder (SUD), examines the persistent gulf between best practices laid out in the scientific literature and what really occurs inside treatment facilities across America. Zach's personal story is just an anecdote, of course, but it is an anecdote that vividly illustrates exactly what the data has repeatedly shown.

Our journalistic analysis draws from a rich body of high-quality evidence from around the world, as well as patients, experts, and scholars whom we've interviewed throughout our careers. In addition to our empirically based approach, our own lived-experience of addiction, treatment, and sustained recovery informs our perspective and analysis. Treatment for OUD is slowly making its way into mainstream medical settings, such as hospitals, primary care, and family medicine practices. However, as Zach's story illustrates, significant portions of the addiction treatment sector remain unregulated and operate without rigorous standards [7]. It is in this environment where group therapy, individual counseling, and educational lectures – largely based on the 12-Steps of Alcoholics Anonymous – are the dominant treatment methods. Far too often, treatment occurs outside the realm of established medical practices, putting patients in danger of fatal overdose after brief periods of abstinence. Within these settings, medications for opioid use disorder (MOUD) – in particular agonist medications like methadone and buprenorphine – are either only briefly used to manage acute withdrawal symptoms or shunned altogether. As previous chapters have demonstrated, this is empirically indefensible. We will have much to say about these harmful practices throughout this chapter.

Here we describe the current landscape of the treatment industry, as experienced by patients. For too long, non-specialist physicians have assumed that the "Minnesota Model" and the 12-step-based approach more generally was supported by evidence; they assumed that if they referred patients to highly respected rehabs with good reputations, they would get evidence-based care – as they would if they went to a center of excellence for cancer treatment. We explore what really happens outside of medical settings, analyzing the mistaken assumptions that reinforce beliefs about the use of medication to treat OUD. Then, we make the case for why proper medical settings (emergency departments, primary care, and hospitals) are the right place to treat OUD. Finally, we argue that a campaign to educate both laypeople and medical professionals about OUD can dramatically change what passes for treatment in the market by educating consumers about choosing the best care. An expanded, more inclusive, and hopeful definition of recovery that goes beyond mere abstinence from substances, one similar to the "any positive change" philosophy born out of the harm reduction movement and articulated by Dr. Kim Sue in Chap. 10, can ensure more people receive the most effective treatment. As with the HIV epidemic over 30 years ago, the medical community today has a duty to use its privilege and knowledge to treat people on the margins of society with the medicine and compassion they deserve.

The fact is that the American addiction treatment system today – both nonprofit and for-profit – is not only overwhelmingly nonmedical, but in certain settings, is decidedly anti-medical. Outmoded ideas, such as "hitting rock bottom," "tough love," "cold turkey," and "codependence" are still promulgated as truth and taught as gospel throughout the addiction treatment sector, despite having no diagnostic criteria or empirical basis. Such concepts stem from twentieth century perspectives that misunderstood compulsive drug use as stemming from character flaws and moral weakness [8]. From this view flows punitive, confrontational, and humiliating methods that further harm and traumatize people in need of medical and therapeutic attention. Though a more modern understanding of addiction is advancing thanks to decades of tireless research and advocacy, the majority of treatment still occurs outside of proper medical settings where antiquated conventions are marketed as "evidence-based" [7, 8]. Intensive outpatient programs and live-in residential facilities continue to deliver a combination of counseling and psychological support without FDA-approved medications. Within the current treatment landscape, it can be difficult for people and their families – "consumers" – seeking help to distinguish between medical and nonmedical treatment.

The problem runs deep and is documented by extensive research. A 5-year analysis of the treatment industry by Columbia University's Center on Addiction concluded, "Of those who do receive treatment, few receive anything that approximates evidence-based care" [7]. "Closing the Gap Between Science and Practice," the 2012 landmark report reveals how the medical system's long neglect of substance use disorder left behind a vacuum that was filled by paraprofessionals and self-help groups. "This neglect by the medical system has led to the creation of a separate and unrelated system of addiction care that struggles to treat the disease without the resources or the knowledge base to keep pace with science and medicine" [7].

The "separate and unrelated system" has flourished despite yielding poor outcomes. More recent analyses of the treatment system reveal that the gap between science and practice identified in the 2012 report remains wide. A 2020 investigation published in *JAMA Network Open* sought to quantify the availability of medications like methadone and buprenorphine among 2863 residential treatment facilities across 232,414 admissions [9]. Across all residential admissions, medication was only used in 34,058 cases, a mere 17%. In states that did not expand Medicaid, the use of medication was even lower, at just under 2% [9]. "A relatively low percentage of the 2,863 residential treatment facilities in this study offered naltrexone (29.8 percent), buprenorphine (33.3 percent), and methadone (2.1 percent)" [9]. These are the three FDA-approved medications to treat opioid use disorder, and they are barely being used. Comparing the outcomes of all three of these medications (as well as behavioral only approaches), another 2020 study of treatment pathways concluded, "only treatment with buprenorphine or methadone was associated with a reduced risk of overdose during 3-month follow-up [10]." Methadone and buprenorphine are the only two treatments that reduce mortality rates by half or more, but the "separate and unrelated" treatment system refuses to use them [11].

The most effective treatment for OUD is hard to come by in American treatment facilities. Only 42% of the nearly 15,000 treatment centers tracked by the Substance Abuse and Mental Health Services Administration (SAMHSA) provide *any* of the three FDA-approved medications for OUD [11]. Fewer than 500 of those facilities (3%) offer *all* three approved medications: methadone, buprenorphine, and naltrexone. Despite OUD being widely recognized as a medical condition, facilities operate without any prescribing physicians on staff. In some states, one can be employed counseling patients without having a high school degree or standardized training [12]. Research has demonstrated unequivocally that this nonmedical approach not only dominates the field, but that it results in higher mortality rates compared to methods that prioritize the use of agonist medications like methadone and buprenorphine [10]. These alarming trends still do not capture the totality of the problems with the field.

For one, medication use is not merely avoided; it is actively attacked and rejected. Narcotics Anonymous, the main 12-step program devoted specifically to opioid addiction, explicitly tells members that they are not "clean" and cannot count their days in recovery while they are on medication [13]. In some meetings, people using MOUD are not even permitted to speak – basically meaning they are not considered to have any time in recovery at all, even if they take no unprescribed drugs. Since there is such strong anti-medication ideology in crucial 12-step programs, the fact that the vast majority of treatment facilities and IOPs rely heavily on these groups and their ideas is a serious flaw in the system that few have even begun to address. While some programs set up "medication friendly" groups for their own patients, this does not reckon with the strong social pressure that exists in these support groups and in much of the field, which can and has been deadly for many.

Moreover, there also are untold numbers of fly-by-night treatment enterprises that SAMHSA does not track, but due to savvy digital advertising, these facilities show up at the top of online search results when people are desperate and seeking help [14]. For example, anyone can hang out a shingle and receive a license to run an addiction treatment facility in California's sprawling, for-profit industry with "no degree, medical or otherwise," according to an investigation by the *Orange County Register*, which was cited in an inquiry investigating fraud and abuse by the House of Representatives Committee on Energy and Commerce [15, 16]. More recently, Senators Elizabeth Warren (D-Mass.) and Tammy Duckworth (D-Ill.) requested the Government Accountability Office investigate the practice of forced-labor at treatment facilities, including those that are faith based [17]. Congress launched these investigations after several journalistic investigations revealed predatory and abusive practices across the industry. On top of offering low-quality treatment, "reports indicate that the facilities may engage in abusive billing practices, including billing insurers several times per week, per patient, for unnecessary urine tests that can cost up to several thousand dollars per test" [16].

While the nonmedical treatment field thrives in an under-regulated environment with little oversight, medications that treat addiction are heavily restricted and *over-regulated*. Strict regulatory structures place a heavy burden on when and where agonist medications can be prescribed. Ironically, any doctor can prescribe methadone or buprenorphine to treat pain, but they cannot prescribe the same medication to treat addiction unless they are practicing within a federally licensed opioid treatment program or hold a special waiver. In the case of buprenorphine, there are nowhere near enough physicians who have completed extra training and filed the proper paperwork required to prescribe it. Less than 7% of physicians in America hold the necessary DEA X-waiver to prescribe buprenorphine, and more than half of the counties in America lack a single buprenorphine prescriber [18]. Despite these obstacles, patients go to great lengths and travel incredible distances to receive the best available treatment. Among 23,141 methadone patients enrolled in 84 methadone clinics across the country, more than half reported traveling over 10 miles to receive their dose, and others reported traveling more than 50 miles [19].

Restrictive regulations have played a critical role in creating the gap between science and practice.

In the midst of a public health emergency with record-breaking overdose deaths, the scarcity of these medications is costing lives. The lack of access to these medications is a situation unlike any other in the medical field: If a medication for cancer, heart disease, or stroke produced the same outcomes that methadone and buprenorphine do for OUD, they would be hailed as wonder drugs. What other factors explain their absence in US addiction treatment?

For decades, burdensome regulations played a significant barrier to the wide use of medications. However, they are not the only hurdle to clear. Stigma and misinformation also play destructive roles. Mistaken beliefs about agonist medications abound; for instance, the notion that these medications do not treat OUD, but merely replace "one addiction with another", are rampant among both laypeople and professionals in the industry [20]. Unfortunately, our colleagues in the media have reinforced this sphere of medical misinformation. Outside of the scientific literature, people seeking help have few places to turn for objective information about the best treatment medicine has to offer. A Johns Hopkins study found that newspaper articles featuring MOUD tend to skew negative, focusing on their potential to be misused or sold in the illicit market while also omitting their life-saving potential [21]. The same analysis also found that "fewer than 40 percent of news stories about the medications mentioned that they are underused" [21]. The dissemination of misinformation and stigma by the press ultimately led us to develop Changing The Narrative, a journalism and communications toolkit that reporters and others could use to avoid repeating harmful mistakes of the past [22]. Inaccurate information about these medications are not only found in the news, but also in marketing materials for treatment facilities that boast their resistance to prescribing medications for their patients. Reviewing marketing materials for treatment facilities, one finds statements such as, "The basic premise of a Suboxone maintenance program is trading one illegal drug for a legal drug" [23].

This idea of "trading one addiction for another" stems from a fundamental misunderstanding of what addiction is and how agonist medications work. Addiction – now called "substance use disorder, severe" in the *Diagnostic and Statistical Manual of Mental Disorders* (DSM) – is defined as compulsive drug use that persists despite negative consequences. Physical dependence, in contrast, is simply a condition in which one takes a drug over time and experiences discomforting symptoms if the drug is abruptly stopped taken. Addiction is always harmful; dependence may not be if the drug's benefits outweigh its risks. For example, selective serotonin reuptake inhibitor (SSRI) antidepressants can cause significant withdrawal symptoms but if they are relieving someone's suicidal depression, the benefit outweighs the risk and the person is in no way "addicted." In fact, the editors of *Diagnostic and Statistical Manual of Mental Disorders, 5th Edition* (DSM-5) dropped the term "substance dependence" as the diagnostic label for addiction in 2013 because they recognized that conflating addiction and dependence generates confusion and does harm.

When patients are on a stable dose of methadone or buprenorphine, they no longer meet DSM-5 criteria for OUD. They remain physiologically dependent and will experience withdrawal symptoms if cut off abruptly from medication, but they are no longer addicted because they are not engaging in compulsive drug use despite ongoing harm. From antidepressants to caffeine, numerous drugs create physical dependence and some also have addiction potential. But physical dependence on opioids should not be conflated with opioid use disorder. Doing so perpetuates the idea that medication use "isn't really recovery" and it also does harm to patients with chronic pain who may lose access to beneficial treatment if they are wrongly seen as addicted.

As with anti-vaccination activists or climate change deniers, a stubborn belief system premised on the negation of scientific research stands in the way of advancing a modern medical approach for treating OUD. In the midst of America's deadliest drug overdose crisis in recorded history, with tens of thousands of people dying annually, unscientific beliefs fill the schism between science and practice [24]. To understand the perils of seeking treatment in an industry that has not kept pace with science and medicine, a closer look at what occurs inside popular residential facilities is especially clarifying.

The Need for Treatment in Medical Settings and a New Definition of Recovery

Zach is lucky to have survived to the kind of treatment he underwent. The painful irony of his experience is that the whole time he was seeking further "treatment," whether at Gateway or Hazelden, he was actually already receiving the standard of care. Although the term "medication-assisted treatment" (MAT) has become a popular way to reference MOUD, it is a misnomer. The treatment proven to reduce mortality *is* the medication; behavioral treatment alone, whether residential or outpatient, does not have this benefit. The term MAT reflects lingering discomfort with the idea of addiction as a medical issue: We don't call depression treatment with SSRIs "medication assisted" because we recognize that antidepressants are themselves treatment.

If anything, counseling and group therapy *assist* the medication. But the treatment industry does not view medications this way, and it nearly cost Zach his life. Experiences like his are not anomalies, which is why we dedicated our careers to this field to prevent others from experiencing harmful, unscientific treatment. Fortunately, without fully knowing it, Zach practiced harm reduction. He avoided situations where he had to use alone, avoided sharing syringes, and carefully dosed as best he could. Meanwhile his parents continued helping him find long-term treatment instead of practicing "tough love." The coda to Zach's story is that his family never gave up on him and he eventually found the path that works for him, which entailed over a year of living within institutions across the treatment spectrum. Few young people are as fortunate to have the time, resources, and support dedicated to their treatment process.

After Zach's stint at Hazelden, which eventually merged with Betty Ford, the institution began to change its stance on medication. Not because of Zach's experience specifically, but because so many others like him over the years relapsed and many died after undergoing treatment devoid of ongoing medication. In November 2012, Hazelden finally incorporated the long-term use of buprenorphine into its program [25]. At the time of the decision, Hazelden's medical director, Dr. Marvin Seppala said, "We believe it's the responsible thing to do."

After merging, Hazelden–Betty Ford became one of the largest and most influential actors in the treatment industry. Many predicted that their new stance on buprenorphine maintenance would convince other facilities rooted in the 12-Steps to follow suit. All these years later, that's not what happened. Rigid and inflexible anti-medication beliefs continue to dominate the industry. And this is precisely why the medical profession must take the lead in treating OUD. Emergency departments, hospitals, primary care, and family medicine practices can, and must, step up to treat OUD, especially at a time when tens of thousands of Americans die from opioid overdoses each year. Writing in the *New England Journal of Medicine*, Dr. Sarah Wakeman and Michael Barnett urge their colleagues in primary care to take on treating OUD: "To have any hope of stemming the overdose tide, we have to make it easier to obtain buprenorphine than to get heroin and fentanyl" [26].

Wakeman and Barnett explain how primary care providers (PCPs) are well situated to take on patients with OUD and ought to mobilize to treat it just as they did during the HIV/AIDS epidemic. They say doctors need not be specialists in addiction in order to make a difference. "Although initially specialists were more likely to prescribe antiretrovirals, by 1990 equal percentages of patients were receiving antiretroviral therapy from PCPs and from specialists" [26]. That's thanks to advocacy and doctors rising to the occasion during a public health emergency in the era of HIV/AIDS, the crisis much like the one we're in now demands a similar response. As we've already discussed, there are regulatory hurdles that stand in the way of every doctor being able to prescribe methadone and buprenorphine. But as Wakeman and Barnett argued, with deliberate education and organizing, these hurdles are surmountable.

A growing chorus of doctors, nurses, physician assistants, and patient advocates are calling on policymakers to eliminate the X-waiver requirement, organizing under the slogan "X the X Waiver" [27]. On April 27, 2021, the U.S. Department of Health & Human Services (HHS) heeded this call and exempted licensed physicians, physician assistants, nurse practitioners, clinical nurse specialists, certified registered nurse anesthetists and certified nurse midwives from federal certification requirements to treat up to 30 patients with buprenorphine. "The need for more accessible medication-based services has never been more urgent than it is today," said Tom Coderre, acting assistant secretary for the Department of Health and Human Services' Substance Abuse and Mental Health Services Administration. https://www.washingtonpost.com/health/biden-administration-eases-restrictions-on-prescribing-treatment-for-opioidaddiction/2021/04/27/9a1c8fa4-a776-11eb-8d25-7b30e74923ea_story.html. While America's drug laws seemingly appear to be ossified and set in stone, recent developments like the sudden X-waiver change are cause for hope that scientific evidence coupled with effective advocacy can result in positive change. While advocates continue working to scale back restrictive regulations, and make agonist medications available to all who need them, it's critical that the medical community continues its concerted effort to step up and treat a stigmatized and misunderstood illness, much the way they've done with HIV/AIDS.

Anecdotally, physicians have told us treating OUD sounds intimidating and complicated. "In our experience," Wakeman and Barnett write, "it is no more burdensome than treating other chronic illnesses. A typical visit includes assessing medication adherence, examining disease control (e.g., cravings and use), titrating doses, and ordering laboratory tests" [26]. With an education campaign to demystify MOUD, and combat stigma, it's possible for more medical professionals to step into the space.

But first they need to understand that people with opioid use disorder are patients like any others – we aren't all liars marred by lifelong "character defects." Research shows that the idea of a single antisocial addictive personality is a myth: While antisocial personality disorder (ASPD) is overrepresented among people with addiction, the majority of us do not have this disorder and treating us as naturally manipulative or dishonest is neither humane nor effective [29, 30].

Far too often, both the public and medical professionals are presented with a hopeless picture of opioid addiction. It is true that OUD can be deadly, and as we've experienced, incredibly painful. However, studies suggest that most people eventually do recover. One study of more than 500 people who had been addicted to opioids like oxycodone found that half of their addictions lasted 5 years or less, and the odds of recovery were 96% [31]. If more people receive appropriate treatment, and have access to medicine and compassion, a much more hopeful and far less stigmatizing perception will emerge. Families trust their doctors to help them and when a loved one is struggling with OUD, a doctor they know and trust ought to be able to assist them. Our hope is that more doctors practicing across various medical settings begin treating people with addiction with the empathy, support, and respect they'd offer if they faced any other life-threatening medical problem.

References

1. Nelson KE, Vlahov D, Cohn S, Lindsay A, Solomon L, Anthony JC. Human immunodeficiency virus infection in diabetic intravenous drug users. JAMA. 1991;266(16):2259–61. PMID: 1920726.
2. Jones CM, McCance-Katz EF. Co-occurring substance use and mental disorders among adults with opioid use disorder. Drug Alcohol Depend. 2019;197:78–82. https://doi.org/10.1016/j.drugalcdep.2018.12.030. Epub 2019 Feb 14. PMID: 30784952.
3. Swedo EA, Sumner SA, de Fijter S, Werhan L, Norris K, Beauregard JL, Montgomery MP, Rose EB, Hillis SD, Massetti GM. Adolescent opioid misuse attributable to adverse childhood experiences. J Pediatr. 2020;224:102–109.e3. https://doi.org/10.1016/j.jpeds.2020.05.001. Epub 2020 May 11. PMID: 32437756.
4. Beetham T, Saloner B, Gaye M, Wakeman SE, Frank RG, Barnett ML. Therapies offered at residential addiction treatment programs in the United States. JAMA. 2020;324(8):804–6. https://doi.org/10.1001/jama.2020.8969. PMID: 32840587; PMCID: PMC7448823.
5. Moyers TB, Miller WR. Is low therapist empathy toxic? Psychol Addict Behav. 2013;27(3):878–84. https://doi.org/10.1037/a0030274. Epub 2012 Oct 1. PMID: 23025709; PMCID: PMC3558610.

6. White W, Miller W. The use of confrontation in addiction treatment history, science, and time for change a history of confrontational therapies. Counselor. 2007;8

7. Addiction medicine: closing the gap between science and practice [Internet]. Center on Addiction. 2017 [cited 2020 Feb21]. Available from: https://www.centeronaddiction.org/addiction-research/reports/addiction-medicine-closing-gap-between-science-and-practice.

8. Szalavitz M. 'Unbroken Brain' explains why 'Tough' treatment doesn't help drug addicts [Internet]. NPR. NPR; 2016 [cited 2020Feb21]. Available from: https://www.npr.org/sections/health-shots/2016/07/07/485087604/unbroken-brain-explains-why-tough-treatment-doesnt-help-drug-addicts.

9. Huhn AS, Hobelmann JG, Strickland JC, Oyler GA, Bergeria CL, Umbricht A, Dunn KE. Differences in availability and use of medications for opioid use disorder in residential treatment settings in the United States. JAMA Netw Open. 2020;3(2):e1920843.

10. Wakeman SE, Larochelle MR, Ameli O, Chaisson CE, McPheeters JT, Crown WH, Azocar F, Sanghavi DM. Comparative effectiveness of different treatment pathways for opioid use disorder. JAMA Netw Open. 2020;3(2):e1920622.

11. Jones A, Honermann B, Sharp A, Millett G. Where multiple modes of medication-assisted treatment are available. Health Affairs Blog. 2018;

12. Szalavitz M. What science says to do if your loved one has an opioid addiction [Internet]. FiveThirtyEight. FiveThirtyEight; 2016 [cited 2020Feb21]. Available from: https://fivethirtyeight.com/features/what-science-says-to-do-if-your-loved-one-has-an-opioid-addiction/.

13. Narcotics Anonymous World Service Board of Trustees, "Bulletin #29: regarding methadone and other drug replacement programs," Narcotics Anonymous, last accessed October 22, 2020, https://na.org/?ID=bulletins-bull29.

14. Ferguson C. How disreputable rehabs game Google to profit off patients [Internet]. The Verge. The Verge; 2017 [cited 2020Feb21]. Available from: https://www.theverge.com/2017/9/7/16257412/rehabs-near-me-google-search-scam-florida-treatment-centers.

15. Sforza T, Saavedra T, Schwebke S, Basheda L, Schauer M, Gritchen J, et al. How some Southern California drug rehab centers exploit addiction [Internet]. Orange County Register. Orange County Register; 2018 [cited 2020Feb21]. Available from: https://www.ocregister.com/2017/05/21/how-some-southern-california-drug-rehab-centers-exploit-addiction/.

16. U.S. House of Representatives. Examining concerns of patient brokering and addiction treatment fraud. https://docs.house.gov/Committee/Calendar/ByEvent.aspx?EventID=106716.

17. Donohue A, Walter S. Rehab work camps appear to violate federal law, senators say. Reveal: The Center for Investigative Reporting; 2020 [cited 2021Jan19]. Available from: https://reveal-news.org/article/rehab-work-camps-appear-to-violate-federal-law-senators-say/.

18. Baylor C. Practitioner and program data [Internet]. SAMHSA. 2019 [cited 2020Feb21]. Available from: https://www.samhsa.gov/medication-assisted-treatment/training-materials-resources/physician-program-data.

19. Rosenblum A, Cleland CM, Fong C, Kayman DJ, Tempalski B, Parrino M. Distance traveled and cross-state commuting to opioid treatment programs in the United States. J Environ Public Health. 2011;2011

20. Karins J. The Landing Place to offer new mental health, addiction treatment options [Internet]. Daily Reporter. 2019 [cited 2020Feb21]. Available from: http://www.greenfieldreporter.com/2019/10/12/the_landing_place_to_offer_new_mental_health_addiction_treatment_options/.

21. Kennedy-Hendricks A, Levin J, Stone E, McGinty EE, Gollust SE, Barry CL. News media reporting on medication treatment for opioid use disorder amid the opioid epidemic. Health Aff. 2019;38(4):643–51.

22. Changing the narrative [Internet]. Northeastern University Law School, Health in Justice Action Lab. 2018 [cited 2021Jan19]. Available from: https://www.changingthenarrative.news.

23. The dangers of long term suboxone use [Internet]. Maryland Addiction Recovery Center. 2014 [cited 2020Feb21]. Available from: https://www.marylandaddictionrecovery.com/the-dangers-of-long-term-suboxone-use/.

24. Understanding the epidemic [Internet]. Centers for Disease Control and Prevention. Centers for Disease Control and Prevention; 2018 [cited 2020Feb21]. Available from: https://www.cdc.gov/drugoverdose/epidemic/index.html.

25. Szalavitz M. Hazelden Introduces anti-addiction medications into recovery for first time [Internet]. Time. Time; 2012 [cited 2020Feb21]. Available from: https://healthland.time.com/2012/11/05/hazelden-introduces-antiaddiction-medications-in-recovery-for-first-time/.

26. Wakeman SE, Barnett ML. Primary care and the opioid-overdose crisis—buprenorphine myths and realities. N Engl J Med. 2018;379(1):1–4.

27. Fiscella K, Wakeman SE, Beletsky L. Buprenorphine deregulation and mainstreaming treatment for opioid use disorder: X the X Waiver. JAMA Psychiat. 2019;76(3):229–30. https://doi.org/10.1001/jamapsychiatry.2018.3685.

28. HHS expands access to treatment for opioid use disorder [Internet]. U.S. Department of Health & Human Services; 2020 [cited 2021Feb9]. Available from: https://www.hhs.gov/about/news/2021/01/14/hhs-expands-access-to-treatment-for-opioid-use-disorder.html.

29. Szalavitz M. Genetics: no more addictive personality. Nature. 2015;522:S48–9. https://doi.org/10.1038/522S48a.

30. Smith RV, Young AM, Mullins UL, Havens JR. Individual and network correlates of antisocial personality disorder among rural nonmedical prescription opioid users. J Rural Health. 2017;33(2):198–207. https://doi.org/10.1111/jrh.12184.

31. Blanco C, Secades-Villa R, Garcia-Rodriguez O, Labrador-Mendez M, Wang S, Schwartz RP. Probability and predictors of remission from life-time prescription drug use disorders: results from the National Epidemiologic Survey on alcohol and related conditions. J Psychiatr Res. 2013;47(1):42–9.

Index